Small Animal Regional Anesthesia and Analgesia

Dedication

I would first like to thank my family for their support and patience while I have worked on this project over the last few years. Emma, thank you for being our family's rock, for inspiring me to be the best version of myself every day, and for challenging me to think of new ways to do things. Grace and Kate, thank you for putting up with the endless hours "on my computer" at the airport and at your horse shows. I am so proud to be your dad and have loved every minute of watching you pursue your passions and succeed in ways we could have never imagined a few short years ago! Our family means everything to me, and I am so thankful to have all of you in my life. Love you guys!

I'd also like to recognize the patients that I get to work with every day. I learn so much from getting to practice anesthesia as part of your medical care and have grown so much as a veterinarian since I have started to see what lies inside and can be better at my job on your behalf.

Finally, I'd like to thank Luis and Berit for years and years of wonderful friendship and their tireless efforts in getting this edition of our book across the finish line. I can't wait to start working on the third edition with you!

Matt Read

At the time of writing this, it feels like we have written and edited a book and a half! It has been a difficult time, filled with unprecedented challenges, and yet, here we are, we made it! During this time, there were many times in which this project was still a big question mark. This is when my partner in crime comes in. Always with encouragement and amazing management skills! Matt Read has guided me through this process all the way to the end! Thank you auld friend!

To Berit Fischer, our new addition to the team and dear friend for many years ... since her Ithaca times! We go back a while, I know ... What a journey! This one will be difficult to forget!

To all the authors in this book and those that were authors and then weren't anymore ... This project went through many stages and many designs ... as I said ... unprecedented times and challenges in making this book a reality. This book is also yours!

To all my workmates, especially Drs. Manuel Martin-Flores, Robin Gleed, and Jordyn Boesch, for allowing me to go into close confinement to "type and read stuff"!

Finally, to my beloved wife and children, Ewa, Kyla, and Kian, for being so patient with me and never asking why...

Luis Campoy

To my mom, my editor growing up in more ways than one, who taught me to always pay attention to the details. To my dad, my running partner, who never let me quit. To my husband, Mike, who smiled and said "Go for it" when I was presented with the opportunity to be an editor for this book. His support throughout my career has been steadfast and in ways I can never repay. To my two amazing daughters, Abigail and Ilse, who continue to inspire me daily with their creativity and thirst for knowledge. I am so incredibly fortunate. And to my co-editors and friends, Matt and Luis, who, having both been mentors at different points in my career, decided to share this journey with me. Until next time...

Berit Fischer

Small Animal Regional Anesthesia and Analgesia

SECOND EDITION

Edited by

Matt Read

Anesthesiologist and Specialty Team Leader

MedVet, Worthington, OH, USA

Luis Campoy

Clinical Professor of Anesthesiology and Pain Medicine

Section Chief of Anesthesiology and Pain Medicine

College of Veterinary Medicine

Cornell University

Ithaca, NY, USA

Berit Fischer

Head of Anesthesia and Pain Management

Eastern Pennsylvania Veterinary Medical Center

Allentown, PA, USA

WILEY Blackwell

For general information on our other products and services or for technical support, please contact our Customer Care Department within the United States at (800) 762-2974, outside the United States at (317) 572-3993 or fax (317) 572-4002.

Wiley also publishes its books in a variety of electronic formats. Some content that appears in print may not be available in electronic formats. For more information about Wiley products, visit our web site at www.wiley.com.

Library of Congress Cataloging-in-Publication Data
Names: Read, Matt, editor. | Campoy, Luis, MRCVS, editor. | Fischer,
   Berit (Berit L.), editor.
Title: Small animal regional anesthesia and analgesia / edited by Matt
   Read, Luis Campoy, Berit Fischer.
Description: Second edition. | Hoboken, New Jersey : Wiley-Blackwell,
   [2024] | Includes index.
Identifiers: LCCN 2023048958 (print) | LCCN 2023048959 (ebook) | ISBN
   9781119514152 (cloth) | ISBN 9781119514145 (adobe pdf) | ISBN
   9781119514138 (epub)
Subjects: MESH: Anesthesia, Conduction–veterinary | Anesthesia,
   Conduction–methods | Nerve Block–veterinary | Ultrasonography,
   Interventional–veterinary | Dogs–surgery | Cats–surgery
Classification: LCC SF914 (print) | LCC SF914 (ebook) | NLM SF 914 | DDC
   636.089/796–dc23/eng/20231208
LC record available at https://lccn.loc.gov/2023048958
LC ebook record available at https://lccn.loc.gov/2023048959

Cover Design: Wiley
Cover Images: © Matt Read, Luis Campoy and Berit Fischer

Set in 9.5/12pt STIXTwoText by Straive, Pondicherry, India

SKY10068721_030424

Contents

List of Contributors

Chiara Adami
Department of Veterinary Medicine
University of Cambridge
Cambridge
United Kingdom

Eric D. Brumberger
Weill Cornell Medicine, Department of Anesthesiology
NewYork-Presbyterian Hospital
New York, NY
USA

Luis Campoy
College of Veterinary Medicine
Cornell University
Ithaca, NY
USA

Tatiana H. Ferreira
School of Veterinary Medicine
University of Wisconsin, Madison
Madison, WI
USA

Berit L. Fischer
Eastern Pennsylvania Veterinary Medical Center
Allentown, PA
USA

Marta Garbin
Department of Clinical Sciences, Faculty of Veterinary Medicine
Université de Montréal
Saint-Hyacinthe, QC
Canada

Augusto Matias Lorenzutti
Facultad de Ciencias Agropecuarias
IRNASUS CONICET-Universidad Católica de Córdoba
Córdoba
Argentina

Stephan Mahler
Bestin'Vet
Saint Grégoire
France

Manuel Martin-Flores
Department of Clinical Sciences, College of Veterinary Medicine
Cornell University
Ithaca, NY
USA

Micheál Ó Cathasaigh
MOC Veterinary Radiology Ltd.
St. Neots, Cambridgeshire
UK

Pablo E. Otero
Division of Anaesthesiology and Pain Management
College of Veterinary Medicine
Buenos Aires University
Ciudad Autónoma de Buenos Aires
Argentina

Peter Pascoe
Department of Surgical and Radiological Sciences
University of California
Davis, CA
USA

Diego A. Portela
Department of Comparative, Diagnostic and Population Medicine
College of Veterinary Medicine
University of Florida
Gainesville, FL
USA

Matt Read
MedVet
Worthington, OH
USA

Marta Romano
Department of Comparative, Diagnostic and Population Medicine
College of Veterinary Medicine
University of Florida
Gainesville, FL
USA

Yael Shilo-Benjamini
Koret School of Veterinary Medicine
The Hebrew University of Jerusalem
Rehovot
Israel

Alexander C. S. Thomson
CityU Veterinary Medical Centre
Sham Shui Po, Kowloon
Hong Kong

Jaime Viscasillas
Anaesthesia Service and Pain Clinic
Silla, Valencia
Spain

Foreword

For many years, the use of local anesthetics in general veterinary practice was largely confined to providing surgical anesthesia for ruminants and performing diagnostic nerve blocks in horses. The first edition of Small Animal Regional Anesthesia and Analgesia, published in 2013, was a driving force behind the widespread adoption of locoregional anesthesia by companion animal practitioners. Since that edition of the book, the practice of locoregional anesthesia has progressed substantially, and this eagerly awaited second edition is an up-to-date reference and learning guide for the small animal practitioner.

Local anesthetic techniques are now used routinely in surgical practice to provide intra- and postoperative analgesia. These techniques allow major surgery to be accomplished at minimal depths of anesthesia and even with procedural sedation. When longer-acting local anesthetics are used, good-quality pain relief can persist well into the postoperative period. Systemic analgesics, such as opioids and nonsteroidal anti-inflammatory drugs (NSAIDs), are beset with adverse side effects and regulatory impediments to their use. The need for opioids and NSAIDs in veterinary practice will be reduced with increasing use of locoregional anesthesia. Some of the procedures described here are of interest to practitioners for relief of chronic pain, e.g., palliative care of patients with limb osteosarcoma.

The chapters are named for the nerves that are to be blocked – and each starts with a section (Block at a Glance) that summarizes the technique and its probable uses. The images include high-quality photographs, dissections, and ultrasonographs that are essential complements to the text. The quality of a nerve block is related directly to the precision with which a local anesthetic is injected. Echolocation is the most precise method available to clinicians for depositing local anesthetic proximate to target nerves – it is superior even to electrolocation. In general, such ultrasound-guided blocks performed by educated operators produce better-quality analgesia than alternative techniques and generate fewer adverse side effects. Fortunately, high-definition ultrasound equipment is now available to the general practitioner, and the editors of this book describe the approach to each block using echolocation.

As was its predecessor, this edition will surely become a primary resource for veterinary students, technicians, general practitioners, surgeons, anesthesiologists, and pain practitioners.

ROBIN D. GLEED, BVSC, MA, MRCVS, DVA, DACVAA, DIPECVAA, MRCA

Professor of Anesthesiology and Pain Management

Senior Associate Chair, Department of Clinical Sciences Cornell University

Preface

2023 marked the ten-year anniversary of the first edition of *Small Animal Regional Anesthesia and Analgesia*, aka "The Green Book", whose success over the last decade was based on the nature of its novel content and practicality. Publication of that book changed our professional lives as well as the lives of many veterinarians and veterinary team members who had an interest in anesthesia and pain management. We are so appreciative of the amazing group of contributors who helped bring that book to fruition and shared their expertise and enthusiasm for this growing area of anesthesia with our readers. We have heard time and again how the information in that edition contributed to the improved comfort and well-being of many pets worldwide and are still somewhat shocked that our book could have made such an impact.

When the first edition of *Small Animal Regional Anesthesia and Analgesia* was published, veterinary locoregional anesthesia was still considered by many to be more "art" than "science" and something that was practiced by few. Over the past ten years, interest in and knowledge of small animal locoregional anesthesia have grown exponentially beyond the scope of the first edition. Blocks have now reached into parts of the body that many of us had never envisioned (or even heard of!) and the field is maturing as a subspecialty thanks to the tireless efforts, thoughtful research, and reporting of clinical experiences of many, many people from around the world. Dissemination of new information pertaining to this exciting area of small animal anesthesia continues to rise through publications, instruction, and casual conversations, and our collective knowledge continues to grow every year for the betterment of the patients we serve.

This new, second edition of *Small Animal Regional Anesthesia and Analgesia* represents a significant revision of our original book, and we are very excited to share it with you. Following a similar path to the one taken by many of our physician counterparts, we have chosen to focus this edition almost exclusively on the use of ultrasound-guided techniques since that is the direction the published literature and clinical practice are taking us. Although we will undoubtedly miss including something, we have tried to be as all-encompassing as we could in terms of summarizing what has been published to date and including as much as is currently known about the anesthetic and analgesic techniques that the use of ultrasound affords us. We have also restructured the presentation of the content to follow a relatively consistent template, making it easier for you, the reader, to find the specific information you might be looking for. We have also tried to include the types of images that will enhance your learning and understanding of the information that is presented in the text, allowing you to appreciate many of the subtle aspects that still fall under the category of "art." This mammoth endeavor led us to add another editor to the project and to invite a dozen new and distinguished colleagues from around the world to share their varied expertise and experiences with us. Together, they have made our vision for the new edition a reality, and we are so very grateful for their support of this project and their continued friendships.

We originally set out on this project with the same goals that we outlined in the first edition of *Small Animal Regional Anesthesia and Analgesia*: to summarize the peer-reviewed and evidence-based literature for our readers, to standardize the techniques and associated nomenclature that are described, to further stimulate interest in this exciting area of veterinary anesthesia, and to improve patient care by creating a resource that would be accessible and helpful to everyone, regardless of their level of experience or training. Although we are confident that this book will be of use to students, veterinarians, technicians, veterinary anesthesiologists, and other veterinary specialists who are interested in improving their understanding of how local and regional anesthesia might fit into their practices, we appreciate that there is still so much for all of us to learn. We hope that we have achieved these goals and that you enjoy and benefit from the information in this book as much as we and our colleagues have enjoyed and benefited from preparing it.

Leave no patient unblocked! But first, do no harm... Let us continue on this journey together.

Matt, Luis, and Berit

January 2024

Acknowledgments

We would first like to acknowledge our amazing collaborators and coauthors, all of whom had great enthusiasm for seeing this new edition of Small Animal Regional Anesthesia and Analgesia come to fruition. So much has been learned and developed since the first edition was published, and it took a village to distill everything that is currently known into a single resource. Thank you all for your time, energy, and passion for sharing what you know with the world!

We also want to thank the exceptional team at Wiley for their support and patience. After many delays, we are all very thankful to see this project finally completed! We would especially like to extend our thanks to Ms. Erica Judisch, Executive Editor, Veterinary Medicine and Dentistry, for her friendship, tireless patience, and understanding over the last ten years. Without her, this edition would never have happened. We are also very grateful for Ms. Vallikkannu Narayanan, Managing Editor, Health Professions and Veterinary Medicine; Ms. Merryl Le Roux, our previous Managing Editor, Health and Life Sciences; and Ms. Susan Engelken, Editorial Publication Coordinator and all that they contributed to the process.

Considerations for Locoregional Anesthesia

PART 1

Ultrasound Guidance

The Inevitable Evolution of Locoregional Anesthesia

CHAPTER 1

Berit L. Fischer

> There's a way to do it better. Find it.
>
> —Thomas Edison

INTRODUCTION

It should come as no surprise that advancements in veterinary medicine often follow those in human medicine, and it is no different with the evolution and use of locoregional anesthesia. This is despite the fact that animals are often used to study and develop new techniques before they are ever used in people. Even Carl Koller, the Austrian ophthalmologist who first used topical cocaine to induce sensory anesthesia of the cornea in a patient for glaucoma surgery in 1884, first experimented with its desensitizing effects on the corneas of dogs and guinea pigs (Calatayud and González 2003).

The interest in, and use of, locoregional techniques has increased significantly. Much of the research up until the mid-1990s focused on the discovery of new drugs (e.g. bupivacaine, ropivacaine, bupivacaine liposome injectable suspension), techniques (e.g. nerve block catheters), and adjuvants (e.g. dexamethasone, clonidine, etc.) that could be used to extend the duration of anesthesia and analgesia provided to patients (Dahl et al. 1988; Eledjam et al. 1991; McGlade et al. 1998). Additionally, methods to assist in nerve location (i.e. paresthesia, electrical nerve stimulation) were sought to provide ways other than anatomic landmarks to target peripheral nerves, and hopefully, improve patient safety and increase success. In 1994, this search culminated in the use of ultrasound guidance when Kapral et al. (1994) published a randomized, controlled trial examining ultrasound-guided brachial plexus blocks in people. A new era in locoregional anesthesia had begun.

ULTRASOUND TECHNOLOGY

A BRIEF HISTORY

The discovery of piezoelectricity by brothers, Jacque and Pierre Curie in 1880, provided the foundation for the development of the modern-day ultrasound transducer. By applying an electric current to quartz crystals, they caused the crystals to vibrate and produce ultrasonic waves. This revolutionary finding became critical to the development of sonar that was used by submarines in World War I, and of ultrasound therapy whereby physicians could use the vibrations that were produced to treat a variety of illnesses (Duck 2021). It was not until 38 years later, in 1928, that Russian physicist SY Sokolov utilized ultrasound for imaging purposes. He invented an ultrasound transducer using a single transmitter and receiver that, when placed on opposite sides of a metal sheet, was able to detect imperfections in the metal and display line images produced from the disruptions in sound wave transmission (Duck 2021).

Ultrasound for medical imaging eventually emerged after several researchers struggled to develop transducers that could work in a hospital setting. In 1956, a predecessor of today's B-mode (i.e. "brightness" mode) ultrasound, the 2-D compound scanner, was developed by obstetrician Ian Donald and engineer Tom Brown to image an unborn fetus (Whittingham 2021) (Figure 1.1). Worldwide advancement of ultrasound technology continued throughout the 1960s and 1970s, culminating in the invention of the linear array transducer that utilized several rows of transducer elements to produce real-time scanning (Whittingham 2021).

USE OF ULTRASOUND FOR LOCOREGIONAL ANESTHESIA

Using ultrasound technology to assist with performing locoregional blockade was first reported by la Grange et al. (1978) who, after identifying the subclavian artery using Doppler ultrasound, performed supraclavicular brachial plexus blocks in 61 patients using anatomy and the presence of paresthesia to determine where to deposit the local anesthetic. It was not until 1994, however, that the use of ultrasound was first described to help guide a stimulating needle toward the target nerve trunks when performing brachial plexus blocks via both axillary and supraclavicular approaches (Kapral et al. 1994).

ULTRASOUND-GUIDED LOCOREGIONAL ANESTHESIA IN VETERINARY SPECIES

As the use of ultrasound guidance in regional anesthesia grew in human medicine, its use slowly started to emerge in the veterinary literature, first with a paper describing the sonographic appearance of canine sciatic nerves in 2007, followed

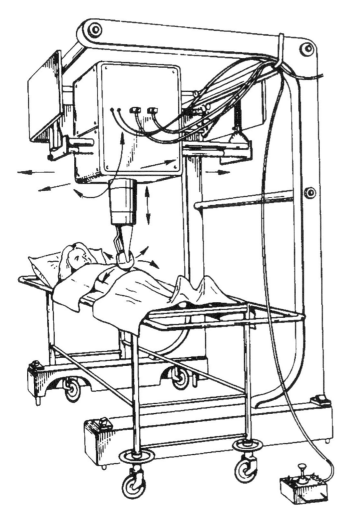

FIGURE 1.1   Drawing of the 2-D compound scanner, developed through the collaborative efforts of Dr. Ian Donald and Tom Brown. Source: McNay and Fleming (1999)/with permission of Elsevier.

shortly thereafter by a similar study that described the use of ultrasound for evaluation of the canine brachial plexus (Benigni et al. 2007; Guilherme and Benigni 2008).

   The first study to describe the use of ultrasound-guided blocks in dogs was accepted for publication in 2009 (Campoy et al. 2010). That study reported using an in-plane needle technique to approach the brachial plexus and the femoral and sciatic nerves in medium- and large-breed dogs. Each approach was followed by deposition of a mixture of lidocaine and methylene blue at the target site, allowing for later identification of nerve staining after euthanasia of the dogs for unrelated purposes. Later that same year, the first efficacy study that documented successful sensory blockade following ultrasound-guided saphenous and sciatic nerve blocks in dogs was submitted for publication by Costa-Farré et al. (2011), and the first description of using ultrasound-guided blocks in cats was published by Haro et al. in 2013. Since then, use of ultrasound guidance for nerve blocks has been reported in a wide range of veterinary species (De Vlamynck et al. 2013; Hughey et al. 2022).

HOW ULTRASOUND GUIDANCE HAS CHANGED LOCOEGIONAL ANESTHESIA

Objective measurement of the impact a new modality or treatment has on an industry, in this case medicine, can be difficult to determine, particularly when it is first being instituted. Fortunately, the impact of ultrasound guidance on regional anesthesia has been established. In 2017, Vlassakov and Kissin (2017) published a study assessing notable advances in regional anesthesia from 1996 through 2015. They evaluated meta-analyses that had been published on a variety of regional anesthesia topics based on their ability to demonstrate measurable clinical benefits. Various topics were analyzed based on their level of academic interest, findings of statistically significant effects, their overall risk of bias, the degree of heterogeneity between the studies within each meta-analysis, and the determination of a minimal clinically important difference (MCID). Of all the topics they analyzed, they concluded that within this 20-year time period, the discovery and development of ultrasound guidance for performing upper and lower limb peripheral nerve blocks was the one of greatest clinical importance.

   This has been supported in practice by several studies that compared the use of ultrasound guidance to other methods of nerve location (i.e. electrostimulation, paresthesia, etc.) for performing regional blocks. A compilation of these findings, published by the American Society of Regional Anesthesia and Pain Medicine (ASRA), provided an objective evidence-based assessment of the literature in order to determine if ultrasound guidance produced a positive effect on the performance, efficacy, and/or safety of regional blocks over other methods of nerve location (Neal et al. 2016). As interest has grown, the feasibility of incorporating ultrasound guidance into large-scale operations and its financial impact have also been investigated and addressed through cost-analysis studies (Liu and John 2010; Ehlers et al. 2012).

PERFORMANCE AND EFFICACY

The ASRA determined that when ultrasound guidance was compared to other methods of nerve location for extremity blocks, it was favored based on fewer needle passes, faster block performance, decreased onset time, and greater block success, with high levels of evidence and minimal differences between upper and lower extremities (Neal et al. 2016). Use of ultrasound guidance for neuraxial blocks also demonstrated superior performance when compared to palpation in terms of determining the correct vertebral interface, requiring fewer needle sticks, and the ability to accurately predict the needle insertion depth to the target ahead of time. Less demonstrable evidence was available at the time of that study to fully evaluate the impact of ultrasound guidance on the performance of truncal blocks, with many of the techniques currently being used still in development and/or lacking methods of comparison to other techniques.

SAFETY

When compared to other methods, one of the most notable benefits of incorporating ultrasound guidance into performance of regional anesthesia is a decreased incidence of local anesthetic systemic toxicity (LAST). Barrington and Kluger (2013) published a landmark study that evaluated the incidence of LAST following peripheral nerve blockade using either ultrasound-guided or non-ultrasound-guided techniques in 20021 patients (25336 blocks). They determined that use of ultrasound guidance reduced the risk of LAST by more than 65% compared to when other techniques were used. This was likely due to being able to visualize and avoid large blood vessels in the target area, recognizing potential intravascular injections earlier by noting the absence of local anesthetic spread in the area of interest, being able to use smaller local anesthetic doses to achieve successful blockade, and requiring fewer repeat blocks because of block failure (Marhofer et al. 1998; Barrington and Kluger 2013). Of particular interest, though not reported in other studies, was that there was no difference in the incidence of vascular puncture between the different groups. Barrington and Kluger postulated that when vascular punctures occurred during performance of ultrasound-guided blocks, they did not result in LAST because the intravascular injections were recognized by the anesthetist and halted before their patients developed clinical signs. With development of newer technologies, such as color power Doppler, the ability to identify smaller, low-flow blood vessels near the area of interest may be further improved, preventing vascular punctures, and accentuating the benefits of ultrasound- over non-ultrasound-guided techniques for preventing LAST to a greater extent (Martinoli et al. 1998).

While several areas within regional anesthesia have been impacted positively by the introduction of ultrasound guidance, the ASRA was unable to find an appreciable difference in the incidence of neurologic complications (i.e. sensorimotor deficits) following peripheral nerve blockade when ultrasound was used versus not (Neal et al. 2016). Several explanations were provided, including lack of technical skill or training of the anesthetist, the inability of ultrasound technology to provide the necessary resolution to allow discrimination between neural and nonneural tissues, and the presence of anatomical barriers that impair visualization of the needle tip.

A retrospective analysis comparing the incidence of neurologic outcomes following interscalene brachial plexus blocks in people before and after the institution of ultrasound guidance was published the same year as the ASRA assessment (Rajpal et al. 2016). Those authors found that the incidence of neurologic complications was significantly lower with ultrasound guidance than the historical rates that were published for the same block using electrostimulation (2% versus 10%, respectively). These results could indicate that ultrasound guidance, when specific blocks are evaluated (particularly those with higher risk of nerve injury), may demonstrate a better risk profile for postoperative neurologic symptoms versus evaluating all blocks as a whole. The potential benefit of using ultrasound to reduce the incidence of neurologic injury has not been definitively proven, so anesthetists need to demonstrate continued diligence when performing blocks, even if ultrasound is being used.

FINANCIAL IMPACT

Incorporation of new modalities is often associated with a price tag. Cost, in many situations, may determine whether a new technique has the ability to be utilized by a larger medical population. Studies in people have investigated the financial impact of using ultrasound guidance for performing locoregional blocks versus other methods. A study that used computer modeling to evaluate cost differences between ultrasound-guided and nerve stimulation for regional anesthesia determined that, when used in an ambulatory setting, ultrasound-guided blocks only became more expensive than using nerve stimulation if the block success rate for nerve stimulation was >96% (Liu and John 2010). This is considerably higher than success rate outcomes for several randomized controlled studies where complete sensory block using nerve stimulation occurred 27–76% versus 87–100% of the time when using ultrasound guidance (Liu 2016).

A prospective clinical study evaluating the cost-effectiveness of ultrasound-guided versus nerve stimulator-guided catheter insertion for continuous sciatic nerve blocks had similar, albeit more relevant, findings (Ehlers et al. 2012). Those authors used the ratio of added cost to the number of additional successful nerve blocks to determine that the use of ultrasound guidance is 84.7% more likely to be effective and less expensive than use of nerve stimulation. It is important to remember, however, that these numbers have the ability to be influenced by several factors, including fluctuating costs of equipment, caseload, and expertise of personnel.

VETERINARY MEDICINE
PERFORMANCE, EFFICACY, AND SAFETY

Only two studies have evaluated the use of ultrasound guidance versus other methods of nerve location in veterinary species, likely a reflection of the relative newness of these techniques and the number of individuals performing them. Both studies compared ultrasound guidance to nerve stimulation in dogs undergoing brachial plexus blocks. Using six Beagles in a crossover study, Akasaka and Shimizu (2017) found that the use of ultrasound guidance resulted in faster block performance, faster onset time, and longer duration of analgesia than when nerve stimulation was used with similar efficacy. Another small clinical study ($n = 32$) sought to determine the differences in complication rates and efficacy in dogs undergoing either ultrasound-guided or nerve-stimulator-guided brachial plexus blocks for thoracic limb surgery. Block success rate in this study was 87% (14/16 dogs) for ultrasound-guided blocks and 75% (12/16 dogs) for nerve stimulator-guided blocks ($P > 0.05$), with similar rates of minor complications (i.e. hypotension, Horner's syndrome) in both groups (Benigni et al. 2019). Unfortunately, these studies do not allow specific metrics or meta-analyses to be performed, leaving veterinary clinicians to rely upon those recommendations produced from studies in people until more data becomes available.

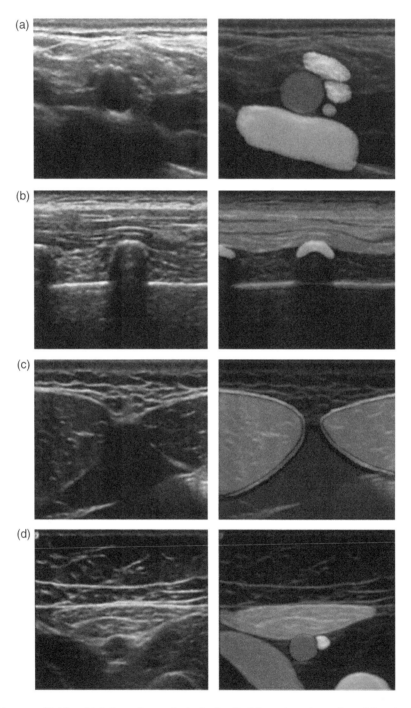

FIGURE 1.2 Ultrasound images of (a) brachial plexus (supraclavicular level); (b) erector spinae plane; (c) rectus sheath; and (d) adductor canal (mid-thigh). Images on the right have artificial intelligence (AI)-assisted identification (ScanNav™ Anatomy PNB) of bone (blue), blood vessels (red), nerves (yellow), fasciae (orange), pleura (purple), and peritoneum (brown). Source: From Bowness et al. (2021)/John Wiley & Sons.

FINANCIAL IMPACT

A recent study by Warrit et al. (2019) compared the financial impact of using ultrasound-guided lumbar plexus and sciatic nerve blocks that were confirmed with nerve stimulation versus no blocks in dogs undergoing tibial plateau leveling osteotomies. Those authors found that dogs that did not receive peripheral nerve blocks had more episodes of hypotension, more interventions to manage hypotension, and more requirements for postoperative rescue analgesia both immediately upon recovery, as well as over the next 12 hours, than dogs that received ultrasound-guided blocks. As a result, dogs in the no-block group had significantly greater and more variable anesthesia costs than the dogs receiving nerve blocks, despite the increased cost of using more advanced equipment such as the ultrasound machine. The authors acknowledged that these cost savings could vary or even be negated in patients that did not develop hypotension or other complications requiring additional interventions. It is worth mentioning that fixed anesthesia costs were not significantly different, with no difference in total anesthesia time being observed between the two groups ($P = 0.4$). This may speak to the use of ultrasound guidance and its ability to decrease the time it takes to perform peripheral nerve blocks, similar to what has been shown in people.

WHAT IS NEXT?

Many of the challenges of performing ultrasound-guided regional anesthesia have primarily been attributed to lack of anesthetist skill and training or technological limitations of currently available ultrasound equipment. These include the inability to identify the needle tip due to anatomic impediments, steep angles or deeper targets, and transducer resolution incapable of allowing identification of structures less than 1 mm in size (e.g. individual fascicles within the nerve) (Abdallah et al. 2016).

These challenges are being addressed, particularly with the advent of artificial intelligence (AI). Recent publications have incorporated AI software capable of identifying and delineating muscles, fasciae, blood vessels, and nerves to assist the anesthetist in image interpretation and subsequent nerve block performance (Figure 1.2) (Bowness et al. 2021). The benefits of such technology, particularly in the training of new regional anesthetists, are just starting to be recognized and appreciated.

SUMMARY

The evolution of ultrasound-guided regional anesthesia has soundly inserted itself into veterinary medicine. With a trajectory in line with its development in human medicine, the expectation can only be to assume that ultrasound guidance will phase out older technologies and become the new standard of care when performing regional anesthesia and analgesia in veterinary patients.

REFERENCES

Abdallah FW, MacFarlane AJ, Brull R (2016) The requisites of needle-to-nerve proximity for ultrasound-guided regional anesthesia: a scoping review of the evidence. Reg Anesth Pain Med 41, 221–228.

Akasaka M, Shimizu M (2017) Comparison of ultrasound- and electrostimulation-guided nerve blocks of brachial plexus in dogs. Vet Anaesth Analg 44, 625–635.

Barrington MJ, Kluger R (2013) Ultrasound guidance reduces the risk of local anesthetic systemic toxicity following peripheral nerve blockade. Reg Anesth Pain Med 38, 289–299

Benigni L, Corr SA, Lamb CR (2007) Ultrasonographic assessment of the canine sciatic nerve. Vet Radiol Ultrasound 48, 428–433.

Benigni L, Lafuente P, Viscasillas J (2019) Clinical comparison of two techniques of brachial plexus block for forelimb surgery in dogs. Vet J 244, 23–27.

Bowness J, Varsou O, Turbitt L et al. (2021) Identifying anatomical structures on ultrasound: assistive artificial intelligence in ultrasound-guided regional anesthesia. Clin Anat 34, 802–809.

Calatayud J, González A (2003) History of the development and evolution of local anesthesia since the coca leaf. Anesthesiology 98, 1503–1508.

Campoy L, Bezuidenhout AJ, Gleed RD et al. (2010) Ultrasound-guided approach for axillary brachial plexus, femoral nerve, and sciatic nerve blocks in dogs. Vet Anaesth Analg 37, 144–153.

Costa-Farré C, Blanch XS, Cruz JI et al. (2011) Ultrasound guidance for the performance of sciatic and saphenous nerve blocks in dogs. Vet J 187, 221–224.

Dahl JB, Christiansen CL, Daugaard JJ et al. (1988) Continuous blockade of the lumbar plexus after knee surgery – postoperative analgesia and bupivacaine plasma concentrations. Anaesthesia 43, 1015–1018.

De Vlamynck CA, Pille F, Hauspie S et al. (2013) Evaluation of three approaches for performing ultrasonography-guided anesthetic blockade of the femoral nerve in calves. Am J Vet Res 74, 750–756.

Duck F (2021) Ultrasound – the first fifty years. Med Phys Int 5, 470–498.

Ehlers L, Jensen JM, Bendtsen TF (2012) Cost-effectiveness of ultrasound *vs* nerve stimulation guidance for continuous sciatic nerve block. Brit J Anaesth 109, 804–808.

Eledjam JJ, Deschodt J, Viel EJ et al. (1991) Brachial plexus block with bupivacaine: effects of added alpha-adrenergic agonists: comparison between clonidine and epinephrine. Can J Anaesth 38, 870–875.

Guilherme S, Benigni L (2008) Ultrasonographic anatomy of the brachial plexus and major nerves of the canine thoracic limb. Vet Radiol Ultrasound 49, 577–583.

Haro P, Laredo F, Gil F et al. (2013) Ultrasound-guided block of the feline sciatic nerve. J Feline Med Surg 14, 545–552.

Hughey S, Campbell D, Rapp-Santos K et al. (2022) Refining the rat sciatic nerve block: a novel ultrasound-guided technique. Lab Anim 56, 191–195.

Kapral S, Krafft P, Eibenberger K et al. (1994) Ultrasound-guided supraclavicular approach for regional anesthesia of the brachial plexus. Anesth Analg 78, 507–513.

la Grange P, Foster PA, Pretorius LK (1978) Application of the Doppler ultrasound bloodflow detector in supraclavicular brachial plexus block. Br J Anaesth 50, 965–967.

Liu SS (2016) Evidence basis for ultrasound-guided block characteristics onset, quality, and duration. Reg Anesth Pain Med 41, 205–220.

Liu SS, John RS (2010) Modeling cost of ultrasound versus nerve stimulator guidance for nerve blocks with sensitivity analysis. Reg Anesth Pain Med 35, 57–63.

Marhofer P, Schrogendorfer K, Wallner T et al. (1998) Ultrasonographic guidance reduces the amount of local anesthetic for 3-in-1 blocks. Reg Anesth Pain Med 23, 584–588.

Martinoli C, Pretolesi F, Crespi G et al. (1998) Power doppler sonography: clinical applications. Eur J Radiol 2, S133-S140.

McGlade DP, Kalpokas MV, Mooney PH et al. (1998) A comparison of 0.5% ropivacaine and 0.5% bupivacaine for axillary brachial plexus anaesthesia. Anaesth Intensive Care 26, 515–520.

McNay MB, Fleming JEE (1999) Forty years of obstetric ultrasound 1957–1997: from A-scope to three dimensions. Ultrasound Med Biol 25, 3–56.

Neal JM, Brull R, Horn JL et al. (2016) The second American society of regional anesthesia and pain medicine evidence-based medicine assessment of ultrasound-guided regional anesthesia: executive summary. Reg Anesth Pain Med 41, 181–194.

Rajpal G, Winger DG, Cortazzo M et al. (2016) Neurologic outcomes after low-volume, ultrasound-guided interscalene block and ambulatory shoulder surgery. Reg Anesth Pain Med 41, 477–481.

Vlassakov KV, Kissin I (2017) Assessing advances in regional anesthesia by their portrayals in meta-analyses: an alternative view on recent progress. BMC Anesthesiol 17, 112.

Warrit K, Griffenhagen G, Goph C et al. (2019) Financial impact of ultrasound-guided lumbar plexus and sciatic nerve blocks with electrostimulation for tibial plateau leveling osteotomy surgery in dogs. Vet Anaesth Analg 46, 682–688.

Whittingham T (2021) The diasonograph story. Med Phys Int 6, 565–601.

Use of Ultrasound for Locoregional Anesthesia

Matt Read, Micheál Ó Cathasaigh, and Luis Campoy

INTRODUCTION

Over the last 20 years, advances in ultrasound technology, including improvements in resolution and enhancements in image processing power and software, have allowed ultrasound-guided locoregional anesthetic techniques to evolve to where we are today in terms of the number of different techniques that are performed and the effects that can be appreciated in terms of efficacy of anesthesia and analgesia, efficiency of performance, and effects on reducing complications and enhancing patient safety (Griffin and Nicholls 2010; Neal 2016; Neal et al. 2016; Wang et al. 2017; Barrington and Uda 2018). Many of the regional anesthetic techniques that have been developed for use in humans are also applicable to veterinary species and can be used effectively and safely in animals to provide anesthesia and analgesia for a variety of painful procedures and conditions (Figure 2.1).

BASIC PHYSICS AND TECHNOLOGY

An ultrasound wave is a form of *acoustic* (mechanical) energy that travels as a longitudinal wave, interfacing with a continuous elastic medium (in the case of medical ultrasound, the body) by compression (areas of high pressure) and rarefaction (areas of low pressure) of that medium's particles. When discussing ultrasound and how it can be used in medical fields, it is useful to understand some basic terminology:

- *Period* – the time for a sound wave to complete one cycle, usually measured in microseconds (μs).

- *Wavelength* – the distance between pressure peaks, usually measured in nanometers (nm), (also referred to as "pulse length").

- *Frequency* – the number of pressure peaks per second, measured in Hertz (Hz).

- *Acoustic velocity* – the propagation velocity by which a sound wave travels through a medium, calculated as the product of frequency and wavelength. In the human body, this speed is fairly constant (~1540 m s^{-1}) (Sites et al. 2007a).

Medical ultrasound uses frequencies of sound (2–15 MHz) that are many times greater than those that are audible to the human ear (20 Hz–20 kHz). These ultrasound waves are created by passing an electric current through rows of piezoelectric crystals that are housed within an ultrasound transducer. Both natural and human-made materials, including quartz crystals and ceramic materials, can demonstrate piezoelectric properties. Recently, lead zirconate titanate has been used as piezoelectric material for medical imaging. By stacking piezoelectric elements into different layers within a transducer, electric energy can be transformed into mechanical oscillations more efficiently.

In order to generate an ultrasound image, these sound waves must bounce off tissues and return to the transducer. After generating an ultrasound wave, the transducer switches to receiving mode and waits until reflected waves return and vibrate the piezoelectric crystals, converting mechanical energy back into electrical energy. This information is then processed by a computer and signal intensity from regions within the area being scanned is converted into pixels whose brightness, based on an arbitrary gray scale, creates a 2-dimensional (2-D) image on the ultrasound screen that displays the cross-sectional anatomy from which the sound waves were returned. This process of transmission and reception is repeated by the transducer thousands of times every second, allowing the resulting images to be displayed in real time.

The number (and timing) of ultrasound waves that return to the transducer depends on the degree to which they are reflected off structures in the body. As ultrasound waves travel through the body, they interact with various tissues through *reflection*, *refraction*, *scatter*, and *attenuation*, depending on the physical properties of the tissues and the degree to which they prevent the transmission of ultrasound waves (Figure 2.2). Structures, such as nerves, are displayed more clearly, and hence, are easier to see when they are surrounded by tissues that have different acoustic impedances since the greater the difference(s), the easier it is for the ultrasound machine to process the information being returned to the

Publications per Year

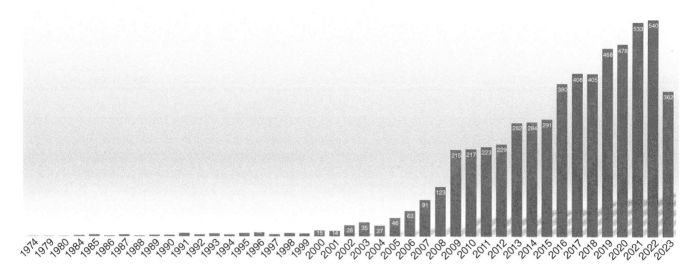

FIGURE 2.1 Graphical representation of the number of publications relating to ultrasound-guided regional anesthesia that enter the human and veterinary literature each year.

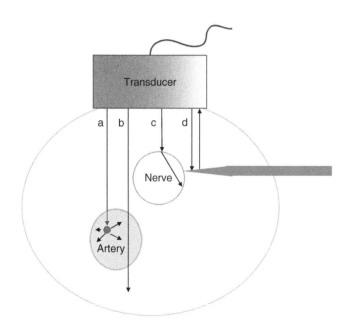

FIGURE 2.2 The many responses that an ultrasound wave produces when traveling through tissue. (a) Scatter reflection: the ultrasound wave is deflected in several random directions both to and away from the probe. Scattering occurs with small or irregular objects. (b) Transmission: the ultrasound wave continues through the tissue away from the probe. (c) Refraction: when an ultrasound wave contacts the interface between two media with different propagation velocities, the ultrasound wave is refracted (bent) depending upon the difference in velocities. (d) Specular reflection: reflection from a large, smooth object (such as a needle) which returns the ultrasound wave toward the probe when it is perpendicular to the ultrasound beam. Based on Sites et al. 2007a.

transducer (Sites et al. 2007a). The overall effect of these interactions is termed "*acoustic impedance*" and determines how many ultrasound waves are ultimately returned to the transducer to be processed.

As sound waves travel into the body, there is a progressive loss of acoustic energy as the waves pass through different tissues. This loss of energy is the result of the conversion of some of the mechanical energy into heat and is referred to as "*attenuation*." Different tissues cause loss of energy differently, which is based on their attenuation coefficient (measured as decibels per centimeter of tissue). The higher the attenuation coefficient of the tissue, the more the energy is lost (Table 2.1). When attenuation occurs, there is a coincident decrease in the intensity of the returning signal.

Higher-frequency waves undergo more attenuation than lower-frequency waves and, therefore, do not penetrate tissues as deeply (Figure 2.3). Settings on the ultrasound machine may need to be adjusted to artificially increase the signal intensity of these returning echoes so they can be

Table 2.1 Attenuation coefficients of different tissues (at 1 MHz).

Material	dB cm^{-1}
Bone	20
Air	12
Muscle	1.2
Fat	0.6
Blood	0.2

Source: Sites et al. (2007a)/BMJ Publishing Group Ltd.

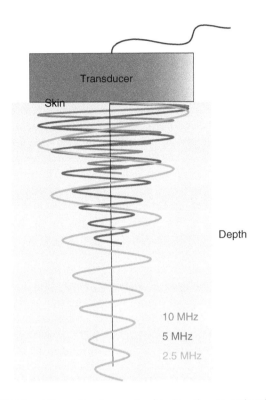

Transducer

Skin

Depth

10 MHz

5 MHz

2.5 MHz

FIGURE 2.3   Attenuation (energy loss) is directly proportional to the frequency of the sound waves and the distance that the sound waves must travel. Note how the lower-frequency US waves are less attenuated compared with the higher-frequency (10 MHz) wave at any given distance (depth). Based on Brull et al. 2010.

processed into useful information for the user (see *image optimization*, below) (Sites et al. 2007a).

The final image that is produced is dependent on the number of waves that are returned to the transducer (which, in turn, is governed by the acoustic impedance of each tissue, as well the differences in impedances between different tissues) and the time it takes for those waves to return (i.e. longer return times are interpreted by the computer as being reflected by objects that are located farther away/deeper in the scan field).

The number and intensity of sound waves that are received by the transducer determine the "*echogenicity*" (brightness) of the reflecting object when it is displayed on the ultrasound screen. Brighter objects (referred to as being "*hyperechoic*") are associated with the return of more waves and, conversely, darker objects (referred to as being "*hypoechoic*") or black objects (referred to as being "*anechoic*") are associated with the return of fewer or no waves, respectively. For example, the acoustic impedance of air and bone (Table 2.1) causes reflection of a large proportion of the sound waves, which creates a bright, hyperechoic structure on the ultrasound screen. Hypoechoic tissues are those that tend to have greater water content, allowing the sound waves to travel through them more easily so fewer waves are reflected and received as echoes by the transducer.

IMAGE QUALITY

Image quality, or "*resolution*," refers to an ultrasound machine's ability to distinguish between different objects and tissues, ultimately determining the amount of detail that can be captured and subsequently displayed as an image. When it comes to performing regional anesthesia, the most important types of resolution to understand are:

- *Spatial* (axial and lateral)
- *Contrast*
- *Temporal*

Spatial Resolution

"*Spatial resolution*" refers to the ability of the ultrasound machine to differentiate between two different, but closely spaced, structures as being separate, discrete objects. This is determined primarily by the *axial* and *lateral* resolutions of the ultrasound beam, which are affected by different aspects of the physics related to use of ultrasonography.

Axial resolution refers to the ability of the ultrasound machine to discern two structures that are located along/parallel to the direction of the ultrasound beam (i.e. overlapping but at different depths from one another) (Brull et al. 2010) (Figure 2.4). Axial resolution is roughly equal to ½ of the pulse length, such that if the distance between the two objects is greater than ½ of the length of the ultrasound pulse, they will appear as two discrete structures on the screen (Sites et al. 2007a).

$$\text{Axial resolution} = \text{Wavelength} \times \text{Number of cycles} \\ \text{per pulse}/2$$

The number of cycles within a pulse is determined by the damping characteristics of the transducer and is usually preset between two and four by the manufacturer of the ultrasound machine. For example, if a 2 MHz ultrasound transducer is used for scanning, the axial resolution would be between 0.8 and 1.6 mm, making it impossible to visualize a 21-gauge needle. Constant acoustic velocity, higher-frequency, ultrasound transducers can detect very small objects and provide images with better resolution. Thankfully, the axial resolution of current ultrasound systems is between 0.05 and 0.5 mm, making needles easier to see than when using earlier machines.

Using high-frequency (shorter pulse lengths) ultrasound waves will result in the highest degree of axial resolution, the most detail, and the best image quality. However, as described above, high-frequency waves are subject to the highest degree of attenuation (i.e. from both scatter and absorption), resulting in overall poor tissue penetration and the inability to provide information about deeper structures. This is why most high frequency (10–15 MHz) transducers,

(a)

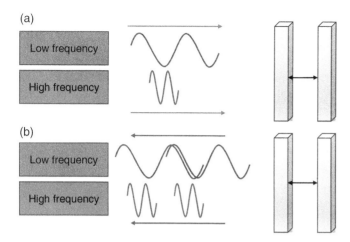

(b)

FIGURE 2.4 Axial resolution is the ability to discern objects in-line with the axis of the ultrasound beam. The axial resolution of an ultrasound wave is dependent upon wavelength, frequency, and the speed of ultrasound in tissue. Axial resolution is roughly described as one-half of the pulse length in mm. (a) A low-frequency and a high-frequency pulse propagating toward two rectangular objects. (b) The waves returning toward the probe following the reflection off of the objects. The blue arrows depict the ultrasound pulse traveling toward the two objects and the red arrows depict the ultrasound traveling back toward the transducer. The lower-frequency ultrasound has a wavelength that is larger than the distance between the objects (indicated by the black arrows), therefore, the returning signal from both objects will overlap and the probe will interpret this signal as coming from a single object. The higher-frequency pulse discerns two separate objects because the wavelength is much shorter than the distance between the two objects and the returning waves will not overlap. Based on Sites et al. 2007a.

while very good at imaging superficial objects at target depths of up to 3–4 cm (such as most peripheral nerves in dogs and cats), are unable to effectively image structures deeper than 6 cm.

When using ultrasound to perform nerve blocks, there is always going to be a trade-off between maximizing the axial resolution of the machine and the depth of penetration of the ultrasound waves. For this reason, it is important for the regional anesthetist to find the optimal balance between using the highest possible frequency, while still obtaining information about the target structures that are located at a particular depth (Brull et al. 2010).

Based on the depth of the target structure(s), the anesthetist should initially choose the appropriate transducer for the intended purpose (i.e. one with a high- [8–15 MHz], medium- [6–10 MHz], or low- [2–5 MHz] frequency ranges], with the next step being selection of the specific frequency of ultrasound waves to be emitted. Many ultrasound machines now allow the user to adjust the transducer frequency during use. For example, on some machines (e.g. Sonosite), the user can select between the low-, mid-, or high-end of the

transducer's stated frequency range by selecting the PEN (penetration), GEN (general), or RES (resolution) settings, respectively (Brull et al. 2010).

Lateral resolution refers to the ability of the ultrasound machine to discern two closely spaced objects as being distinct from each other when they lie perpendicular to the beam direction (i.e. beside each other at the same depth) (Sites et al. 2007a) (Figure 2.5). Even though the user sees a 2-D image on the screen, the ultrasound waves that are generated by the transducer are actually being emitted in three dimensions. These waves have a self-focusing effect, which refers to the natural narrowing of the ultrasound beam at a certain distance/depth where the waves converge toward each other slightly before diverging as they transmit further into the body (Figure 2.6). Conceptually, targets could be missed if they were small enough to "slip in between" the incoming ultrasound waves if the beam was divergent. By using the concept of "*focus*," the user can minimize the chances of this occurring and make sure that lateral resolution is maximized in the area of interest.

Since the emitted waves are closest together at the narrowest part of the ultrasound beam, this area has the highest degree of lateral resolution and is referred to as the "*focal*" or "*transition zone*." The relative position of the focal/transition zone leads to the commonly used terms of "*near field*" (also called the Fresnel zone) and "*far field*" (also called the Fraunhofer zone). Some ultrasound machines allow the user to manually adjust and set the focal zone (as indicated by a marker/arrow on the side of the screen) to match the depth of the structure(s) they are most interested in. In the case of

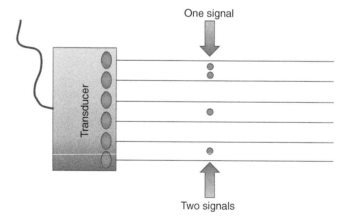

FIGURE 2.5 Lateral resolution is demonstrated here for a hypothetical linear ultrasound transducer. The ability of the ultrasound machine to correctly display two objects as separate structures depends on the relative distance between individual piezoelectric crystals versus the distance between the objects. The top two structures in this example will be imaged as one structure because each falls within surrounding crystal beams. The red ovals indicate individual piezoelectric crystals. For illustration purposes, this figure represents a fictitious situation in which there is no focal zone or divergence of the ultrasound beam. Based on Sites et al. 2007a.

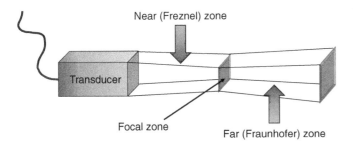

FIGURE 2.6   Characteristics of an ultrasound beam. The focal zone is where the ultrasound beam width is narrowest and demarcates the near zone (Fresnel zone) from the far zone (Fraunhofer zone). It is also the area with the best lateral resolution because the beam width is the narrowest at this location. Once the beam extends beyond the focal zone, lateral resolution begins to deteriorate due to divergence. This figure represents a prototypical electronically focused ultrasound beam. Based on Sites et al. 2007a.

many newer ultrasound machines, the focal zone is automatically set to be in the center of the screen so manual adjustments are not necessary. Instead, when using these ultrasound machines, the user simply needs to adjust the depth controls to position the area of interest (i.e. the target nerve in the case of regional anesthesia) in the center of the screen where the lateral resolution would be expected to be the highest. This way, very small objects will be more easily seen as discrete structures and the anesthetist will be able to better visualize important structures related to the block.

Contrast Resolution

"*Contrast resolution*" refers to the various shades of grey that are seen on the screen and is the ability of the ultrasound machine to distinguish between the different echo amplitudes that are returned from adjacent structures or tissues that have different characteristics. The more shades of gray that are able to be displayed on the screen, the higher the quality of the image.

Temporal Resolution

"*Temporal resolution*" relates to the inherent frame rate of the ultrasound machine, which is a measure of how quickly it can produce consecutive images (Sites et al. 2007a). The higher the frame rate, the more easily the machine will be able to accurately distinguish between events that are closely spaced in time, such as movements of a structure in real time (e.g. movement of a needle or a local anesthetic being injected). If frame rate is slow, there will be more blurring when motion is observed in the scan field, leading to a vaguer image.

Frame rate is related to the sweep speed of the ultrasound beam since sound waves are generated as adjacent/neighboring crystals are activated across the face of the transducer. The speed with which a sound wave transmits through the body's tissues and is reflected back to the transducer limits sweep speed since deeper tissues will reflect the beam

after more of a delay than shallower structures, and the next wave cannot be generated by a crystal until the preceding crystal receives its echo (Sites et al. 2007a). This is another good reason for the user to set the scan depth just below the target of interest – if beams are able to be reflected sooner, temporal resolution can be maximized.

Based on the same principle, if the local anesthetic solution is injected too quickly, movement in the surrounding tissues will be detected, resulting in blurring of the image around the target. Injections should be performed slowly to avoid this artifact. Images reconstructed in real time can have a temporal resolution of approximately 30 frames per second. Modern scanners collect multiple scan lines simultaneously with frame rates of approximately 70–80 frames per second.

COLOR DOPPLER

The "*Doppler effect*" describes the change in the frequency of a sound wave that results from the wave being reflected back to a stationary listener (in this case the transducer) from an object that is in motion (e.g. blood). Ultrasound machines utilize this principle by assessing the change(s) in frequency as sound waves are reflected back from moving red blood cells and superimposing this additional information on the existing real-time 2-D image, allowing the user to identify and quantify the direction and velocity of blood flow in the area being assessed (Brull et al. 2010) (Figure 2.7).

If red blood cells are moving toward the transducer, the frequency of the reflected echoes will be higher than the original sound wave (the sound waves have to be squeezed) and the received sound will have a higher pitch ("*positive* Doppler shift"). If the red blood cells are moving away from the transducer, the frequency of the reflected echoes will be lower than the original sound wave (the sound waves have to be stretched) and the received sound will have a lower pitch ("*negative* Doppler shift"). This is the reason behind the

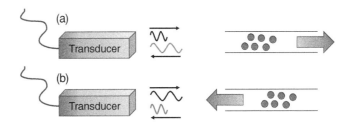

FIGURE 2.7   The Doppler effect. Doppler is used to measure velocity and directionality of objects. In the body, Doppler is most commonly used to measure velocity of blood flow. (a) The signal from fluid moving away from the probe will return at a lower frequency than the original emitted signal. (b) The signal contacting fluid moving toward the probe will return at a higher frequency than the original emitted signal. It is also important to note that the cosine of 0° is 1 and the cosine of 90° is 0. Therefore, as the angle approaches 90°, large errors are introduced into the Doppler equation.Based on Sites et al. 2007a.

sound of a siren changing as it first approaches a listener and then passes by and moves away from them. The Doppler equation states:

$$\text{Frequency shift} = \left(2 \cdot V \cdot F_1\right)\left(\text{cosine}\,\theta\right)\big/ c$$

where V is the velocity of the moving object, F_1 is the frequency of the transmitted ultrasound waves, θ is the angle of incidence of the ultrasound waves and the direction of blood flow, and c is the speed of the ultrasound waves in the tissues of interest. Since the magnitude of a Doppler shift depends on the incident angle between the emitted ultrasound beam and the moving reflectors (e.g. red blood cells when imaging a blood vessel), if the transducer is oriented nearly perpendicular or perpendicular to the vessel (i.e. at a 90° angle), there will be no Doppler shift since the cosine of 90° is zero. As a result, there will not appear to be any flow through the vessel and it will appear on the ultrasound screen as being black. When the angle is 0° or 180° (i.e. the beam is nearly parallel to the movement of the object), the largest degree of Doppler shift will be detected. For this reason, when imaging an area for suspected vessels, the transducer should be manipulated through the use of tilting (see *image optimization*, below) in order to change the angle of incidence and make sure that an error is not inadvertently made in missing the presence of a vessel in the area of the needle's planned trajectory.

Although the Doppler shift can be used to calculate both the speed of blood flow as well as the direction of blood flow (i.e. during echocardiography), these measurements are less of a priority during the performance of regional anesthesia. For the regional anesthetist, the most important use of color Doppler (also referred to as color velocity Doppler) is the ability to confirm the absence of blood flow within their planned needle path (Sites et al. 2007a; Brull et al. 2010). For this reason, color Doppler is commonly used to scan for vessels within the area of the anticipated needle trajectory since small, hypoechoic vessels look very similar to small, hypoechoic nerves when using the standard gray scale.

It is a common misconception of novices that, when using color Doppler, *red* denotes arterial flow and *blue* denotes venous flow, however, this is not always the case (Figure 2.8). Instead, the common convention has it that blood flow moving toward the transducer is assigned shades of red, while blood flow moving away from the transducer is assigned shades of blue. For this reason, if the transducer is facing "down" the direction of arterial flow, movement within the vessel will still appear blue, even though it is an artery. When using color Doppler before performing a nerve block (e.g. on a limb), it can be useful to tilt the transducer toward the heart slightly, ensuring that pulsatile arterial flow appears red, and making it easier to correlate the color of the flow with the structure it is expected to relate to.

A second form of Doppler, known as *"Color Power Doppler,"* (CPD) is up to five times more sensitive in detecting blood flow than traditional color Doppler, but it does not

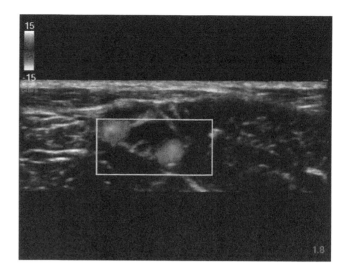

FIGURE 2.8 Ultrasonographic image of the relevant area following administration of local anesthetic for a proximal RUMM block in a dog. Color Doppler is being used to assess the intensity and direction of blood flow in order to identify the axillary artery (red) and axillary vein (blue).

provide information on the direction of flow. For this reason, CPD is particularly useful for assessing an area of the patient for very small vessels that would otherwise be difficult or impossible to see using standard color Doppler. As described above, while one limitation of using traditional color Doppler is the relationship between the angle of the ultrasound beam relative to the direction of blood flow, CPD functions almost independent of this limitation and the angle of incidence does not affect signal strength.

Since CPD does not provide information about the direction of movement (i.e. using red and blue), it uses an orange scale to indicate the intensity of the Doppler signal (Figure 2.9). Since CPD is so acutely sensitive to movement, to prevent artifacts from being introduced due to motion, the

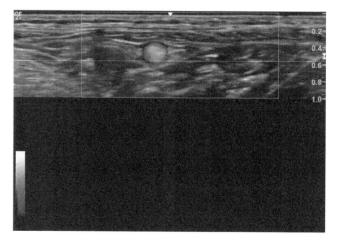

FIGURE 2.9 Ultrasonographic image demonstrating the use of CPD to indicate blood flow in the femoral artery during performance of a saphenous nerve block in a dog. Source: Berit Fischer.

transducer needs to be kept as still as possible on the patient in order for a clear image to be obtained. Other movements, such as patient respirations, can also add to the noise that is observed when CPD is being used.

IMAGE OPTIMIZATION

Image optimization (sometimes referred to as "knobology") refers to the understanding of an ultrasound machine's various settings and the adjustments that can be made to enhance image quality, and hopefully, contribute to improved efficiency and patient safety. For this reason, it is important that the anesthetist familiarize themselves with their ultrasound machine prior to use. Although many current ultrasound machines have factory-ready settings that will optimize the image for various different applications (including nerve blocks), it is useful to know how to manually make adjustments, nonetheless. With the wide range of patients that are encountered (i.e. species, breed, patient size, and body condition) and the variety of locoregional techniques that can be performed, no "one-size-fits-all" setting is likely to be effective for the small animal regional anesthetist.

DEPTH AND FOCAL POINT

As discussed previously in relation to the principles of axial and lateral resolution, to optimize an image, the depth setting on the machine should be adjusted based on the depth of the area or structure of interest in the patient. Once the target is located on the screen, it may be necessary to adjust the default depth setting of the machine so that the target appears in the center of the screen (Figure 2.10). As mentioned above, maximal lateral resolution occurs in the focal zone, so if the machine does not center this automatically, the focal zone will need to be manually adjusted.

It should be noted that altering the depth of the image will affect temporal resolution (frame rate) and potentially result in blurring and artifacts. Increasing depth reduces the temporal resolution/frame rate since it takes longer for sound waves to be reflected back to the transducer, resulting in a slight delay before the next wave can be transmitted. One way that ultrasound machines have been designed to preserve temporal resolution as depth is increased is to reduce the width of the sector beam (i.e. as opposed to it being the entire width of the transducer). This way, fewer sound waves need to be emitted and returned to the transducer, creating less delay before the image can be refreshed and displayed (Brull et al. 2010). As a result, changing the depth will change the aspect ratio of the image – increasing the depth will make the image narrower and the target structure smaller, whereas, decreasing the depth will make the image wider and the target structure larger (Figure 2.10). By appreciating this basic principle of ultrasound function, a balance between optimal depth and image quality can be obtained.

In some patients (e.g. small breed dogs or cats for RUMM or TAP blocks), very superficial structures will not be able to be placed in the focal zone, no matter how shallow the depth is set to. In this situation, the use of a "stand-off" pad may be necessary. A standoff is a custom-made silicone covering for the ultrasound transducer (Figure 2.11). Placing a standoff on the transducer will increase the distance from the face of the transducer to the patient's skin, effectively adding several mm to the distance the sound waves need to travel before they interact with the target area. This way, superficial structures that may have otherwise been too shallow to be shown in good detail are able to be imaged in the focal zone and displayed with much higher resolution.

GAIN

"*Gain*" refers to how bright (hyperechoic) or dark (hypoechoic) the overall image appears (Figure 2.12). Since the mechanical energy of returning sound waves is converted back into an electrical signal, the intensity of this signal can be manipulated by the user to adjust the brightness of all the points in the displayed image, analogous to turning up the volume on a speaker – the information being broadcast is the same, it is just louder. Increasing the gain will amplify the electrical signal produced by all of the echoes, which will increase the overall brightness of the entire image, including any background noise and any artifacts that have been generated (Brull et al. 2010). Conversely, decreasing the gain too much can negate real echo information, making the image darker and potentially making it harder to see the structures being imaged. In this situation, poor visualization could possibly result in medical errors and patient injury. Ideally, gain should be adjusted so vessels appear jet black, resulting in other structures appearing as they should.

"*Color Gain*" refers to the ability of most ultrasound machines to increase or decrease the gain of the color Doppler or CPD signal, helping to increase the conspicuity of flow within a vessel.

TIME GAIN COMPENSATION

Time gain compensation (TGC) is a selective type of gain control that compensates for the fact that, due to attenuation, echoes returning from deeper structures (i.e. those located in the far field) are weaker, and therefore, are interpreted by the machine as being darker than those returning from more superficial structures. By the same principle, the decreased attenuation of echoes returning from superficial structures (i.e. those located in the near field) can result in objects appearing relatively bright. Most modern ultrasound machines automatically compensate for these differences in attenuation, but the final image may not always be accurate so manual adjustments using TGC can be helpful for image optimization.

Using the TGC controls that are available on their machine, the anesthetist can specifically amplify the far-field echoes and reduce the intensity of the near-field echoes so that the brightness and appearance of the image can be balanced. This can be achieved using individual "slide pot" controls or

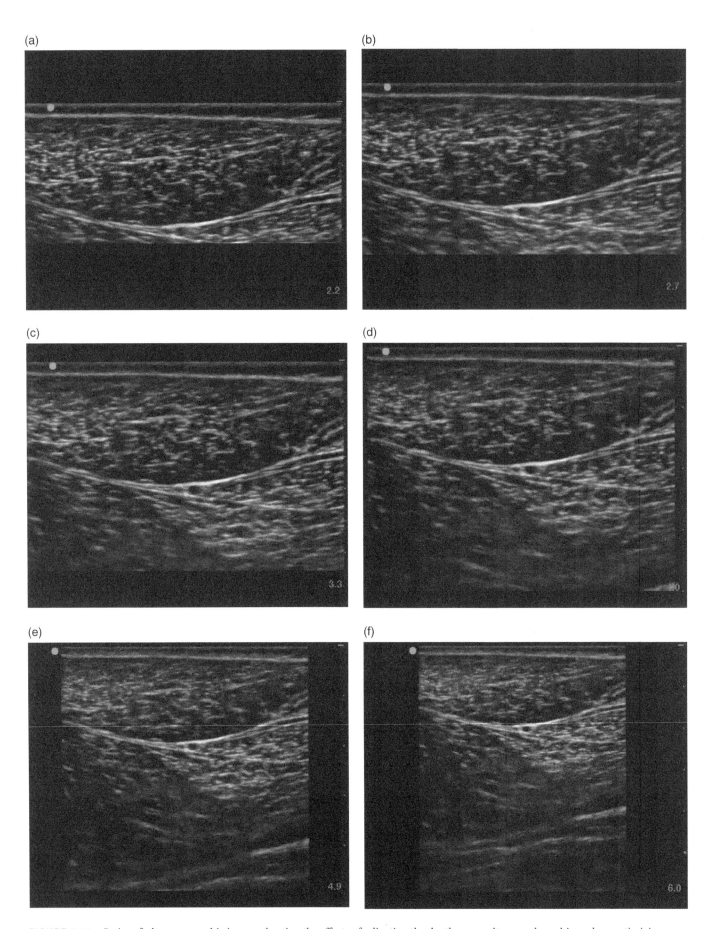

FIGURE 2.10 Series of ultrasonographic images showing the effects of adjusting the depth on an ultrasound machine when optimizing an image. Note the resolution/focus of the image when the sciatic nerve (two small adjacent circles) is positioned in the center of the image (c, d), as opposed to when the nerve is positioned outside of the ultrasound machine's focal zone (i.e. too deep (a, b) or too shallow (e and f)). Also note the changes in lateral resolution and the width of the image as depth is adjusted, with deeper settings resulting in narrower scan fields on the image (d, e, f). See text for details.

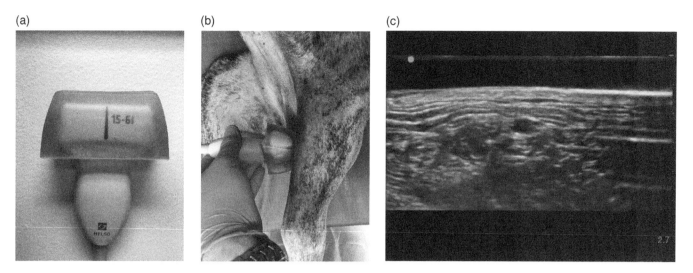

FIGURE 2.11   (a) Example of a silicone standoff pad and the corresponding ultrasonographic image (b) when it is being used to assist with centering the saphenous nerve during performance of a **saphenous nerve** block (c). Note the 0.5 cm black area at the top of the image (proximal scan field) that represents the standoff pad. The use of this tool allows the area of interest to be positioned more toward the transducer focal zone in the center of the image. Incidentally, an example of mirror artifact can be seen on the right side of the image. See Figure 2.21 and text for details.

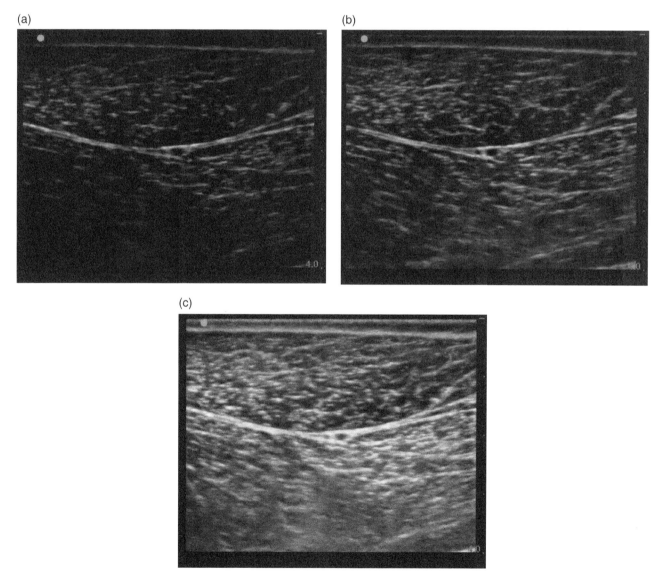

FIGURE 2.12   Series of ultrasonographic images showing the effects of adjusting the gain on an ultrasound machine when optimizing an image. (a) shows an inappropriately low gain setting ("undergain") where there is an apparent absence of existing structures, (b) is ideal, and (c) shows an inappropriately high gain setting ("overgain") where existing structures are obscured.

(a)

(b)

(c)

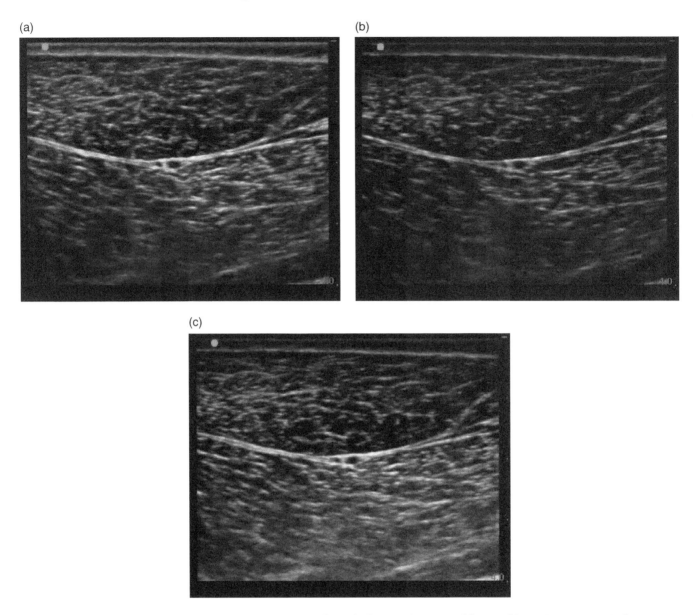

FIGURE 2.13   Series of ultrasonographic images showing the effects of adjusting the near and far gain (time gain compensation) on an ultrasound machine when optimizing an image. (a) shows the near gain turned up so the top half of the image (near field) is brightest, (b) is the neutral setting that the machine automatically set, and (c) shows the far gain turned up so the bottom half of the image (far field) is brightest.

simple "near" and "far" gain controls or dials (Figure 2.13). TGC is analogous to adjusting the equalizer on a stereo – by altering the bass and treble, the user can fine-tune the final sound to obtain the desired effect.

POWER

The *power* control is associated with the regulation of the intensity of sound *output* from the transducer, which it does by modifying the voltage being applied to pulse the piezoelectric crystals. Increasing the power has the effect of uniformly increasing the amplitude of the returning echoes. The lowest possible power setting should be used to ensure the best resolution and prevent artifacts, while still maintaining sufficient penetration of tissues. As described previously, selecting a transducer that transmits the appropriate frequency for the anticipated tissue depth and then altering the gain to increase the displayed amplitude of the returning echoes are the typical steps for optimizing image quality, with adjustments to power being less commonly made.

ZOOM

The *zoom* function can be used to focus on a specific region within an image. Zooming does not improve image quality, but simply increases the size of a specific section of the image that has already been obtained. If a sharper image is desired, it is important that other parameters, particularly depth and focal point, be adjusted prior to using the zoom feature in order to get the best possible image.

TRANSDUCER MANIPULATION

Although ultimately based on personal preference, when performing ultrasound-guided nerve blocks, most people will feel more comfortable holding and manipulating the ultrasound transducer with their nondominant hand and placing and manipulating the needle with their dominant hand. Since the dominant hand is usually better for performing movements that involve fine motor control, it is easier for most people to use this hand to hold the needle and make the small adjustments that are necessary to safely advance and position the needle tip at the target location. The nondominant hand is used to control the relatively gross movements of the transducer to improve the image, described further below. For novices, this arrangement works well as hand–eye coordination is being honed and blocks are being learned. Once a certain level of expertise is achieved, some anesthetists will choose to work on becoming ambidextrous so they can hold and manipulate the transducer and needle with either hand, though this is not necessary for performing most block techniques.

In many cases, it is easiest to visualize peripheral nerves (when they are large enough to be imaged) when they are in a "short-axis" view, that is, when they are imaged in cross section. If the ultrasound transducer is oriented so they are imaged in a long-axis view, nerve may appear very similar to structures such as veins or layers of fascia and can be harder to identify. For this reason, many block techniques for areas such as the limbs involve initially placing the transducer perpendicular to the long axis of the expected nerve trajectory in order to increase the likelihood of identifying the target nerve(s) more easily. Once the nerve(s) and other relevant structures are identified, the image should be optimized.

There are several different ways that the transducer can be manipulated to improve the image and obtain more information. When holding the transducer, the hand should ideally be positioned low down on the transducer and can even be rested on the patient to ensure that there is an even distribution of pressure on the skin and the image will remain stable on the screen. The New York School of Regional Anesthesia teaches the mnemonic PARTH to help remind the anesthetist of the specific, but complimentary, ways that the transducer can be manipulated when obtaining an image (Figure 2.14).

Pressure – As long as a coupling agent is being used and the transducer is being applied to the skin with enough force,

a clear image should be obtained and no "drop-out" (see artifacts, below) will occur. However, it can sometimes be useful to apply more pressure to the skin to compress (or, conversely, to apply less pressure to expand) structures under the transducer to help confirm their identity and/or verify their location. For example, applying more pressure can compress veins in the scan field, helping to identify them as vessels as opposed to a small, hypoechoic nerve. Conversely, letting pressure off may help to identify a vein that has inadvertently been compressed as the initial scanning was taking place. This is a common occurrence when performing certain superficial blocks, such as saphenous nerve blocks, where the vein lies just under the skin and is easy to inadvertently collapse. Use of color Doppler can help to further confirm the presence of blood flow through these structures.

Alignment – After the transducer is placed on the patient, it can be moved across the surface of the skin using an "alignment" technique. This refers to maintaining the transducer in the same orientation (i.e. perpendicular to the patient) and then gliding/sliding it in two dimensions across the skin, forward and/or backward and/or side to side. Using this technique, additional anatomy can be imaged in the general area of interest prior to needle placement. It is important to not change the orientation of the transducer, otherwise, the angle of insonation will be altered and the observed image will change.

Rotation – Rotation refers to turning the transducer clockwise or counterclockwise around its long axis. This maneuver is particularly useful when a nerve is already being imaged and the anesthetist uses small rotational manipulations to fine-tune its short-axis view (i.e. cross-sectional view). Rotation is typically used to alter the orientation of the image between 0° and 90° (i.e. so a short-axis view can be turned into a long-axis view). It is commonly used when performing thoracic paravertebral blocks and erector spinae plane blocks to change the orientation from sagittal to slightly off sagittal in order to get a better image of the target bony structures.

Tilt – Tilting (also referred to as "rocking") refers to the particular manipulation whereby the faceplate of the transducer remains on the skin and the handle is fanned back and forth to change the angle of insonation. This maneuver is very useful when looking for nerves that lie within muscles (e.g. the femoral nerve in the ***m. psoas major***) or to change the angle of the ultrasound beam relative to a vessel when trying to identify it using color Doppler.

Heel – This maneuver, referred to as "heeling," involves tipping the transducer from side to side while the faceplate stays in contact with the patient. This is a useful manipulation to improve contact on the patient (e.g. to prevent "drop out" – see artifacts, below) and/or to image structures from a slightly different angle (e.g. to look "under" a rib when performing intercostal nerve blocks).

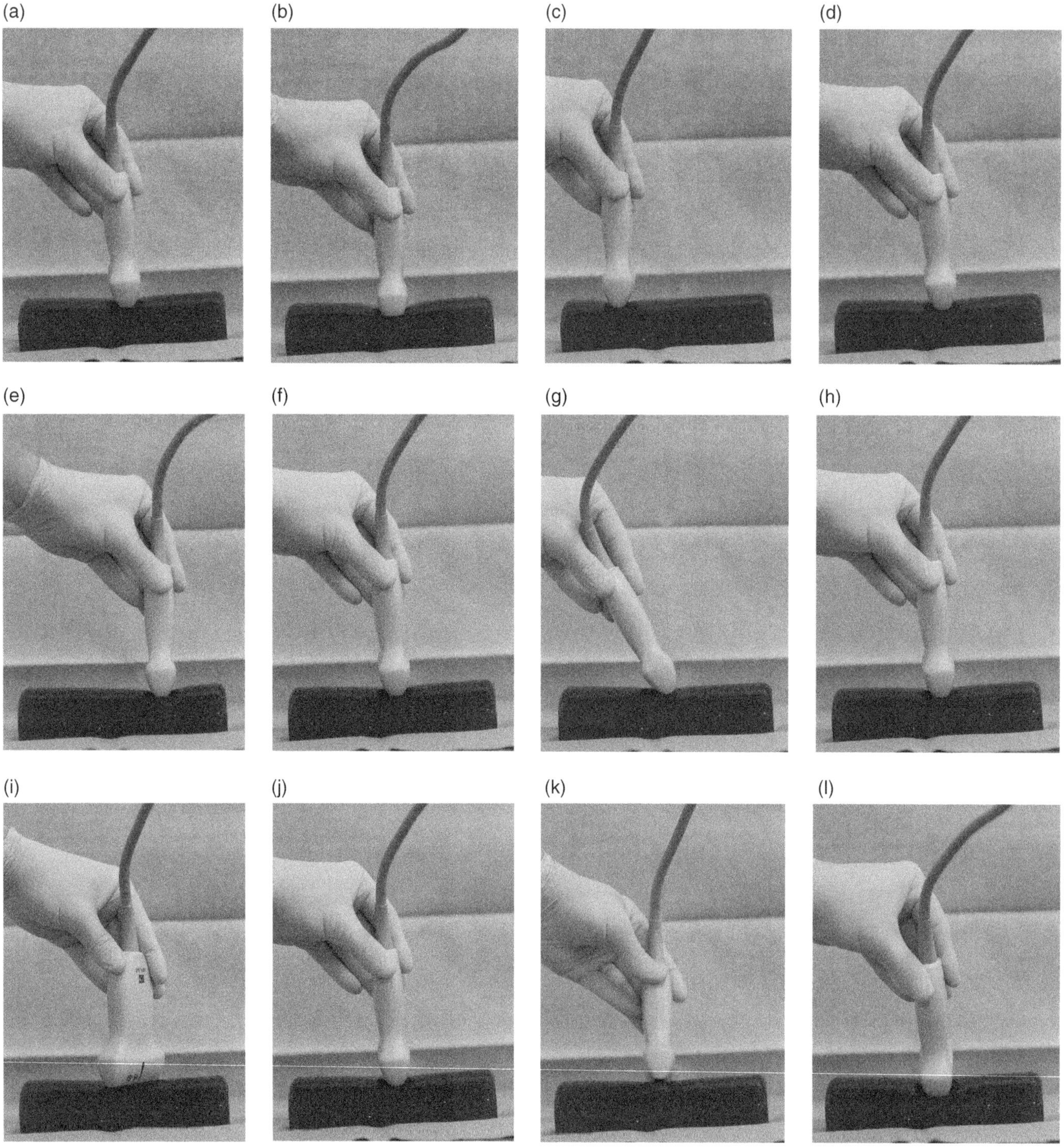

FIGURE 2.14   Series of ultrasonographic images to demonstrate the different types of transducer manipulations that can be utilized when imaging a patient. (a) neutral position. (b) applying increased pressure; (c, d, and e) sliding/gliding the transducer for alignment; (f) neutral position; (g) tilting/rocking the transducer; (h) neutral position; (i) rotation; (j) neutral position; and (k, l) heeling the transducer.

ARTIFACTS

In routine diagnostic ultrasound, numerous artifacts may develop or be present during the course of performing the study. Although many of these artifacts are disruptive and may contribute to image inaccuracies, others can be useful. For example, reverberation artifacts can indicate the presence of air, and shadowing artifacts can help identify the presence of bony structures. Additionally, some ultrasound artifacts can intentionally be used to improve the assessment of certain organs. For example, since the lungs contain air which makes it impossible for ultrasound waves to travel through them, artifacts are almost entirely relied upon to assess lung tissue. There are many different types of artifacts that may be encountered during the course of performing regional anesthesia, the most common of which will be detailed below.

CONTACT ARTIFACT (TRANSDUCER-SKIN ARTIFACT)

This artifact is encountered when there is inadequate contact and/or coupling between the transducer and the patient's skin (Figure 2.15). When this occurs, because air does not conduct ultrasound waves, they are prevented from traveling from the transducer into the patient and back again and a shadow (also called "drop-out") will appear on the screen. To prevent this from occurring, coupling agents such as alcohol or ultrasound gel should be used to remove air and improve contact between the surface of the transducer and the patient's skin. In the case of peripheral nerve blocks, the most common coupling agent is isopropyl alcohol since it is inexpensive, readily available, and usually provides enough contact for the block to be performed before it evaporates and needs to be reapplied.

To further reduce the chances of experiencing contact artifacts, the user must apply sufficient pressure to the transducer as it contacts the skin. If areas of light contact are present, "drop-out" may be seen on the screen if the sound waves encounter air and do not penetrate the body. A needle should not be advanced through an area of drop-out since it is impossible to observe the patient's anatomy or see the needle in this area. To remedy this situation, the anesthetist might consider selecting a transducer with a smaller footprint/faceplate (e.g. choosing a 35 mm linear transducer instead of 50 mm linear

transducer), adjusting the orientation of the transducer (e.g. through rotation, alignment, pressure, or heeling), and/or adding more coupling agent so the entire area of interest can be visualized.

ANISOTROPY

"*Anisotropy*" relates to changes in the appearance of soft tissues that are dependent on the angle of insonation (i.e. the angle of the ultrasound beams relative to the object(s) being imaged) (Figure 2.16). For example, certain tissues (e.g. muscles and some nerves) may appear hypoechoic when the transducer is at an oblique angle, whereas they may appear more hyperechoic when it is oriented perpendicular to them. Although the anesthetist can take advantage of this principle in many situations, it is especially useful when looking for nerves that are located within muscles, such as the **femoral nerve** in the ***m. psoas major*** when performing a psoas compartment block. To make it easier to identify the nerve within the muscle, the anesthetist can slowly tilt the transducer back and forth, which results in more attenuation and makes the muscle fibers darker and the nerve easier to identify within the muscle. Unlike muscles, most nerves can still be visualized when the transducer is not in a perpendicular orientation, so tilting the transducer to use a different angle of insonation is a useful technique to use when initially scanning the area of interest.

ACOUSTIC SHADOWING

"Acoustic shadowing" occurs deep to the shallow border of a highly attenuating structure, such as bone or gas, where sound waves are almost completely absorbed or reflected (Figure 2.17). Although the highly attenuating structure will appear as a bright object and can be easily identified, a black

(a)

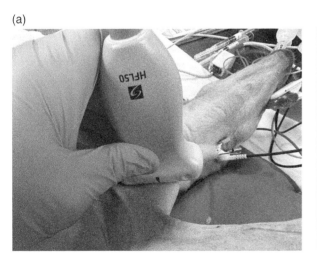

(b)

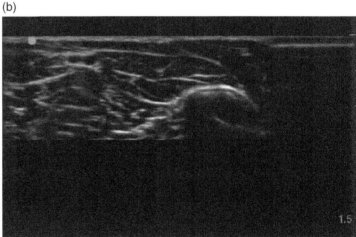

FIGURE 2.15   (a) A proximal RUMM block is being performed on a canine patient. Note that the transducer is relatively wide compared to the size of the patient's limb, resulting in part of the transducer not being in contact with the patient. (b) Corresponding ultrasonographic image showing the effect of the transducer not being in contact with the skin ("drop out" on the right side of the image).

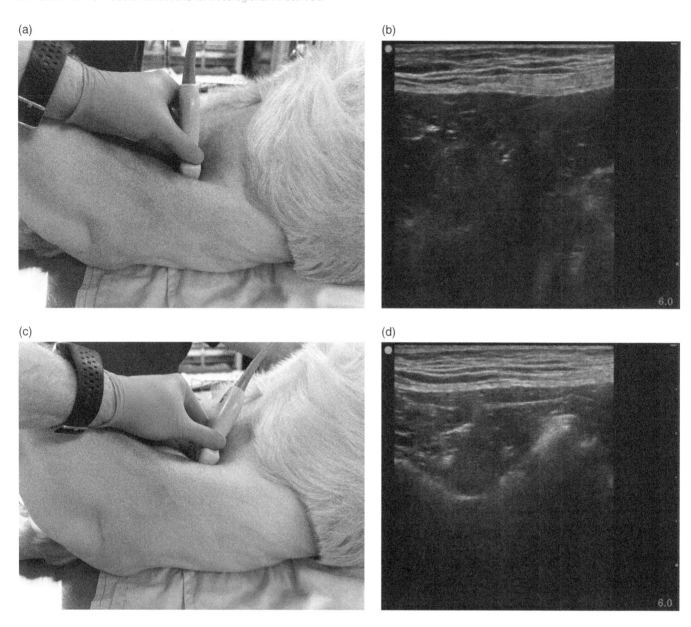

FIGURE 2.16 Example of using tilt to change the angle of insonation to change the appearance of soft tissues. (a) The psoas muscle is being imaged to identify the location of the **femoral nerve**. (b) Corresponding ultrasonographic image showing hypoechoic rim of the nerve in the center of the muscle. (c) The ultrasound transducer has been tilted caudally to change the angle of insonation. (d) Corresponding ultrasonographic image demonstrating how the nerve is now more easily identified in the center of the muscle than in (b).

"shadow" will appear deep to it, making it difficult or impossible to see any structures that lie deep to the highly attenuating structure.

This artifact is useful for identifying certain anatomical structures in the scan field, such as ribs (e.g. during performance of intercostal or serratus plane blocks), vertebra (during performance of thoracic paravertebral or erector spinae plane blocks), or long bones of the limbs (e.g. the humerus during performance of RUMM blocks, the femur during performance of **sciatic nerve** blocks), but can also make it more difficult to see the target area, depending on the angle that the sound waves encounter the bone. This is especially important when performing blocks where the target nerves lie

in close contact with a bony structure, such as intercostal nerves that lie behind (and slightly under) the ribs. In this situation, the transducer may need to be "heeled" slightly so the beam is directed under the side of the bony structure, allowing the target to be visualized in the area that was initially located under the shadow of the bone.

Acoustic shadowing can also be useful for visualizing the needle and identifying the needle tip as it is guided toward the area of interest. Even if the needle itself cannot be seen (e.g. when it is being introduced on an acute angle as opposed to perpendicular to the ultrasound beam), the needle should create a shadow that can be identified, making it easier to extrapolate where the needle tip is located.

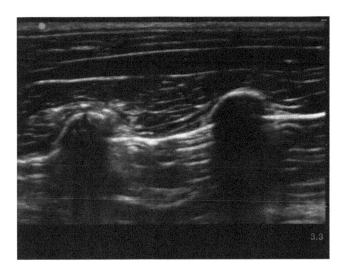

FIGURE 2.17   Ultrasonographic image of the lateral thoracic body wall of a canine patient. The ribs do not allow ultrasound waves to pass through, resulting in shadows that obscure the detail of the image distal (deep) to the ribs.

ACOUSTIC ENHANCEMENT

Attenuation of the ultrasound beam is greater when it encounters soft tissues than when it encounters fluids (Table 2.1). As a result, tissues that are located deep to a fluid-filled structure such as a large artery or vein will appear more echogenic than the same tissues that are located adjacent to the fluid-filled structure on either side (Figure 2.18). Although it may appear as though there is a discrete hyperechoic structure located deep to the vessel, this is simply an enhancement artifact and should not be mistaken for a nerve or other object.

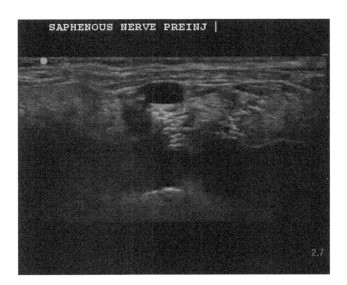

FIGURE 2.18   Ultrasonographic image of the femoral artery of a canine patient demonstrating enhancement artifact. This effect results from ultrasound waves passing more easily through the artery and having more energy when they are reflected back from the tissues immediately deep into the artery, giving the impression of a hyperechoic structure being located there.

REVERBERATION ARTIFACT

"*Reverberation artifacts*" occur when ultrasound waves bounce back and forth between two highly reflective specular interfaces (such as the block needle and the transducer), leading to multiple linear, equally spaced hyperechoic densities emanating deep to the reflective surface. For example, in the case of *needle reverberation artifact*, the hyperechoic lines represent ultrasound waves bouncing back and forth within the lumen of the needle before returning to the transducer (Figure 2.19) (Sites et al. 2007b). Because there is a slight delay in the reflected waves returning to the transducer to stimulate the crystals, the machine processes this information as coming from separate, but identical structures, hence the identical, but slightly deeper images that are displayed. Due to attenuation of the energy of these waves, these reverberation artifacts appear slightly less bright with each reflection (Figure 2.20). This artifact can make the needle itself appear larger than it really is, and obscure the position of the needle tip. When multiple reverberation artifacts merge, the artifact can look like a comet tail (Sites et al. 2007b).

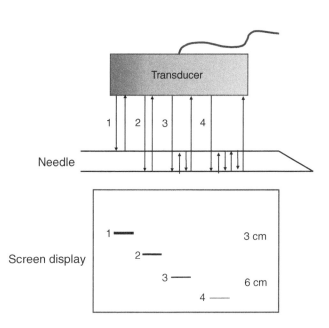

FIGURE 2.19   Reverberation artifact, detailed in a stepwise manner. Each number above the needle (top) has a corresponding number on the ultrasound screen (bottom) to graphically represent the result of different reverberation events. The original ultrasound beam contacts the needle and is reflected back to the transducer correctly (1). In addition, part of the ultrasound beam penetrates the hollow needle and is reflected back to the transducer from the distal wall of the needle (2). However, a component of the ultrasound beam becomes "stuck" within the needle lumen because the needle walls are highly reflective barriers. This signal component is reflected between the needle walls several times before "escaping" back to the transducer (3), (4). Thus, the transducer interprets these later occurring signals as objects distal to the needle at intervals which are multiples of the needle diameter. Based on Sites et al. 2007b.

(a)

(b)

(c)

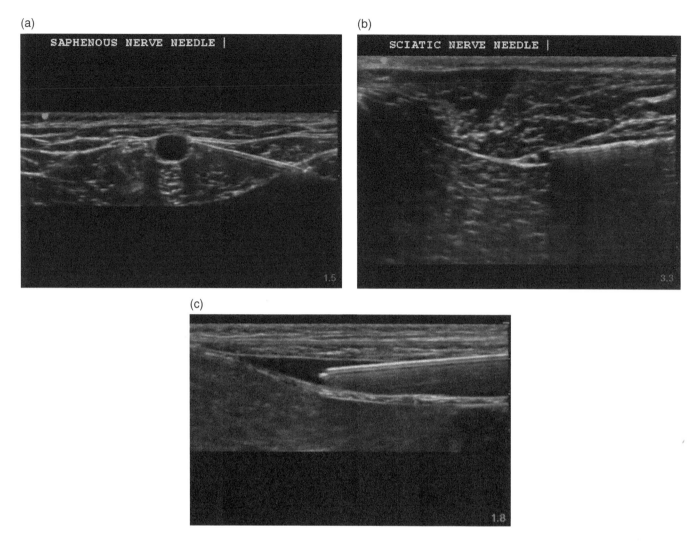

FIGURE 2.20   Examples of reverberation artifact resulting from reflection of ultrasound waves off of, and inside, the shaft of the needle when performing a variety of blocks. (a) **saphenous nerve** block; (b) **sciatic nerve** block; (c) transversus abdominis plane (TAP) block. Note the shadow under the needle in (b), representing a degree of dropout as a result of the needle reflecting the majority of the ultrasound waves. This artifact can be useful for helping to identify the location of the needle tip when it is "in-plane" since the shadow always starts at the tip of the needle.

MIRRORING ARTIFACT

Similar to needle reverberation artifacts, "*mirroring artifacts*" are a type of reverberation artifact that occur when sound waves interact with perpendicularly orientated, strongly reflective surfaces such as air, a fascial plane, or the peritoneum (Romano et al. 2020). When this occurs, the ultrasound is "fooled" and does not recognize that the beam has been reflected off a reflective surface. Instead, it interprets the information it is receiving back from the echoes as coming from different structures and produces a mirror image of the superficial structures, deep to the highly reflective surface (Figure 2.21). The actual (superficial) and artifactual (deep) structures appear in equal size and distance from the mirroring object, however, the artifactual structures appear dimmer.

This artifact can occur in a variety of different situations. Recently, a case report described performance of Transversus Abdominis Plane (TAP) blocks postoperatively in two dogs when the air in their abdomens created dramatic examples of mirroring that could have contributed to the needles being advanced into dangerous locations had the anesthetist not been aware of the potential for this artifact (Romano et al. 2020).

(a)

(b)

(c)

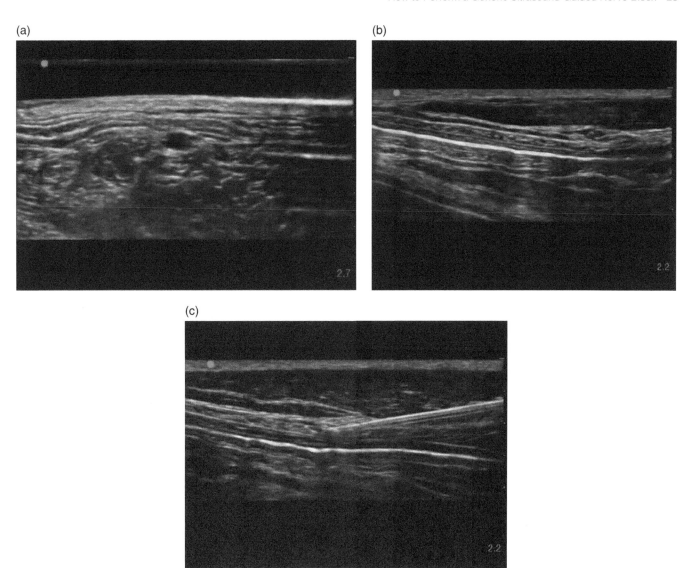

FIGURE 2.21 Examples of mirror imaging artifacts resulting from strong return of ultrasound waves off reflectors. (a) The use of a standoff pad (see Figure 2.11) without perfect coupling to the skin resulted in a thin layer of air existing between the standoff pad and the skin on the right side of the image. Ultrasound waves are reflected off the air and are processed incorrectly by the ultrasound machine, creating artifacts that appear as discrete structures below/deep to the reflector. The anesthetist should appreciate that these objects are evenly spaced below the reflector and appear identical, suggesting that they are artifacts and not actual structures. (b) Ultrasonographic image of the ventral abdominal body wall of a dog undergoing a TAP block and (c) with the needle being advanced into its final position. The hyperechoic peritoneum is acting as a strong reflector, resulting in mirror image artifact deep to the peritoneum where reflections of the ***mm. rectus abdominis*** and ***transversus abdominis***, and needle, can be observed. These reflections interfere with the anesthetist's ability to identify actual structures deep to the peritoneum.

HOW TO PERFORM A GENERIC ULTRASOUND-GUIDED NERVE BLOCK

In order to perform an ultrasound-guided nerve block, the patient should first be sedated or anesthetized and positioned on a flat surface in the recumbency that will allow the block to be performed easily and safely. This positioning will vary based on the block being performed. The hair over the surgical field and area where the ultrasound transducer and needle will contact the patient's skin should be clipped and prepared aseptically (e.g. using chlorhexidine and alcohol).

The anesthetist should think about the planned needle trajectory and position themselves accordingly. In most cases, for right-handed anesthetists, it is best if the needle appears on the screen and moves from right to left as it does in the patient, allowing the brain to process the information it is seeing on the screen more easily. The opposite is true for left-handed anesthetists. This is especially important for novices who tend to have enough trouble orienting the transducer, finding the nerve, optimizing the image, manipulating the needle into the correct location, etc. If the anesthetist is advancing the needle from right to left in the patient but it appears to be moving from left to right on the screen, their brain will need to "flip" the image and relate it to the patient's anatomy, contributing to cognitive load and making learning slower. For this reason, the anesthetist should plan to stand (or sit) on the side of the patient that will allow them to advance the needle along its planned path most easily.

To ensure that the orientation of the transducer on the patient relates to the image on the screen, make sure that the marker on the transducer matches the orientation of the marker on the ultrasound screen (Figure 2.22). It should be noted that, for consistency, most of the ultrasound images in this book have been oriented for a right-handed anesthetist. As such, the marker was set to appear on the left side of the ultrasound screen and the transducer was oriented so that the marker on the side of the transducer was on the left side of the anesthetist who was capturing the images related to performing the blocks described herein.

To have the most control, most experts will hold the needle between their index finger and thumb using a "palm-up" approach with their hand resting on the patient so as to have more stability, as opposed to holding the needle between their index finger and thumb but having their palm facing down and their hand "floating" in the air (Figure 2.23).

Ideally, the patient should be positioned at a height and location on a flat surface (e.g. table, gurney) beside which the anesthetist can comfortably stand or sit adjacent to the patient so they are not leaning over or are otherwise uncomfortable. This is especially important when someone is learning how to perform a block and may require an extended period of time to perform it.

The ultrasound machine should be positioned on the opposite side of the patient so the anesthetist can look up and down between their hands, the needle, and the ultrasound screen quickly and easily. This is a very important consideration for novices since they may have underdeveloped hand–eye coordination and will need to look back and forth frequently to "find the needle" and check its position when they are first learning to perform the block. However, even after mastery is achieved, ergonomics are important for efficiency, comfort, and to minimize the risk of developing long-term musculoskeletal injuries – if the machine is positioned beside the anesthetist, they will need to turn their head to watch the screen, making it less efficient (and awkward) to look down at their hands and the needle.

Using the optimization and transducer manipulation techniques described above, the area of interest should be scanned and the relevant structures identified. Normal and abnormal anatomy (and possible artifacts) should be evaluated and vessels along the planned needle trajectory accounted for. A preinjection image of the target area should be saved for documentation purposes to show the appearance of the nerve and associated structures before the needle has been introduced and any drug(s) have been injected.

Once the target has been identified, the needle can be placed. Before use, the needle (and extension set) should be primed with the local anesthetic to displace air and fill the dead space with a liquid. This step is crucial because air reflects ultrasound waves and the injection of even a small volume of air from an unprimed needle can obscure the area of interest (Figure 2.24).

In most cases, an "*in-plane*" needle technique will be used, referring to a needle that is oriented in-line with the face of the linear transducer (Figure 2.25). Even if it is being advanced on an angle (from shallow to deep or vice versa) and is not directly parallel with the face of the transducer on the

(a)

(b)

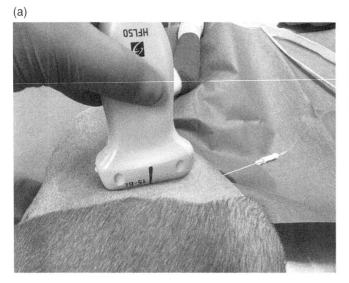
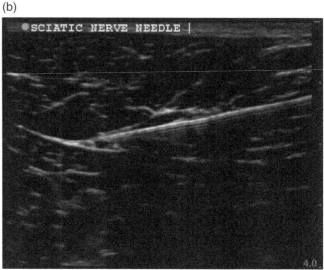

FIGURE 2.22   (a) An ultrasound transducer has been positioned for a **sciatic nerve** block in a dog. The small marker on the side of the transducer is on the cranial aspect of the limb, corresponding to the blue dot on the upper left side of the accompanying ultrasonographic image. (b) When these are aligned, the needle orientation on the ultrasound screen will match that of the needle "*in situ*".

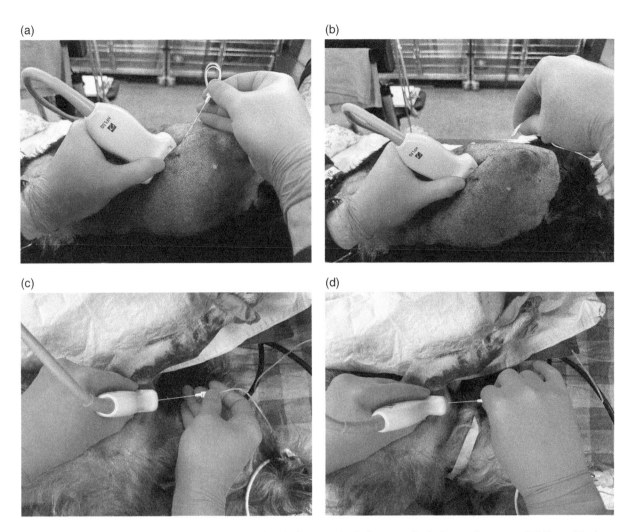

FIGURE 2.23   Examples of how to stabilize the dominant hand when manipulating a needle during performance of different blocks. (a) TAP block being performed with hand resting lightly on the patient to provide more motor control and stability than when hand is floating (b). (c) Proximal RUMM block being performed with hand resting lightly on the patient to provide more motor control and stability than when hand is floating (d).

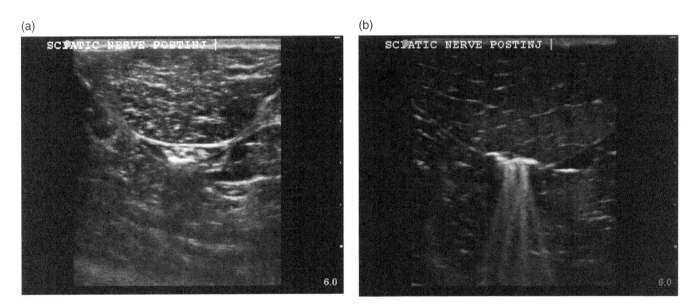

FIGURE 2.24   Series of ultrasonographic images to demonstrate the appearance of air following injections. (a) A small volume of air has been injected deep to the **sciatic nerve**, creating an area of hyperechoic reflection but not obscuring the nerve itself. (b) A small volume of air has been injected superficial to the **sciatic nerve**, creating an area of hyperechoic reflection that completely obscures the nerve. For this reason, it is helpful to always start injections deep to the target nerve so that any air that may inadvertently be injected will not interfere with the ability to visualize the nerve. Initially injecting superficial to the target nerve risks administration of air, resulting in the inability to continue the block at that location due to the nerve not being able to be visualized appropriately.

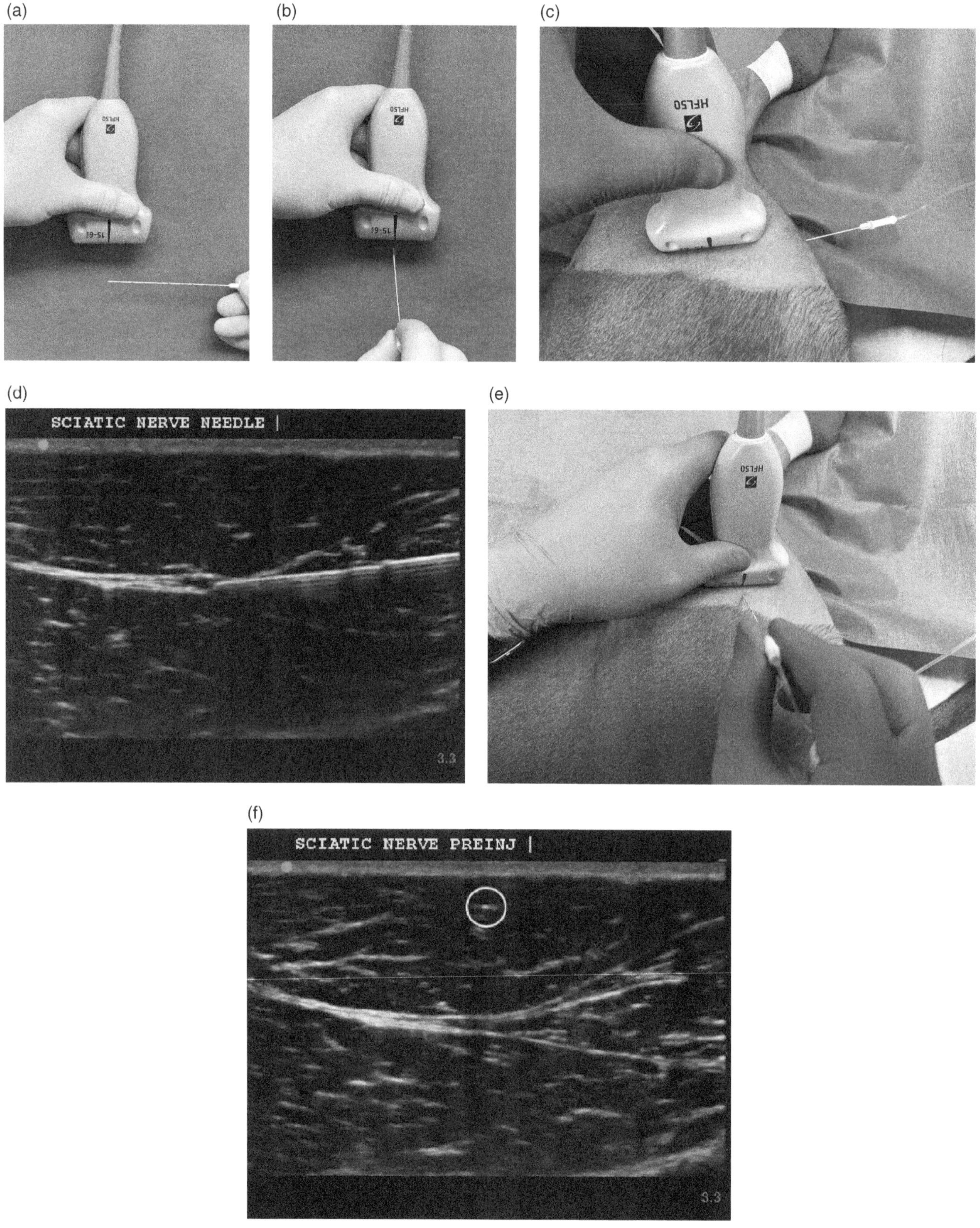

FIGURE 2.25   (a) In-plane and (b) out-of-plane needle techniques. (c) A needle has been positioned in-plane during performance of a sciatic nerve block in a dog, with corresponding ultrasonographic image showing reflection of the needle along its entire length (d). (e) A needle has been positioned out-of-plane for demonstration purposes, with corresponding ultrasonographic image to show the appearance of the needle in cross section (inside circle) (f).

skin, a needle is still considered to be in-plane as long as its entire length can be visualized. *"Out-of-plane"* refers to a needle that is oriented perpendicular to the face of the transducer so the needle is imaged in cross section and appears as a bright "dot" on the screen. Although out-of-plane techniques have their uses and may be called upon for a variety of situations, in-plane techniques are those that are used for the vast majority of locoregional anesthetic blocks since the needle and all of the anatomic structures it will encounter along its planned trajectory can be visualized on the screen in real-time together.

The tip of the needle should be visible at all times as it is being advanced toward the target location. One of the most important rules of performing ultrasound-guided blocks is to never move the needle if the tip cannot be seen. Moving the needle when it cannot be seen risks causing patient injury since the tip might encounter structures such as blood vessels, the pleura, etc. Whenever the needle tip cannot be seen, stop moving the needle and manipulate the ultrasound transducer via tilting, gliding, or rotation until the needle is found. Once the tip can be visualized, the needle can again be moved.

Electrolocation can optionally be used in conjunction with ultrasound guidance to perform certain blocks where there is a motor component to the target nerve. In these cases, the anesthetist should monitor for contractions of appropriate muscles that indicate the needle is in proximity to the nerve(s) of interest. Unlike its use when performing blind techniques, when using nerve stimulation together with ultrasound guidance, the use of a low-intensity current (less than 0.6 mA) and a low frequency (1 Hz instead of 2 Hz) will help to minimize the strength and frequency of muscle contractions that interfere with the image being displayed on the ultrasound screen.

In the case of ultrasound-guided regional anesthesia, it is better to think of nerve stimulation as being used not for *"electrolocation,"* but for *"electroconfirmation."* Instead of using nerve stimulation to provide indirect information about the possible position of the needle relative to a target nerve as it has traditionally been used for, in the case of ultrasound-guided regional anesthesia where the target nerve is likely already being imaged, nerve stimulation is simply used to confirm the identity of the structure as being a nerve (as opposed to being something else). Once the needle is in its final position, an image of the needle tip and other structures should be saved for documentation purposes to show where the needle was located before injection and what the surrounding structures appeared like prior to any drug(s) being administered.

Before injecting the local anesthetic, the syringe should be aspirated to ensure that it is not in an intravascular location. Although a negative aspiration test does not preclude the needle tip from being in a vessel, it is considered good practice to make sure an obvious intravascular injection will not be made. Color Doppler or CPD can be used to further look for vessels when there is uncertainty. If desired, a small air bubble can be aspirated into the syringe to help provide the anesthetist with a visual and tactile indicator of resistance to injection (see Chapter 28). If this technique is being used, to avoid introduction of air into the area being scanned, make sure to stop injecting before the air bubble enters the extension line or needle.

If no blood is observed on aspiration, the local anesthetic can be injected slowly. The spread of the injection should be monitored, making sure that the local anesthetic is distributed in the desired area (i.e. around the nerve, along a fascial plane, etc.). Following completion of the injection, the needle should be removed from the patient and an image of the relevant area should be saved for documentation purposes to show the appearance of the nerves and related structures following drug administration.

The three images (at a minimum – more can be documented if desired, see Chapter 3) that are saved are very useful, beyond the expected necessity for simply documenting performance of a medical procedure in a patient's medical record. These images can be used to revisit the block later if it failed (i.e. to decide if something could have been done better or differently), to share with colleagues to solicit feedback on technique, to guide personal reflection when someone is learning how to perform a new block, to contribute to teaching and learning by being used in presentations, to be used for prospective or retrospective research, or to be referred to in medicolegal situations. The anesthetist may even want to review these images after having attained mastery to look at how far they have come in terms of optimizing their images, how long it takes for them to perform the block (there is usually a time stamp on the images), etc. As the old adage says, *"if it isn't written down, it didn't happen"* and documenting performance of locoregional anesthetic techniques with strong visuals such as ultrasound images should be part of the routine for anyone using ultrasound guidance to perform their blocks.

REFERENCES

Barrington MJ, Uda Y (2018) Did ultrasound fulfill the promise of safety in regional anesthesia? Curr Opin Anaesthesiol 31, 649–655.

Brull R, Macfarlane AJR, Tse CCH (2010) Practical knobology for ultrasound-guided regional anesthesia. Reg Anesth Pain Med 35, S68–S73.

Griffin J, Nicholls B (2010) Ultrasound in regional anaesthesia. Anaesthesia 65, S1–12.

Neal JM (2016) Ultrasound-guided regional anesthesia and patient safety: Update of an evidence-based analysis. Reg Anesth Pain Med 41, 195–204.

Neal JM, Brull R, Horn JL et al. (2016) The second american society of regional anesthesia and pain medicine evidence-based medicine assessment of ultrasound-guided regional anesthesia: executive summary. Reg Anesth Pain Med 41, 181–194.

Romano M, Portela DA, Otero PE et al. (2020) Mirroring artefact during postoperative transversus abdominis plane (TAP) block in two dogs. Vet Anaesth Analg 47, 727–728.

Sites BD, Brull R, Chan VWS et al. (2007a) Artifacts and pitfall errors associated with ultrasound-guided regional anesthesia. Part I: understanding the basic principles of ultrasound physics and machine operations. Reg Anesth Pain Med 32, 412–418.

Sites BD, Brull R, Chan VWS et al. (2007b) Artifacts and pitfall errors associated with ultrasound-guided regional anesthesia. Part II: a pictoral approach to understanding and aviodance. Reg Anesth Pain Med 32, 419–433.

Wang ZX, Zhang DL, Liu XW et al. (2017) Efficacy of ultrasound and nerve stimulation guidance in peripheral nerve block: a systematic review and meta-analysis. IUBMB Life 69, 720–734.

How to Document the Use of Locoregional Anesthesia in the Medical Record

Eric D. Brumberger and Luis Campoy

CHAPTER 3

DOCUMENTATION AT A GLANCE

Record keeping and patient documentation are requirements of any successful regional anesthetic procedure. Detailed records can be useful in determining the success rate of a given block for a given procedure, or whether a particular block procedure requires adjustments to refine it in the future. Detailed records may also be helpful in the event of an adverse outcome by outlining the procedure and demonstrating adherence to an accepted standard of care. Records also provide references for returning patients having a similar procedure by providing useful information such as needle depth, response to dose/volume, and duration of block. Minimum required information that should be recorded in the patient's chart when receiving a locoregional block should include:

- Type of block;

- Drug(s) administered (dose, concentration, and volume);

- Verification of absence of resistance to injection;

- Verification of negative aspiration prior to injection;

- If electrolocation was used, what motor responses were elicited and what was the minimum current to elicit a motor response;

- Ultrasound images that document the different steps performed (i.e. initial appearance of the target nerve(s) and local anatomy, needle tip position prior to injection, neural integrity following injection, local anesthetic solution surrounding the nerve, etc.).

Other information with regards to preparation for, and response to, performed blocks provides additional value and, though not required, is strongly recommended.

WHY?

As an increasingly important component of modern anesthesiology, regional anesthesia merits comprehensive documentation of its practice in the patient's medical record. Similar to the meticulous notation of vital signs, pertinent medical history, and administered anesthetic drugs, utilizing a structured and rigorous approach to the documentation of regional anesthesia procedures is considered best practice. Thorough documentation of all interventions in the medical record is consistent with complete and comprehensive care and provides several benefits.

STANDARDIZATION

A detailed and descriptive account of the procedure allows it to be both recreated by another trained practitioner when successful, as well as learned from and improved upon when failures or other obstacles are encountered.

COMPLETE WRITTEN RECORDS PREVENT MISREPRESENTATION OF PROCEDURAL EVENTS

In human medicine, there are increasingly sophisticated and ever-changing documentation requirements that make it prudent for regional anesthesia practitioners to develop meticulous charting skills. From a medicolegal standpoint, many would argue that if the information is not charted, it did not occur. Detailed documentation, while important for all interventions regardless of the outcome, is especially useful in cases where outcomes are less than desirable. When misguided accusations of wrongdoing are levied against a defendant, robust testimony guided by the medical record, sometimes obtained years after the fact, can debunk a challenger's claims, or at the very least create enough opportunity for an alternative explanation to invalidate the challenge.

Small Animal Regional Anesthesia and Analgesia, Second Edition. Edited by Matt Read, Luis Campoy, and Berit Fischer.
© 2024 John Wiley & Sons, Inc. Published 2024 by John Wiley & Sons, Inc.

HOW?

Most important to the successful documentation of regional anesthesia procedures in the medical record is that it is done legibly, timely, and with as much detail as possible. Illegible, incomplete, and/or disorganized notes add little value to information transfer between practitioners, let alone to legal proceedings, and, in some situations, may cause more harm than having no documentation at all.

Specifics regarding equipment, medications, and positive and negative events (whether routine or unexpected) help to recreate events for practitioners attempting to replicate care, as well as for a legal team defending a clinician should a patient have an undesirable outcome. Even seemingly insignificant details such as the presence of other individuals, the location in the hospital where the procedure took place, and detailed timestamps can all be useful.

Timeliness and accuracy are critical with regard to any documentation. Coordination of care across departments is greatly facilitated when practitioners reflect the care they have given as close to the intervention as possible. Memory fades quickly, and the fidelity of an accurate representation of what was done decreases as the time between performing a procedure and charting that event increases. There may be situations where a clinician needs to amend a record. If there is a reason to alter an error or an omission, it is important to document the date and time of the change as well as provide justification for the edit.

RECORD-KEEPING SYSTEMS

More and more, clinicians are reaping the benefits of electronic recordkeeping platforms or anesthesia information management systems (AIMSs). These electronic systems have several features, including templates and "fill-in-the-box" checklists with frequently used phrases and procedures used in regional anesthesia. While beneficial in its time-saving capabilities, it is possible that selecting items from a list could increase the likelihood of inadvertently omitting any number of details in a "*de-novo*" note (manufacturer, drug, negative aspiration, etc.). Therefore, preserving additional sections to edit and free-type text remains an important feature. Paper-charting or handwritten records continue to be adequate, as long as they are neat and detailed. Checklist-style forms and large freeform boxes for notes are both readily available. Many practitioners utilize the ability to store digital ultrasound images within the electronic medical record to document their locoregional procedures. Following performance of a block, an additional image utilizing text features allows a description to be cataloged directly with the images before they are sent to the archive system (e.g. Picture Archiving and Communication System [PACS]) (Figure 3.1a, b).

(a)

(b)

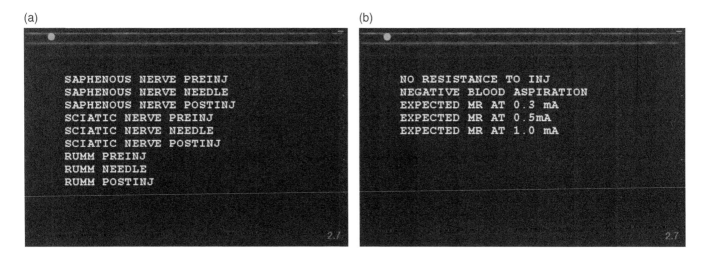

FIGURE 3.1 Examples of text labels that can be pre-populated using the "annotation" feature on an ultrasound machine. (a) shows examples of prepopulated labels for different techniques and (b) shows qualifers and descriptors that can be used to characterize technique. Selecting from these labels can allow the anesthetist to quickly document and describe key components of an ultrasound-guided nerve block that can be saved with the patient's other images in the electronic archive system. Source: Images from Matt Read. Used with permission.

WHAT?

When documenting locoregional procedures, more information is better. In 2005, based on the available literature at that time, an expert consensus group from North American academic institutions produced both peripheral nerve block and neuraxial anesthesia procedural notes (Gerancher et al. 2005). More recently, Moran et al. (2017) also contributed to establish a minimum standard of documentation. The best procedural notes logically and chronologically present a complete story from start to finish, beginning with the indication for the intervention and documentation that informed consent (i.e. discussion of the risks, benefits, and alternatives to the procedure) was obtained either verbally or in writing. Prior to performing the actual block, the correct patient, procedure, body part, and side should be verified and documented by completing a time-out with appropriate personnel. Following this, the record should include any other preparatory items of note: who performed and/or supervised the procedure, where the procedure was performed (e.g. operating room, anesthesia induction area, ICU, etc.), what the patient's position was, when the block was completed, and how long it took to perform. Additionally, whether the block was performed under sedation or anesthesia, and if there were any responses from the patient during performance of the procedure, can also be documented.

The regional anesthesia procedural note should continue with a description of the method used: anatomic/landmark-based, nerve stimulator, ultrasound (or any combination of the three) in conjunction with the type/name of the block and the orientation (e.g. landmark-based epidural or ultrasound-guided, in-plane, axillary brachial plexus block). It is also suggested that information regarding the antiseptic practice implemented (e.g. sterile/semi-sterile, alcohol, chlorhexidine, betadine, etc.) and specifics regarding equipment (e.g. brand, type, style, and size of needle) be cataloged. A description of relevant anatomy, with associated coordinates, is useful to demonstrate proper technique and avoidance of complications. For example, "... the entire shaft of the needle was visualized throughout as was the femoral artery, vein, and nerve which was noted to be two centimeters deep. Local anesthetic was visible around the femoral nerve and the femoral nerve was noted to be undisturbed and grossly intact upon completion of the injection." When using a nerve stimulator, it is standard practice to describe the amount and range of applied current as well as the obtained motor response: "... radial nerve stimulation observed as a triceps muscle twitch was obtained between 1.0 and 0.4 milliamperes (mA)" indicating both appropriate equipment use, as well as twitch onset and offset. Details about medications administered, including generic name, concentration, and dose are required.

Description of the injection of local anesthetic itself should detail that it was performed in a safe manner by including comments regarding confirmation of negative aspiration prior to injection, as well as the absence of pain/sympathetic response, and lack of resistance during injection. Any comments regarding the degree of difficulty encountered while performing the block should also be detailed. In the unfortunate circumstance that an unexpected complication (e.g. intravascular injection, local anesthetic systemic toxicity, accidental dural puncture, etc.) occurs during or following a block, it should be detailed in the record along with any treatments or interventions that were administered. While not a specific requirement, it is also recommended to record the quality and duration (sensory +/− motor) of the block. This may be demonstrated by patient stability under anesthesia and various tests of motor and sensory function, including the presence of neurologic deficits and patient response to incisional palpation in the postoperative period. Chronicling these types of metrics can help practitioners who perform locoregional blocks to better communicate expectations to colleagues and owners.

SUMMARY OF WHAT TO DOCUMENT

- Technique name*

- Type of guidance (ultrasound versus electrolocation versus landmark-based)*

- Motor response obtained (if applied)*

- Verified negative aspiration test*

- Verified absence of resistance to injection*

- Medications administered (local anesthetic +/− additives)*

- Complications*

- Comments: Brief description of the technique, including needle depth**

- Equipment used: Type of needle, brand of peripheral nerve stimulator, and ultrasound machine . . .**

*Essential information to document
**Recommended (but not essential) (Figure 3.2)

(a)

(b)

(c)

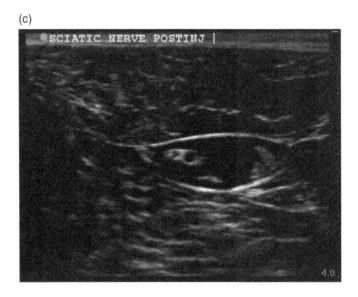

FIGURE 3.2 Example of three key images to save when performing an ultrasound-guided nerve block, in this case, a **sciatic nerve** block in a dog. (a) The "Pre-" image documents the appearance of the regional anatomy before the needle is placed and the local anesthetic is administered. (b) The "Needle" image documents the final position of the needle prior to the local anesthetic being administered. (c) The "Post-" image documents the appearance of the regional anatomy after the needle has been removed from the patient and shows the distribution of the local anesthetic immediately following administration. Source: Images from Matt Read. Used with permission.

REFERENCES

Gerancher JC, Viscusi ER, Liguori GA et al. (2005) Development of a standardized peripheral nerve block procedure note form. Reg Anesth Pain Med 30, 67–71.

Moran PJ, Fennessy P, Johnson MZ (2017) Establishing a new national standard for the documentation of regional anaesthesia in Ireland. BMJ Open Qual 6, e000210.

Local Anesthetic Pharmacology

Manuel Martin-Flores and Augusto Matias Lorenzutti

Local anesthetics interrupt the generation and propagation of action potentials in neural tissue, resulting in transient loss of sensory, motor, and/or autonomic functions. This conduction blockade is segmental, limited in proximity to where the drug was deposited, and it is completely reversed once the agent is removed from the site of action.

PHYSIOCHEMICAL PROPERTIES OF LOCAL ANESTHETICS

A number of agents are commonly used for regional anesthesia techniques, and, although they differ in terms of potency, duration of action, risk for toxicity, and chemical structure, they all share the same mechanism of action: Na^+ channel blockade (Table 4.1).

CHEMICAL STRUCTURE

All local anesthetics share a common chemical structure. Briefly, a lipophilic unit is linked to a hydrophilic unit by an intermediate hydrocarbon chain that contains either an ester or an amide group. The lipophilic group is typically an unsaturated ring (such as a benzene) and provides local anesthetic molecules with the ability to cross nerve cell membranes. The intermediate chain containing either an ester or an amide group determines the synthesis and metabolism of the drug. It is the makeup of the intermediate chain that serves as the primary basis for local anesthetic classification (Figure 4.1).

Ester local anesthetics (aminoesters) are hydrolyzed by the cholinesterase enzyme in the plasma and liver. Amide local anesthetics (aminoamides) undergo hepatic metabolism by microsomal enzymes. Compared with ester-linked anesthetics, the metabolism of amide-linked drugs involves more steps and is more complex. As a result, amide agents are more likely to accumulate and produce elevated plasma concentrations, thereby increasing the risk of local anesthetic toxicity (for further information, the reader is referred to the previous edition of this book).

DEGREE OF IONIZATION

The diffusion of a molecule across a biological membrane following a concentration gradient is explained by Fick's law, whereby the molecular weight, the partition coefficient, and the degree of ionization of the drug determine the rate of diffusion of that substance. Biological membranes, because of their lipid nature, are more permeable to nonionized molecules than to ionized ones; hence, only the nonionized fraction is available to diffuse across the membrane. The degree of ionization of a substance is determined by its pK_a, which is a measure of the tendency of the substance to dissociate in aqueous solution. pK_a is defined as the pH at which 50% of the drug is present in its ionized form. When the pH of the environment is different from the pK_a, the degree of ionization of the substance will vary: for weak basic drugs such as local anesthetics, a decrease in pH below the pK_a will result in a proportionally higher ionized fraction of the drug. Local anesthetics typically have pK_a values ranging from 7.72 to 9.06 (Tables 4.1 and 4.2), and therefore, a higher proportion of the molecules exist in their ionized cationic form at physiological pH (7.4).

Therefore, changes in pH can affect the onset of action and potency of local anesthetics. Figure 4.2 depicts how the ionized fraction of the local anesthetic changes with decreases in pH value as it may occur during inflammation and infection. In this graph, for pH values lower than 7.2, the ionized fraction exceeds 70% for all agents, which delays onset and decreases potency of the drug. This is to say, an acidic environment, such as might be associated with infected tissues, will negatively affect the speed and effect of local anesthetics.

MODE OF ACTION
MEMBRANE POTENTIAL

Like many other cells in the body, a neuron's resting membrane potential (RMP) is negative as a result of the disequilibrium of charged ions across its membrane. The Na^+-K^+-ATPase pump, a membrane protein, moves K^+ into the cell and Na^+ out of the cell in an active process that consumes energy (Butterworth and Strichartz 1990). An intracellular-to-extracellular gradient is created, with approximately 30 times more K^+ inside the cell and 10 times more Na^+ outside the cell. Two-pore domain K^+ channels (K2P), also known as "leak channels," are present within the cell membrane and allow facilitated diffusion of K^+ out of the cell along its concentration gradient during its resting state. There are three K^+ leak channels per one Na^+ channel, making the membrane more

Small Animal Regional Anesthesia and Analgesia, Second Edition. Edited by Matt Read, Luis Campoy, and Berit Fischer.
© 2024 John Wiley & Sons, Inc. Published 2024 by John Wiley & Sons, Inc.

Table 4.1 Characteristics of commonly use local anesthetics.

Drug	pK_a	Ionization (%) at pH = 7.4	Partition coefficient (lipid solubility)	Protein binding (%)	Relative potency
Lidocaine	7.77 ± 0.04	57.34	366 ± 31	64	4
Bupivacaine	8.10 ± 0.02	80.05	3420 ± 263	95	8
Levobupivacaine	8.10 ± 0.02	80.05	3420 ± 263	97	8
Ropivacaine*	8.16 ± 0.02	82.62	775 ± 53	94	4.8

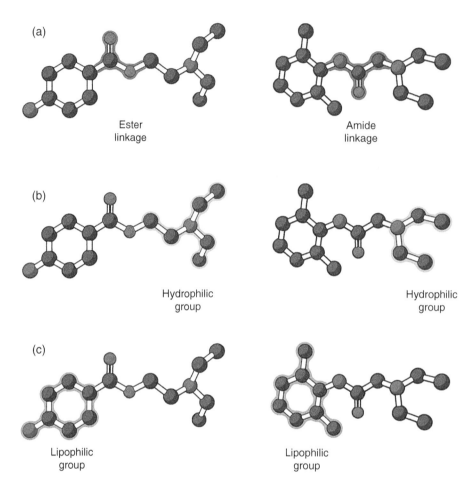

FIGURE 4.1 Diagrams of the chemical structures of an ester (left) and amide (right) local anesthetic. The intermediate chain (ester or amide) is highlighted in purple (a), the hydrophilic unit is highlighted in light blue (b), and the lipophilic ring is highlighted in orange (c).

Table 4.2 Summary of nerve fiber characteristics and functions.

Fiber	Diameter (μm)	Myelin	Conduction velocity (m s^{-1})	Innervation	Function	Nerve block onset
Aα	6–20	+++	75–120	Afferent: Spindle proprioceptors Efferent: skeletal muscle	Motor and reflex functions	+
Aβ	5–12	+++	30–75	Afferent: cutaneous mechanoreceptors	Touch and pressure	++
Aγ	3–6	++	12–35	Efferent: muscle spindle	Muscle tone	+++
Aδ	1–5	++	5–30	Afferent: pain and temperature	Fast pain, touch, and temperature	++++
B	‹ 3	+	3–15	Efferent: sympathetic	Autonomic	+++++
C	0.2–1.5	–	0.5–2	Afferent: pain and temperature	Slow pain, temperature	++++

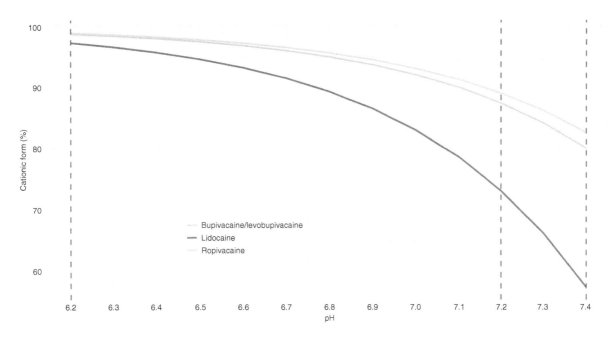

FIGURE 4.2   The fraction of a local anesthetic that is ionized changes as pH is altered. Local anesthetics are weak bases so a decrease in the pH of the environment will result in an increase in their ionized forms, and hence, a decrease in their ability to permeate membranes.

permeable to K^+ than to Na^+ and thus producing a net negative charge inside the cell, with a resulting RMP of −60 to −70 mV.

Activation of voltage-gated Na^+ channels is necessary for the generation of an action potential (Figure 4.3). A stimulus (mechanical, chemical, or electrical) from a sensory cell causes a neuron to depolarize via ligand-gated channels. If the

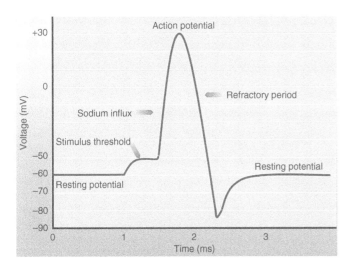

FIGURE 4.3   When the change in voltage is sufficiently large, voltage-gated Na^+ channels open, and an influx of Na^+ into the cell triggers an action potential. At the same time, K^+ exits the cell. After the action potential is generated, the different ions are pumped across the membrane to restore the initial concentrations and the resting membrane potential.

threshold potential is reached (−55 mV) at the axon hillock, located where the body and the axon of a neuron meet, voltage-gated Na^+ channels open, and the neuron completely depolarizes to a membrane potential of +20–40 mV. An influx of Na^+ through these channels results in further depolarization of the cell membrane through a positive feedback loop that ensures the propagation of the action potential. Activation of voltage-gated Na^+ channels is very short-lived, and after only a few milliseconds, these channels become inactive. The process of inactivation is also triggered by the depolarization itself; after a slight delay, K^+ channels open, leading to an efflux of K^+ ions along their concentration gradient and eventual hyperpolarization of the cell. The hyperpolarized membrane enters a refractory period where it cannot be depolarized. Once the K^+ channels close and the Na^+/K^+ transporter restores the RMP, the channels are available to open again.

Voltage-gated Na^+ channels progress through three different states during the cycle described above. During the resting state, these channels are closed but can be activated. When the membrane depolarizes, these channels undergo a conformational change and "open" to allow ion flow across the cell membrane. Almost immediately after they are activated, voltage-gated Na^+ channels become inactive; that is, they close and cannot be activated again until they revert to their resting state. This period, as indicated previously, is referred to as "refractory." Voltage-gated Na^+ channels are either fully opened or fully closed, with no intermediate conductance level (Butterworth and Strichartz 1990; Wann 1993). After an action potential is successfully generated, adjacent

Na+ channels respond in similar fashion, and the impulse is propagated along the nerve cell membrane.

Local anesthetics reversibly bind to sodium channels that are in their resting/inactive state. Binding of the agent with the receptor prevents activation so that no sodium influx occurs. Hence, cell depolarization is prevented, a threshold potential is not attained, and the action potential is not propagated.

The affinity of the local anesthetic agent to the voltage-gated Na+ channel increases markedly with the depolarization rate of the neuron, meaning that a resting nerve is less sensitive to a local anesthetic than a nerve that is repeatedly stimulated. When action potentials are occurring at a high frequency, there is rapid opening and closing of sodium channels. The affinity of the local anesthetic for the sodium channel, therefore, increases strictly because there are more opportunities to encounter a channel in an accepting state.

SELECTIVE BLOCK

The characteristics of the nerve fiber size and the presence or absence of myelin have been shown to correlate with conduction velocity and function. Most peripheral nerves that transmit information to the central nervous system are composed of a combination of myelinated and nonmyelinated cells. These nerve cells can be classified into three groups depending on their diameter and conduction velocity.

- **Group A** are large, myelinated somatic fibers that are responsible for transmitting information about touch and pressure (obtained from mechanoreceptors), as well as modulating muscle tone and motor/reflex activity. Specifically, Aδ fibers transmit information about nociception (pain) and temperature.

- **Group B** are small, myelinated autonomic fibers that are involved in modulating autonomic functions such as altering smooth muscle tone in the vascular system.

- **Group C** are small, nonmyelinated fibers that carry information about temperature and pain. Whereas Aδ fibers (above) carry information at a high velocity (i.e. fast, sharp, "first" pain), C fibers do so more slowly (i.e. slow, dull, "second" pain).

In 1929, Gasser and Erlanger (1929) first described the ability of a local anesthetic agent to block some nerve fibers while sparing others, what is now referred to as "differential" or "selective" block. They documented that cocaine induced a reduction in action potential amplitude more rapidly in smaller myelinated fibers than in larger ones. This evidence has been confirmed many times, and it is now widely accepted that small, myelinated fibers (Aδ) are more susceptible to local anesthetic blockade than larger, myelinated ones (Aα and Aβ) (Matthews and Rushworth 1957; Franz and Perry 1974; Ford et al. 1984; Gokin et al. 2001). This "size principle" is not, however, without exceptions. Small, myelinated

B fibers are less susceptible to blockade than larger Aβ fibers (Heavner and de Jong 1974). In addition, C fibers, which lack myelin but are of a smaller diameter than A or B fibers, appear to be either as susceptible or less susceptible than the myelinated but larger A fibers (Rosenberg and Heinonen 1983; Fink and Cairns 1984; Gokin et al. 2001).

The ability of different agents to produce differential block varies and is not based entirely on the "size principle." Experience and scientific observations provide evidence of differential blockade and suggest that Aδ and C fibers are commonly desensitized before Aα fibers. As a result, a preferential sensory block is possible with minimal motor block. For example, bupivacaine and ropivacaine are frequently used at low concentrations (0.0625–0.125%) to provide analgesia while sparing motor block during labor in women. This technique has also been implemented in the veterinary field to alleviate postoperative pain in dogs after cesarean section, with minimal motor impairment (Martin-Flores et al. 2019). However, this effect depends not only on the agent but also on the dose that is administered, as larger doses or higher concentrations will generally block all nerve fibers that are exposed to the drug.

COMMONLY USED LOCAL ANESTHETICS
LIDOCAINE

Lidocaine is one of the most frequently used local anesthetics and is considered the "prototype" of the aminoamide family. Lidocaine provides quick onset and an intermediate duration of action. It is commonly used for local anesthesia of peripheral nerves, neuraxial anesthesia, local infiltration, intravenous regional anesthesia (IVRA), and even for topical desensitization of mucosa or skin. For surgical anesthesia, concentrations of 1–2% are commonly used. In addition, lidocaine is used systemically as an intravenous agent for its analgesic, anti-inflammatory, and antiarrhythmic effects.

BUPIVACAINE

Since its introduction into clinical practice in the early 1960s, bupivacaine has become one of the most commonly used local anesthetic agents. Bupivacaine has a relatively slow onset of action, but its anesthetic and analgesic effects extend for a significantly longer time than that of lidocaine. However, bupivacaine is significantly more cardiotoxic than other local anesthetic agents. Bupivacaine is frequently used for nerve blocks and neuraxial anesthesia in a wide range of concentrations (0.06–0.75%), allowing for the development of differential blockade (sensory without motor block) when lower concentrations are used.

LEVOBUPIVACAINE

Levobupivacaine is a formulation that includes one of the two enantiomers of bupivacaine, and therefore its actions are similar to the standard racemic mixture. The main advantage of its use is a markedly reduced risk of cardiotoxicity when compared to use of standard bupivacaine. The onset and duration of levobupivacaine do not differ from those of bupivacaine.

ROPIVACAINE

Ropivacaine is a long-lasting amide-type of local anesthetic, with a lower potential for inducing cardiovascular and central nervous system (CNS) toxicity than bupivacaine. At low concentrations (0.25–0.5%), ropivacaine has a relatively slow onset similar to bupivacaine. At higher concentrations (0.75%), its onset may be as fast as that of lidocaine. In general, ropivacaine produces sensory blockade similar to that obtained with bupivacaine, but there is less chance of inducing motor blockade (Hadzic 2004). As a result of these favorable characteristics, ropivacaine has gained wide acceptance and is frequently used for conduction and neuraxial anesthesia.

MIXTURES OF LOCAL ANESTHETIC AGENTS

Local anesthetics have been combined prior to use with the intention of maximizing the desirable characteristics of the individual drugs. As an example, lidocaine (for its quick onset) and bupivacaine (for its longer duration) have been frequently mixed in equal parts. There are few data available regarding the safety, efficacy, or potentially altered pharmacokinetics of mixing local anesthetics. The onset of a mixture of agents may be unpredictable, as the resulting pK_a of the mixture is unknown. In addition, a 50 : 50 mixture will reduce the concentration of each drug by half (i.e. lidocaine 2% and bupivacaine 0.5% would become lidocaine 1% and bupivacaine 0.25%). Since concentration of local anesthetic is positively correlated with duration of action, there is concern that lower concentrations of the fast-acting drug and long-lasting drug will result in a shorter duration than the long-acting drug by itself with minimal effect on onset of action (Fenten et al. 2015). This was shown in a study where a mixture of equal parts of chloroprocaine 2% and bupivacaine 0.5% was administered to rats and produced anesthesia with characteristics similar to those of chloroprocaine (Galindo and Witcher 1980). A study that investigated femoral and sciatic peripheral nerve blocks in people combined bupivacaine 0.5% or ropivacaine 0.75% with equal volumes of lidocaine 2%. Their results showed that when each of the long-acting local anesthetics was mixed with lidocaine, the onset of the block was faster, but there was a significantly decreased duration of both sensory and motor blockade than when they were administered alone (Cuvillon et al. 2009). In other words, the available data suggest that combination of agents may result in some reduction in the time of onset at the expense of a shorter duration of block. Due to the lack of evidence showing a consistent advantage of mixing local anesthetics, a better approach is to select a single agent based on its desired predictable characteristics (such as onset time, duration of action, or potential for differential block) and to use it as appropriate to the patient and the procedure.

ADJUVANTS COMMONLY USED TO ENHANCE LOCOREGIONAL ANESTHESIA AND ANALGESIA

Adjunct agents are often combined with local anesthetics to exploit desirable characteristics such as prolonged duration of sensory blockade and earlier onset of action than the local anesthetic alone.

α_2 ADRENOCEPTOR AGONISTS

Alpha 2 (α_2) agonists are commonly used to enhance the analgesia offered through both epidural anesthesia and peripheral nerve blocks. Dexmedetomidine produces analgesia through supraspinal and spinal mechanisms via adrenergic receptors and has inhibitory effects on conduction of nerve impulses (Butterworth and Strichartz 1993; Eisenach et al. 1996). Dexmedetomidine enhances local anesthetic action via the $\alpha_2 A$ receptor (Yoshitomi et al. 2008) and may prolong the duration of ropivacaine by blocking the hyperpolarization-activated cation current, a modulator of action potential generation (Brummett et al. 2011; Brummett and Williams 2011).

Clinical benefits of the addition of dexmedetomidine to amide-type local anesthetic agents have been shown in dogs with the duration of hindlimb peripheral nerve blocks with either lidocaine or ropivacaine being prolonged when dexmedetomidine was added to the local anesthetic solution (Acquafredda et al. 2021; Marolf et al. 2021).

Fewer systemic effects are observed with perineural administration than when an equivalent dose of dexmedetomidine is used systemically, even if systemic administration also contributes to providing analgesia (Pavlica et al. 2022). Dexmedetomidine has also been used as an adjuvant for fascial plane blocks, such as the transversus abdominis plane block, in dogs undergoing ovariohysterectomy (Campoy et al. 2022a).

Epidural administration of α_2 agonists has also been shown to improve the quality of anesthesia. In children, the addition of dexmedetomidine to bupivacaine prolonged the analgesic duration from 5 to 16 hours, and from 6 to 18 hours in 2 separate studies (El-Hennawy et al. 2009; Saadawy et al. 2009). No urinary retention was observed, unlike that seen following epidural administration of opioids.

OPIOIDS

The addition of opioids to local anesthetics for neuraxial anesthesia is widely practiced. When deposited in the epidural space, opioids exert their analgesic actions through a variety of supraspinal and spinal mechanisms, including attenuation of C fiber-mediated nociception that is independent of its spinal actions (Niv et al. 1995). Morphine, fentanyl, and other opioids are commonly added to local anesthetics in order to enhance epidural analgesia without affecting motor blockade. Morphine is the most commonly used epidural opioid in veterinary medicine, either alone or in combination with local anesthetics. Numerous reports have documented the use of morphine as part of a solution administered epidurally in dogs (Hoelzler et al. 2005; Kona-Boun et al. 2006; Campoy et al. 2012). The addition of morphine to lidocaine for epidural anesthesia in dogs results in prolonged analgesia, without changing the duration of motor blockade (Almeida et al. 2010). Documentation of the use of epidural fentanyl in dogs is scarce but has been used combined with local anesthetics (Martin-Flores et al. 2019).

Administration of epidural morphine can result in urine retention. The incidence of urinary retention following epidural opioid administration in humans ranges between 30% and 60% (Liang et al. 2010; O'Neill et al. 2012). Campoy et al. (2012) reported that approximately half of their dogs developed urine retention following epidural morphine. In addition, a case report of urinary retention in a dog has been described (Herperger 1998). Other opioids, such as tramadol and buprenorphine, have been successfully used via the epidural route in animals (Pypendop et al. 2008; Almeida et al. 2010; Martin-Flores et al. 2019).

Although opioids are primarily used for neuraxial block, some have also been used as adjuncts for peripheral nerve blockade. Buprenorphine specifically may enhance the quality of the nerve block through a local anesthetic-like mechanism of action involving Na^+ channel block, a property that other μ agonists do not share (Leffler et al. 2012). Addition of buprenorphine to bupivacaine has been reported to enhance analgesia following sciatic nerve block in people (Candido et al. 2010), and it has been suggested that duration of analgesia may be increased in dogs when combined with bupivacaine (Snyder et al. 2016).

CORTICOSTEROIDS

In recent years, attention has been focused on the use of corticosteroids as local anesthetic adjuvants. In particular, dexamethasone has been increasingly adopted as an additive in order to extend the duration of analgesia. Corticosteroids can reduce transmission through C-fiber activity, thereby decreasing conduction of painful stimuli. This effect has been observed shortly after administration, suggesting a direct effect on the cell itself, rather than an anti-inflammatory effect. Moreover, no observable cytotoxic effects have been observed with use of preservative-free formulations (Johansson et al. 1990; Knight et al. 2015). In people, dexamethasone has been used clinically for a variety of blocks, including but not restricted to adductor (Ibrahim et al. 2019), transversus abdominis plane (TAP) (Chen et al. 2018), and brachial plexus blocks (Knezevic et al. 2015). In these instances, dexamethasone increases the duration of analgesia of local anesthetics.

Evidence of the clinical use of dexamethasone as an adjuvant to local anesthetics in animals is scarce. At the time of preparing this chapter, no reports of the use of steroids as adjuvants for peripheral nerve blocks were found. Epidural administration of methylprednisolone and dexamethasone

has been reported in dogs (Aprea and Vettorato 2019; Gomes et al. 2020). A dose–response effect in the duration of analgesia provided by lidocaine and dexamethasone given epidurally was established in dogs following ovariohysterectomy (Hermeto et al. 2017). Given the well-known potential side effects of corticosteroids in small animals and the absence of information regarding any potential complications when used in animals receiving nonsteroidal anti-inflammatory agents, studies are needed before this technique can be recommended for routine practice.

BUPIVACAINE LIPOSOME SUSPENSION

Sustained-release formulations of bupivacaine are currently available for humans and small animals. Exparel® (for humans) and Nocita® (for veterinary use) are commercially available multivesicular liposomal formulations of bupivacaine that are Food and Drug Administration approved for specific uses in the United States. Patented technology uses microscopic, bilayered vesicles to release encased, aqueous bupivacaine over approximately 96 hours. As these vesicles break down over time, bupivacaine is released and available to produce Na^+ blockade locally before ultimately being taken up by the systemic circulation and eliminated through normal mechanisms. These vesicles, however, do not diffuse across tissues in the same way as aqueous bupivacaine does, and hence, infiltration with a "moving needle" technique is recommended so that the formulation is deposited over all layers of tissues that are to be desensitized.

A number of studies in humans have evaluated the efficacy of Exparel® for postoperative pain relief, with variable results. Exparel® reduced postoperative pain scores and opioid consumption in patients after hemorrhoidectomy or orthopedic surgery when compared with a saline-treated control, with the improvements lasting 36–72 hours (Golf et al. 2011; Gorfine et al. 2011). Intercostal liposomal bupivacaine was also as effective as thoracic epidural for patients undergoing thoracotomies (Rice et al. 2015) and was effective in providing analgesia after application via TAP block for abdominal surgery (Feierman et al. 2014). Other studies have failed to show clear advantages of using liposomal bupivacaine over aqueous local anesthetics (Alijanipour et al. 2017; Zamora et al. 2019). In particular, recent meta-analyses have failed to identify any benefit of this formulation over perineural aqueous local anesthetics when the liposomal formulation was administered by infiltration or perineurally (Hussain et al. 2021; Ilfeld et al. 2021).

Data on the use of Nocita® in small animals are still scarce. A multicenter study reported an advantage of liposomal bupivacaine over placebo in dogs undergoing stifle surgery, with these benefits extending over a 72-hour period (Lascelles et al. 2016). Reader et al. (2020) reported the effects of liposomal bupivacaine versus 0.5% bupivacaine hydrochloride for postoperative pain control in 28 dogs undergoing tibial plateau leveling osteotomy (TPLO), administered by periarticular soft tissue injection. Dogs that received liposomal bupivacaine were less likely to need rescue analgesia (21% versus 71% for bupivacaine hydrochloride), required fewer doses, and had a lower total amount of opioids. Rescue analgesia was administered at 6–8 hours in those dogs that received bupivacaine hydrochloride and at 8 and 16 hours in dogs with liposomal bupivacaine. A more recent study evaluated the use of the perineural application of this agent (off-label) in dogs. Interestingly, peaks and valleys in the magnitude of conduction blockade were observed, suggesting that the rate of release of bupivacaine from the vesicles is not constant (Campoy et al. 2022b).

FUTURE OF LOCAL ANESTHETICS/ADJUVANTS?

Several controlled delivery systems are under investigation and development with the objective of increasing the duration of the analgesic effect of local anesthetics. Liposomes, microparticles, and nanoparticles systems were used for long-acting local anesthetic formulations. New investigations have focused on responsive hydrogel systems for development of controlled delivery local anesthetics formulations that will be useful in several scenarios (Tan et al. 2010; Bagshaw et al. 2015). A hydrogel is a drug delivery system with controlled release properties, constituted by cross-linked hydrophilic polymers with a high-water content. A responsive hydrogel is a hydrogel that can undergo structural transitions (changes) in response to changes in the local environment; the releasing properties of the hydrogel are thus affected by external factors.

Most responsive hydrogels are sensitive to changes in temperature, pH, ions, proteins, DNA, or electromagnetic radiation, with thermosensitive hydrogels being the most studied systems because of their potential utility *in vivo*. These hydrogels have a critical solution temperature near 37 °C. Below this temperature, the polymers exist in a soluble state, while above this temperature, the polymers become more hydrophobic. The decrease in solubility that occurs results in a transition from an aqueous solution to a gel (referred to as sol–gel transition), resulting in the prolonged release of the local anesthetic contained within (Bagshaw et al. 2015; Klouda 2015; Akkari et al. 2016).

Although there is a growing body of research related to hydrogel-based controlled-release systems for local anesthetics, there are only a few studies that evaluate the clinical efficacy and toxicity of these systems by different routes of administration *in vivo*. Kim et al. (2015) reported that a 1.25% bupivacaine thermosensitive delivery system resulted in analgesic effects that lasted for two days in an induced osteoarthritic knee model in rats (Kim et al. 2015). A different study showed that a hydrogel extended-release formulation of 4% bupivacaine administered by peri-incisional subcutaneous injection or by wound instillation significantly reduced allodynia for up to 96 hours (versus control) in a porcine skin and muscle incision model, with subcutaneous injection being superior to wound instillation. Moreover, this formulation showed an acceptable local and systemic toxicity profile (Heffernan et al. 2023).

Qiao et al. (2022) reported that, compared with ropivacaine hydrochloride, sciatic nerve blocks performed with a thermosensitive hydrogel combined with hyaluronan controlled delivery system containing 2.25% ropivacaine, induced longer sensory blockade (17.7 ± 0.7 hours versus 5.7 ± 0.8 hours) and longer motor blockade (6.8 ± 0.8 versus 3.5 ± 0.8 hours) in a hot plate rat model without significant side effects. Similar results were observed in dogs following sciatic and femoral nerve blocks in which a thermo-responsive hydrogel controlled-release formulation of 0.5% bupivacaine resulted in significantly longer sensory blockade (8.0 ± 1.6 and 10.9 ± 1.6 hours for femoral and sciatic blocks, respectively) compared with 0.5% bupivacaine hydrochloride (3.7 ± 2.0 and 8.0 ± 1.4 hours for femoral and sciatic block, respectively) (Kim et al. 2023). The formulation also resulted in longer-lasting motor blockade (9.3 ± 1.6 and 12.7 ± 1.5 hours versus 4.6 ± 1.9 and 9.6 ± 1.5 hours, respectively). No adverse effects were reported. Clinical evidence suggests that controlled-release systems for local anesthetics based on thermo-responsive hydrogels could be a good strategy for the development of long-lasting formulations that allow effective and safe postsurgical pain control.

REFERENCES

Acquafredda C, Stabile M, Lacitignola L et al. (2021) Clinical efficacy of dexmedetomidine combined with lidocaine for femoral and sciatic nerve blocks in dogs undergoing stifle surgery. Vet Anaesth Analg 48, 962–971.

Akkari ACS, Papini JZB, Garcia GK et al. (2016) Poloxamer 407/188 binary thermosensitive hydrogels as delivery systems for infiltrative local anesthesia: physicochemical characterization and pharmacological evaluation. Mater Sci Eng C Mater Biol Appl 68, 299–307.

Alijanipour P, Tan TL, Matthews CN et al. (2017) Periarticular injection of liposomal bupivacaine offers no benefit over standard bupivacaine in total knee arthroplasty: a prospective, randomized, controlled trial. J Arthroplast 32, 628–634.

Almeida RM, Escobar A, Maguilnik S (2010) Comparison of analgesia provided by lidocaine, lidocaine-morphine or lidocaine-tramadol delivered epidurally in dogs following orchiectomy. Vet Anaesth Analg 37, 542–549.

Aprea F, Vettorato E (2019) Epidural steroid and local anaesthetic injection for treating pain caused by coccygeal intervertebral disc protrusion in a dog. Vet Anaesth Analg 46, 707–708.

Bagshaw KR, Hanenbaum CL, Carbone EJ et al. (2015) Pain management via local anesthetics and responsive hydrogels. Ther Deliv 6, 165–176.

Brummett CM, Hong EK, Janda AM et al. (2011) Perineural dexmedetomidine added to ropivacaine for sciatic nerve block in rats prolongs the duration of analgesia by blocking the hyperpolarization-activated cation current. Anesthesiology 115, 836–843.

Brummett CM, Williams BA (2011) Additives to local anesthetics for peripheral nerve blockade. Int Anesthesiol Clin 49, 104–116.

Butterworth JF, Strichartz GR (1990) Molecular mechanisms of local anesthesia: a review. Anesthesiology 72, 711–734.

Butterworth JF, Strichartz GR (1993) The alpha 2-adrenergic agonists clonidine and guanfacine produce tonic and phasic block of conduction in rat sciatic nerve fibers. Anesth Analg 76, 295–301.

Campoy L, Martin-Flores M, Boesch JM et al. (2022a) Transverse abdominis plane injection of bupivacaine with dexmedetomidine or a bupivacaine liposomal suspension yielded lower pain scores and requirement for rescue analgesia in a controlled, randomized trial in dogs undergoing elective ovariohysterectomy. Am J Vet Res 83, ajvr.22.03.0037.

Campoy L, Martin-Flores M, Gleed RD et al. (2022b) Block duration is substantially longer with a liposomal suspension of bupivacaine than with 0.5% bupivacaine HCl potentiated with dexmedetomidine following an ultrasound-guided sciatic nerve block in Beagles. Am J Vet Res 83, ajvr.22.01.0007.

Campoy L, Martin-Flores M, Ludders JW et al. (2012) Comparison of bupivacaine femoral and sciatic nerve block versus bupivacaine and morphine epidural for stifle surgery in dogs. Vet Anaesth Analg 39, 91–98.

Candido KD, Hennes J, Gonzalez S et al. (2010) Buprenorphine enhances and prolongs the postoperative analgesic effect of bupivacaine in patients receiving infragluteal sciatic nerve block. Anesthesiology 113, 1419–1426.

Chen Q, An R, Zhou J et al. (2018) Clinical analgesic efficacy of dexamethasone as a local anesthetic adjuvant for transversus abdominis plane (TAP) block: a meta-analysis. PLoS One 13, e0198923.

Cuvillon P, Nouvellon E, Ripart J et al. (2009) A comparison of the pharmacodynamics and pharmacokinetics of bupivacaine, ropivacaine (with epinephrine) and their equal volume mixtures with lidocaine used for femoral and sciatic nerve blocks: a double-blind randomized study. Anesth Analg 108, 641–649.

Eisenach JC, De Kock M, Klimscha W (1996) Alpha(2)-adrenergic agonists for regional anesthesia. A clinical review of clonidine (1984–1995). Anesthesiology 85, 655–674.

El-Hennawy AM, Abd-Elwahab AM, Abd-Elmaksoud AM et al. (2009) Addition of clonidine or dexmedetomidine to bupivacaine prolongs caudal analgesia in children. Br J Anaesth 103, 268–274.

Feierman DE, Kronenfeld M, Gupta PM et al. (2014) Liposomal bupivacaine infiltration into the transversus abdominis plane for postsurgical analgesia in open abdominal umbilical hernia repair: results from a cohort of 13 patients. J Pain Res 7, 477–482.

Fenten MG, Schoenmakers KP, Heesterbeek PJ et al. (2015) Effect of local anesthetic concentration, dose and volume on the duration of single-injection ultrasound-guided axillary brachial plexus block with mepivacaine: a randomized controlled trial. BMC Anesthesiol 15, 130.

Fink BR, Cairns AM (1984) Differential slowing and block of conduction by lidocaine in individual afferent myelinated and unmyelinated axons. Anesthesiology 60, 111–120.

Ford DJ, Raj PP, Singh P et al. (1984) Differential peripheral nerve block by local anesthetics in the cat. Anesthesiology 60, 28–33.

Franz DN, Perry RS (1974) Mechanisms for differential block among single myelinated and non-myelinated axons by procaine. J Physiol 236, 193–210.

Galindo A, Witcher T (1980) Mixtures of local anesthetics: bupivacaine-chloroprocaine. Anesth Analg 59, 683–685.

Gasser HS, Erlanger J (1929) The role of fiber size in the establishment of a nerve block by pressure or cocaine. Am J Physiol Legacy Content 88, 581–591.

Gokin AP, Philip B, Strichartz GR (2001) Preferential block of small myelinated sensory and motor fibers by lidocaine: in vivo electrophysiology in the rat sciatic nerve. Anesthesiology 95, 1441–1454.

Golf M, Daniels SE, Onel E (2011) A phase 3, randomized, placebo-controlled trial of DepoFoam(R) bupivacaine (extended-release bupivacaine local analgesic) in bunionectomy. Adv Ther 28, 776–788.

Gomes SA, Lowrie M, Targett M (2020) Single dose epidural methylprednisolone as a treatment and predictor of outcome following subsequent decompressive surgery in degenerative lumbosacral stenosis with foraminal stenosis. Vet J 257, 105451.

Gorfine SR, Onel E, Patou G et al. (2011) Bupivacaine extended release liposome injection for prolonged postsurgical analgesia in patients undergoing hemorrhoidectomy: a multicenter, randomized, double-blind, placebo-controlled trial. Dis Colon Rectum 54, 1552–1559.

Hadzic A (2004) Peripheral Nerve Blocks: Principles and Practice. McGraw-Hill Professional.

Heavner JE, de Jong RH (1974) Lidocaine blocking concentrations for B- and C-nerve fibers. Anesthesiology 40, 228–233.

Heffernan JM, McLaren AC, Glass CM et al. (2023) Extended release of bupivacaine from temperature-responsive hydrogels provides multi-day analgesia for postoperative pain. Pain Med 24, 113–121.

Hermeto LC, Rossi R, Bicudo NA et al. (2017) The effect of epidurally administered dexamethasone with lignocaine for post-operative analgesia in dogs undergoing ovariohysterectomy. A dose-response study. Acta Cir Bras 32, 307–318.

Herperger LJ (1998) Postoperative urinary retention in a dog following morphine with bupivacaine epidural analgesia. Can Vet J 39, 650–652.

Hoelzler MG, Harvey RC, Lidbetter DA et al. (2005) Comparison of perioperative analgesic protocols for dogs undergoing tibial plateau leveling osteotomy. Vet Surg 34, 337–344.

Hussain N, Brull R, Sheehy B et al. (2021) Perineural liposomal bupivacaine is not superior to nonliposomal bupivacaine for peripheral nerve block analgesia. Anesthesiology 134, 147–164.

Ibrahim AS, Aly MG, Farrag WS et al. (2019) Ultrasound-guided adductor canal block after arthroscopic anterior cruciate ligament reconstruction: effect of adding dexamethasone to bupivacaine, a randomized controlled trial. Eur J Pain 23, 135–141.

Ilfeld BM, Eisenach JC, Gabriel RA (2021) Clinical effectiveness of liposomal bupivacaine administered by infiltration or peripheral nerve block to treat postoperative pain. Anesthesiology 134, 283–344.

Johansson A, Hao J, Sjolund B (1990) Local corticosteroid application blocks transmission in normal nociceptive C-fibres. Acta Anaesthesiol Scand 34, 335–338.

Kim T, Seol DR, Hahm SC et al. (2015) Analgesic effect of intra-articular injection of temperature-responsive hydrogel containing bupivacaine on osteoarthritic pain in rats. Biomed Res Int 2015, 812949.

Kim J, Kim D, Shin D et al. (2023) Effect of temperature-responsive hydrogel on femoral and sciatic nerve blocks using bupivacaine in Beagle dogs. Vet Med Sci 9, 91–97.

Klouda L (2015) Thermoresponsive hydrogels in biomedical applications: a seven-year update. Eur J Pharm Biopharm 97, 338–349.

Knezevic NN, Anantamongkol U, Candido KD (2015) Perineural dexamethasone added to local anesthesia for brachial plexus block improves pain but delays block onset and motor blockade recovery. Pain Physician 18, 1–14.

Knight JB, Schott NJ, Kentor ML et al. (2015) Neurotoxicity of common peripheral nerve block adjuvants. Curr Opin Anaesthesiol 28, 598–604.

Kona-Boun JJ, Cuvelliez S, Troncy E (2006) Evaluation of epidural administration of morphine or morphine and bupivacaine for postoperative analgesia after premedication with an opioid analgesic and orthopedic surgery in dogs. J Am Vet Med Assoc 229, 1103–1112.

Lascelles BD, Rausch-Derra LC, Wofford JA et al. (2016) Pilot, randomized, placebo-controlled clinical field study to evaluate the effectiveness of bupivacaine liposome injectable suspension for the provision of post-surgical analgesia in dogs undergoing stifle surgery. BMC Vet Res 12, 168.

Leffler A, Frank G, Kistner K et al. (2012) Local anesthetic-like inhibition of voltage-gated Na+ channels by the partial mu-opioid receptor agonist buprenorphine. Anesthesiology 116, 1335–46.

Liang CC, Chang SD, Wong SY et al. (2010) Effects of postoperative analgesia on postpartum urinary retention in women undergoing cesarean delivery. J Obstet Gynaecol Res 36, 991–995.

Marolf V, Ida KK, Siluk D et al. (2021) Effects of perineural administration of ropivacaine combined with perineural or intravenous administration of dexmedetomidine for sciatic and saphenous nerve blocks in dogs. Am J Vet Res 82, 449–458.

Martin-Flores M, Anderson JC, Sakai DM et al. (2019) A retrospective analysis of the epidural use of bupivacaine 0.0625–0.125% with opioids in bitches undergoing cesarean section. Can Vet J 60, 1349–1352.

Matthews PB, Rushworth G (1957) The relative sensitivity of muscle nerve fibres to procaine. J Physiol 135, 263–269.

Niv D, Nemirovsky A, Rudick V et al. (1995) Antinociception induced by simultaneous intrathecal and intraperitoneal administration of low doses of morphine. Anesth Analg 80, 886–889.

O'Neill P, Duarte F, Ribeiro I et al. (2012) Ropivacaine continuous wound infusion versus epidural morphine for postoperative analgesia after cesarean delivery: a randomized controlled trial. Anesth Analg 114, 179–185.

Pavlica M, Kržan M, Nemec A et al. (2022) Cardiopulmonary effects and pharmacokinetics of dexmedetomidine used as an adjunctive analgesic to regional anesthesia of the oral cavity with levobupivacaine in dogs. Animals (Basel) 12, 1217.

Pypendop BH, Siao KT, Pascoe PJ et al. (2008) Effects of epidurally administered morphine or buprenorphine on the thermal threshold in cats. Am J Vet Res 69, 983–987.

Qiao Q, Fu X, Huang R et al. (2022) Ropivacaine-loaded, hydroxypropyl chitin thermo-sensitive hydrogel combined with hyaluronan: an injectable, sustained-release system for providing long-lasting local anesthesia in rats. Reg Anesth Pain Med 47, 234–241.

Reader RC, McCarthy RJ, Schultz KL et al. (2020) Comparison of liposomal bupivacaine and 0.5% bupivacaine hydrochloride for control of postoperative pain in dogs undergoing tibial plateau leveling osteotomy. J Am Vet Med Assoc 256, 1011–1019.

Rice DC, Cata JP, Mena GE et al. (2015) Posterior intercostal nerve block with liposomal bupivacaine: an alternative to thoracic epidural analgesia. Ann Thorac Surg 99, 1953–1960.

Rosenberg PH, Heinonen E (1983) Differential sensitivity of A and C nerve fibres to long-acting amide local anaesthetics. Br J Aneasth 55, 163–167.

Saadawy I, Boker A, Elshahawy MA et al. (2009) Effect of dexmedetomidine on the characteristics of bupivacaine in a caudal block in pediatrics. Acta Anaesthesiol Scand 53, 251–256.

Snyder LB, Snyder CJ, Hetzel S (2016) Effects of buprenorphine added to bupivacaine infraorbital nerve blocks on isoflurane minimum alveolar concentration using a model for acute dental/oral surgical pain in dogs. J Vet Dent 33, 90–96.

Tan JP, Tan MB, Tam MK (2010) Application of nanogel systems in the administration of local anesthetics. Local Reg Anesth 3, 93–100.

Wann KT (1993) Neuronal sodium and potassium channels: structure and function. Br J Anaesth 71, 2–14.

Yoshitomi T, Kohjitani A, Maeda S et al. (2008) Dexmedetomidine enhances the local anesthetic action of lidocaine via an alpha-2A adrenoceptor. Anesth Analg 107, 96–101.

Zamora FJ, Madduri RP, Philips AA et al. (2019) Evaluation of the efficacy of liposomal bupivacaine in total joint arthroplasty. J Pharm Pract 34, 403–406, 897190019872577.

Locoregional Anesthetic Blocks for Small Animal Patients

The Eye

Yael Shilo-Benjamini and Peter Pascoe

CHAPTER 5

OVERVIEW

Surgery on and around the eye ranges from superficial skin procedures (lacerations and entropion) to the removal of the eye and adnexa. These procedures are considered to produce moderate to severe pain, due to the rich innervation of the globe and orbit (Murphy and Pollock 1993; Giuliano 2008; Giuliano and Walsh 2013). Postoperative pain of the globe or orbit can lead to self-trauma, such as facial rubbing, and possible dehiscence of the surgical site, that can result in further inflammation and pain (Ploog et al. 2014).

Most ophthalmic procedures in people are performed using local anesthetics and minimal or no sedation (Jaichandran 2013; Palte 2015). In children undergoing general anesthesia, it is recommended to add regional techniques (Deb et al. 2001; Gupta et al. 2007; Jaichandran 2013; Palte 2015). Similarly, in small animals, where most ophthalmic procedures are performed under general anesthesia, the use of regional anesthetic techniques in conjunction with general anesthesia can also be advantageous (Shilo-Benjamini 2019).

In addition to the analgesic effect, and therefore, the reduction in the need for intraoperative general anesthetics and perioperative systemic opioids, there are several specific benefits of using regional techniques during ocular surgery. First, regional techniques produce akinesia of the extraocular muscles, which results in globe centralization, and therefore, the need for administration of neuromuscular blocking agents and positive pressure ventilation is minimized (Hazra et al. 2008; Ahn et al. 2013c). Second, regional techniques produce mydriasis, which provides better surgical conditions for several ophthalmic procedures (Accola et al. 2006; Ahn et al. 2013c). Lastly, regional techniques may reduce the incidence of the oculocardiac reflex, initiated at the **trigeminal nerve**, via the ciliary ganglion and the **vagus nerve**, which can result in severe bradyarrhythmias, and asystole (Short and Rebhun 1980; Fayon et al. 1995; Shende et al. 2000; Deb et al. 2001; Morel et al. 2006; Gupta et al. 2007; Ghali and El Btarny 2010; Oel et al. 2014; Vezina-Audette et al. 2019; Vezina-Audette 2020).

FUNCTIONAL ANATOMY

The sensory innervation of the eyelids comes from the **ophthalmic** and **maxillary branches** of the **trigeminal nerve** (cranial nerve V_1 and V_2, respectively). The **ophthalmic branch** within the periorbita divides into three branches: the **frontal**, the **lacrimal**, and the **nasociliary nerves**. The **frontal nerve** supplies the sensory fibers to the superior eyelid. It passes between the periorbita and the fascia of the extraocular muscles and exits the orbit at the most dorsal part of the orbital rim where there is a small notch (Figure 5.1). The **lacrimal nerve** is a branch of the **frontal nerve** but has also been described as arising from the **maxillary nerve**. It may provide some sensory fibers to the lateral portion of the superior eyelid and the conjunctiva (Oduntan and Ruskell 1992). The **infratrochlear nerve** is a branch of the **nasociliary nerve** and supplies some sensory innervation to the medial commissure of the eyelids as well as the third eyelid. The **zygomatic nerve**, a branch of the **maxillary nerve**, supplies the lateral part of the upper eyelid (zygomaticotemporal branch), the lower lid, and the lateral canthus. There is some overlap in innervation between these branches (Figure 5.2). The cornea, the sclera, and the conjunctiva have sensory innervation supplied by the **long ciliary nerves**, which branch off the **ophthalmic nerve** (Figure 5.3). The neurons in the **long ciliary nerves** are myelinated up to the junction of the sclera and the cornea but are unmyelinated in the cornea. There is extensive branching and overlap in the nerve supply to the cornea and the bare nerve endings are within the superficial epithelium of the cornea.

The **auriculopalpebral nerve** is a branch of the **facial nerve** (cranial nerve VII) and supplies the motor fibers to the *m. orbicularis oculi* that close the eyelids. In the dog, the palpebral and auricular branches separate early in the course of the nerve and the palpebral branch runs over the zygomatic arch where the arch begins to curve ventrally, moving rostrally along the arch. The **palpebral nerve** forms the rostral auricular plexus between the eye and the ear and **superior** and **inferior branches** supply the dorsal and ventral parts of the *m. orbicularis oculi*, respectively. In cats, the division of the **auriculopalpebral nerve** occurs after it emerges from the caudal border of the zygomatic arch and it runs dorsally along the base of the ear before dividing into the **palpebral** and **rostral auricular branches**. The superficial temporal artery and vein run alongside this nerve. The dorsal branch of the **oculomotor nerve** innervates the *m. levator palpebrae superioris*, which retracts the upper eyelid.

The extraocular muscles that provide movement for the eye originate in the orbital fissure and insert on the sclera. These four muscles are contained within a fascial sheath and

Small Animal Regional Anesthesia and Analgesia, Second Edition. Edited by Matt Read, Luis Campoy, and Berit Fischer.
© 2024 John Wiley & Sons, Inc. Published 2024 by John Wiley & Sons, Inc.

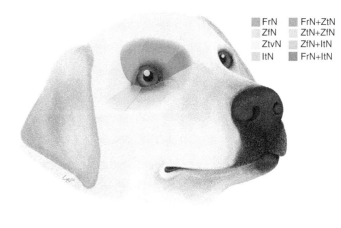

FIGURE 5.1   Diagram showing the **frontal**, **lacrimal**, **zygomaticotemporal**, and **zygomaticofacial nerves** as they exit the orbit in the dog.

FIGURE 5.2   Diagram showing the overlapping innervation of the **frontal**, **lacrimal**, **zygomaticotemporal**, and **zygomaticofacial nerves** in the dog. Source: Adapted from Whalen and Kitchell (1983).

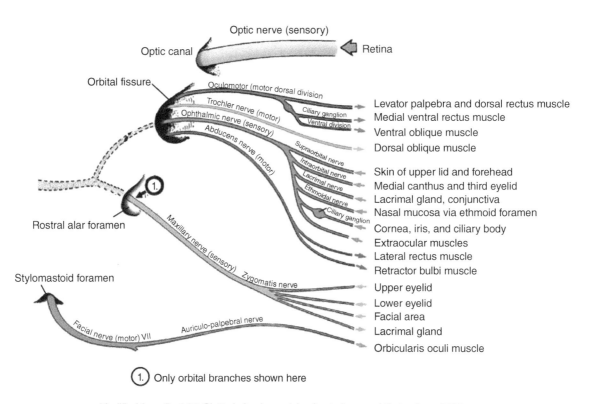

Modified from fig 1-22, Slatter's fundamentals of veterinary ophthalmology, 2008

FIGURE 5.3   Diagram of the nerves supplying innervation to ocular structures. The arrows indicate efferent (pointing to the right) and afferent (pointing to the left) directions.

this conical sheath is often referred to as the "extraocular muscle cone." This leads to descriptions of nerves or injections being either *intraconal* or *extraconal*. The **frontal**, **infratrochlear**, **zygomaticotemporal**, and **zygomaticofacial nerves** all run outside this fascial sheath but lie within the periorbita, which is the dense fibrous capsule that contains all the ocular structures. The globe is also encased in a further

fascial layer, known as the vagina bulbi or Tenon's capsule. This inserts on the sclera at the limbus and encircles the globe caudally to the insertion of the **optic nerve**. The vagina bulbi is also penetrated by the extraocular muscles and the **short** and **long ciliary nerves**. Injection of local anesthetics into this capsule will block corneal and conjunctival sensation with low volumes, and the drug can spread into the eyelids and back into the cone around the extraocular muscles if larger volumes are injected (Ripart et al. 1998; Ripart et al. 2000; Stadler et al. 2017).

TOPICAL CORNEAL ANESTHESIA

BLOCK AT A GLANCE

What is it used for?

- Corneal surgeries (e.g. conjunctival flap).

Landmarks:

- Cornea

What equipment and personnel are required?

- N/A

When do I perform the block?

- Several minutes prior to surgery; no preparation is required.

What volume of local anesthetic is used?

- One to two drops 0.5% proparacaine or 0.4% oxybuprocaine.

Goal:

- To deposit a small volume of local anesthetic onto the cornea.

Complexity level:

- Basic

WHAT DO WE ALREADY KNOW?

Proparacaine 0.5% has been tested in both dogs and cats (Herring et al. 2005; Binder and Herring 2006). Those studies showed a rapid onset of action with corneal insensitivity being demonstrated by one minute after application of the solution. The duration of complete insensitivity was approximately 20 minutes in dogs and 5 minutes in cats, with decreased sensation lasting for approximately 55 minutes in dogs and 30 minutes in cats. In dogs, there was a difference between applying one or two drops (1 minute apart), with the latter increasing the duration of insensitivity from 15 to 25 minutes. In Europe, another drug, oxybuprocaine (0.4%), has been used. When compared with tetracaine (1%) in dogs, the onset was rapid (1 minute for both drugs) and the duration of insensitivity was approximately 20 minutes for both drugs (Douet et al. 2013). There was more conjunctival hyperemia and edema with tetracaine and in people, it is reported to sting for 10–30 seconds following application (Khatatbeh and Qubain 2012). Oxybuprocaine in cats had a similar onset and

duration of analgesia (Giudici et al. 2015). Viscous tetracaine (0.5%) produced insensitivity within a minute and this lasted for about 35 minutes in dogs (Venturi et al. 2017). There was no blepharospasm but conjunctival hyperemia was noted in some dogs lasting for 15 minutes.

Lidocaine injectable solution has been tested topically in dogs and people and it does not seem to be as effective as the other drugs (Borazan et al. 2008; Costa et al. 2014). Several lidocaine gels have been produced and these seem to be more effective and last longer in the species where they have been tested. In a study in people with a 2% lidocaine gel, patients had lower pain scores than those with topical lidocaine solution (Bardocci et al. 2003). In horses using a similar 2% gel product, there was significantly decreased corneal sensitivity from 5–75 minutes, although maximal intensity (mean corneal touch threshold ≤0.5 cm) was from 10–45 minutes (Regnier et al. 2018). A 3.5% lidocaine gel (Akten™) has been used widely in people with minimal ocular irritation and excellent analgesia (Shah et al. 2010). In a study in dogs, this 3.5% gel produced insensitivity within a minute and a duration of about 20 minutes (similar to proparacaine) (Venturi et al. 2017). There was some blepharospasm that resolved quickly (1 minute) and conjunctival hyperemia lasting for about 15 minutes. Ropivacaine drops (1%) produced corneal insensitivity in dogs within a minute with analgesia lasting about 20 minutes (Costa et al. 2014). Application of the ropivacaine was associated with mild blepharospasm and mild hyperemia, which resolved within a minute. Bupivacaine (0.5%) in dogs did not produce corneal insensitivity but did decrease response to a noxious stimulus for about 25 minutes (Costa et al. 2014). In horses, bupivacaine produced corneal insensitivity with a rapid onset and this lasted longer than for lidocaine, proparacaine, or mepivacaine (Pucket et al. 2013).

Studies with lidocaine and bupivacaine have shown that increasing the pH of the solution improves the uptake of the drug into the cornea (Liu et al. 1993; Fuchsjager-Mayrl et al. 2002). Contrarily, increasing the pH of a tetracaine solution from 4.54 to 7.2 worsened the pain associated with instillation in human volunteers (Weaver et al. 2003) The formulated drug should not cause ocular irritation and it should have an osmolality of 200–400 mOsm kg^{-1} (Trolle-Lassen 1958) (Table 5.1). Low osmolalities can lead to corneal edema and high osmolalities can dehydrate the cornea.

In a clinical study comparing culture rates from corneal ulcers in dogs before and after proparacaine (with preservative), no differences were detected (Fentiman et al. 2018). The local anesthetics do not have any effect on corneal healing when administered once but tend to delay healing if applied repeatedly. This has led to investigations into other analgesics such as opioids. Both mu and delta receptors have been found in the canine cornea although there appear to be more of the latter (Stiles et al. 2003). The use of a topical 1% morphine solution (every eight hours) on surgically created corneal ulcers in dogs decreased corneal sensitivity and blepharospasm but did not interfere with corneal healing (Stiles et al. 2003). However, in clinical cases, a single application of topical morphine did not show any benefit in dogs or cats with

Table 5.1 Characteristics of drugs used for topical ocular anesthesia.

Drug	Concentration (%)	Preservative	Other ingredients	pH	Osmolality (mOsm kg⁻¹)	Systemic CNS toxic dose (estimated) (mg kg⁻¹)
Proparacaine	0.5	0.01% benzalkonium chloride	Glycerin, HCl, Na HCO₃	5–6	300	2.9
Oxybuprocaine or benoxinate	0.4	None	HCl	4.5–6	N/A	14.4
Tetracaine	0.5–1	None	NaCl, sodium acetate trihydrate, acetic acid	4.5	N/A	3.4
Lidocaine	2	None		4.5–6	270–320	20
Lidocaine gel	2, 3.5	None	Hypromellose, NaCl	5.5–7.5	N/A	20
Bupivacaine	0.5, 0.75	None	NaCl, KCl	6.5–6.7	280–290 (McLeod 2004)	4.3
Levobupivacaine	0.75	None	NaCl, KCl	5.85	334	8.6
Ropivacalne	1	None	NaCl, KCl	6.2	291	4.9

corneal ulceration or corneal surgery (Thomson et al. 2013). An opioid agonist/antagonist, nalbuphine, also did not provide a benefit in research dogs with a corneal wound. The most recent approach is to use topical enkephalinase inhibitors thereby allowing endogenous enkephalins to persist and provide analgesia and enhanced corneal healing (Reaux-Le Goazigo et al. 2019).

PATIENT SELECTION
INDICATIONS FOR THE BLOCK

Indicated for any corneal procedure.

CONTRAINDICATIONS

Epitheliopathy, which is an acquired inflammatory process affecting the retinal pigment epithelium, has been reported in people following short-term use, and even after a single use (Ansari et al. 2013; Patel and Fraunfelder 2013). Therefore, some authors recommend that topical anesthesia agents should be used cautiously in patients with dry eyes where the integrity of the ocular surface may be compromised (Ansari et al. 2013).

POTENTIAL SIDE EFFECTS AND COMPLICATIONS

Ophthalmic topical local anesthetics are generally safe (Waldman et al. 2014); however, ocular complications can arise from both short-term and long-term use. Prolonged use of topical ocular anesthetics in experimental animals and in people can lead to superficial punctate keratitis, persistent epithelial defects, stromal/ring infiltrates, corneal edema, endothelial damage, and ocular inflammation. It is thought that local anesthetics cause direct toxicity to corneal tissues, which leads to release of antigens and an inflammatory

response. Preservatives in anesthetic drops may play a further role in the development of ocular toxicity (Patel and Fraunfelder 2013).

Local anesthetics have some bactericidal activity, so the use of a local anesthetic prior to obtaining samples for culture could alter the results. For example, proparacaine inhibited the growth of *Staph. epidermidis* at 0.25% but not of three other *Staph.* spp. at 0.5%, whereas oxybuprocaine and tetracaine inhibited growth of *Staph. epidermidis* at 0.1% and 0.0625%, and the minimum inhibitory concentrations were below the clinically applied concentrations for the other *Staph.* spp. (Pelosini et al. 2009). However, it is important to recognize that any drug applied to the cornea is diluted in the tear film and the concentration that the cornea is exposed to is less than that applied.

GENERAL CONSIDERATIONS
EXPECTED DISTRIBUTION OF ANESTHESIA

Deposition of local anesthetics onto the cornea will lead to desensitization of nociceptors, desensitizing the corneal surface.

LOCAL ANESTHETIC: DOSE, VOLUME, AND CONCENTRATION

The ester local anesthetics have been the most commonly used drugs for topical application, with proparacaine being the most popular (Table 5.1). The solution causes minimal irritation or pain on application to the cornea.

The size of the drop is important as it only takes about 20 µl to get a full effect and any more volume than this will spill over into the lacrimal system. If a second drop is administered it should be placed at least one minute after the first drop to prevent spillage from the eye and dilution of the drug with increased tear production (Novack 2011). If two drugs are to be administered, the second one should be dropped into the eye after the peak effect of the first drug so that dilution and spillover do not reduce its effectiveness.

PATIENT PREPARATION AND POSITIONING

Lateral or sternal recumbency.

STEP-BY-STEP PERFORMANCE

ADMINISTRATION OF LOCAL ANESTHETIC – WHAT TO LOOK FOR, WHAT TO FEEL FOR, AND DECISION POINTS

The eyelids should be held open with the nondominant hand while a single drop is applied from the highest point so that it runs down over the cornea.

BLOCK EFFECTS AND PATIENT MANAGEMENT

Desensitization of the cornea.

COMPLICATIONS AND HOW TO AVOID THEM

Transient blepharospasm is common. Conjunctival hyperemia has been reported following administration of certain drugs (see above). These effects tend to be of short duration and do not require treatment.

Local toxicity may be associated with the administration of some of these local anesthetics. Since these drugs alter sensation, they decrease the feedback that stimulates lacrimation. This results in a decreased tear production rate of about 30% as determined by Schirmer's tear test in dogs (Williams 2005). Therefore, a Schirmer's tear test should not be performed until the local anesthetic has worn off. With the decreased tear production and blink rate there is a deterioration of the tear film and the ocular surface. Many of these local anesthetics have been shown to be toxic to the corneal epithelium and they may delay healing of corneal wounds if applied chronically. The mechanism is thought to be from disruption of the vinculin-based epithelial motility complexes which affects motility of the cells (Dass et al. 1988). However, there is very little suggestion that a single application of any of the drugs leads to significant changes because of the rapid clearance of the drug from the eye (Sun et al. 1999). Toxicity to the endothelium is more likely to occur with intracameral administration but can be the result of topical application. Direct exposure of the endothelium to benzalkonium chloride (preservative used in proparacaine) concentrations of 0.025–0.05% caused irreversible corneal edema in rabbits (Britton et al. 1976).

In people, it has been shown that there is no irritation when the pH of the solution is between 7.3 and 9.7 (Trolle-Lassen 1958). Drugs with pH values as low as 4 do not appear to damage the eye but will be more likely to sting on instillation.

Systemic toxicity with the local anesthetics is unlikely if a single drop of the ophthalmic solution is used in each eye. A standard drop is 20–50 µL so this would be, at most, 0.25 mg of proparacaine (the most toxic of the local anesthetics listed for topical administration) or 0.5 mg if both eyes were treated. This would be lower than the toxic dose for a 200 g animal, assuming total uptake of the drug (which would be unlikely from topical ocular administration).

Allergy to proparacaine and tetracaine has been reported in people, manifesting as contact dermatitis but this has rarely been reported in animals (Dannaker et al. 2001). Marked chemosis and hyperemia were observed in two dogs in response to tetracaine (0.5%) and in one dog the response was prevented by prior instillation of an antihistamine (Koch and Rubin 1969).

Limiting the amount of drug applied will also reduce systemic uptake of the drug and potential systemic toxicity. Some local anesthetics contain preservatives and it is important to recognize that these may affect the response of the animal.

If multidose bottles of drugs are used, there is the possibility of getting bacterial contamination of the tip of the bottle or the drug itself (Tsegaw et al. 2017).

AURICULOPALPEBRAL NERVE BLOCK

BLOCK AT A GLANCE

What is it used for?

- To treat blepharospasm in conjunction with other treatments for the root cause.

- In conjunction with topical anesthesia and subconjunctival local anesthetic, it can be used in placement of a third eyelid flap surgery in dogs.

Landmarks:

- Zygomatic arch

What equipment and personnel are required?

- Hypodermic needle 25 Ga 16 mm (5/8 in) or 26–27 Ga 12 mm (1/2 in.)

- Syringe of drug(s)

- Gloves

When do I perform the block?

- Prior to surgery, after skin preparation with alcohol 70%, with or without clipping the hair at the zygomatic arch level.

What volume of local anesthetic is used?

- Lidocaine 2% 0.025–0.05 ml kg^{-1}; with a minimum volume of 0.2 ml.

Goal:

- To block the **auriculopalpebral nerve** with a local anesthetic, resulting in the patient's inability to completely close the eyelids.

Complexity level:

- Basic

WHAT DO WE ALREADY KNOW?

Park et al. (2009b) is the only published study that has examined this block to date. Those authors reported 100% success within five minutes of injection of 0.4 ml lidocaine 2% in 47 dogs, with return of the palpebral reflex approximately one hour later (Park et al. 2009b).

A slight variation to the approach, blocking the **dorsal** and **ventral branches** of the **auriculopalpebral nerve** separately has been published (Westhues and Fritsch 1964). The dorsal branch of the nerve was blocked by advancing a needle above the lateral limit of the dorsal orbit, caudal to the rim of the orbit, and injecting a local anesthetic solution at this location. The ventral branch of the nerve was blocked by injecting a local anesthetic along the lower orbital rim in a similar fashion (Westhues and Fritsch 1964).

PATIENT SELECTION
INDICATIONS FOR THE BLOCK

An auriculopalpebral block can be used to treat blepharospasm, in conjunction with treatments more specific to the root cause of the ocular irritation. This block has also been used in conjunction with topical proparacaine and subconjunctival lidocaine to carry out placement of a third eyelid flap (nictitating membrane-to-superotemporal bulbar conjunctival flap construction surgery) in dogs where general anesthesia was avoided (Park et al. 2009b).

CONTRAINDICATIONS

This block should not be used where the lack of blinking may contribute to further ocular damage.

POTENTIAL SIDE EFFECTS AND COMPLICATIONS

Due to lack of blinking, it is possible that the animal will injure its own eye, therefore, the animal should be placed with a protection where it is unlikely to injure the blocked eye until the block wears off.

GENERAL CONSIDERATIONS
CLINICAL ANATOMY

In the dog, the **auriculopalpebral nerve** can be palpated under the skin as it crosses the zygomatic arch, making it easy to determine the location where the tip of the needle ultimately needs to be positioned.

EXPECTED DISTRIBUTION OF ANESTHESIA

The **auriculopalpebral nerve** is a motor nerve to the **m. orbicularis oculi** so blocking this nerve will affect the movement of the eyelids. A successful nerve block will result in the animal's inability to completely close the eyelids and there will be an absent palpebral reflex.

The auriculopalpebral block does not stop movement of the third eyelid, which is controlled by contraction of the **m. retractor bulbi**.

LOCAL ANESTHETIC: DOSE, VOLUME, AND CONCENTRATION

Lidocaine 2% 0.025–0.05 ml kg^{-1} with a minimum volume of 0.2 ml.

PATIENT PREPARATION AND POSITIONING

The patient should be positioned in sternal or lateral recumbency.

STEP-BY-STEP PERFORMANCE
SURFACE ANATOMY AND LANDMARKS TO BE USED

The zygomatic arch should be identified. During palpation of the zygomatic arch at the level of the lateral canthus, the **auriculopalpebral nerve** can usually be palpated under the skin where the zygomatic arch curves ventrally near its caudal aspect. The needle is inserted dorsal to the zygomatic process at its caudal one-third and the local anesthetic is injected subcutaneously (Park et al. 2009b).

NEEDLE INSERTION TECHNIQUE

A small-gauge hypodermic needle is inserted under the skin in the vicinity of the nerve, directing it subcutaneously parallel to the dorsal aspect of the zygomatic arch. Usually, the needle is advanced in a rostral to caudal direction (Figure 5.4).

An older approach is to block the dorsal and ventral branches of the **auriculopalpebral nerve** separately. In the dog, this can be achieved by inserting a needle above the lateral aspect of the dorsal orbit, a few millimeters caudal to the orbital rim. The needle is advanced subcutaneously and, following negative aspiration, the local anesthetic solution is injected as the needle is withdrawn. The ventral branch of the

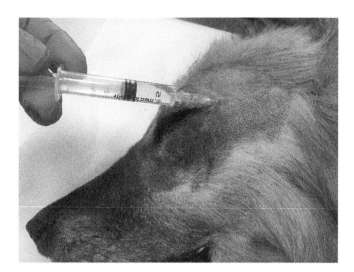

FIGURE 5.4   Administration of an **auriculopalpebral nerve** block in a dog. This nerve can often be palpated as it crosses the zygomatic arch. A small gauge needle is directed subcutaneously towards the nerve, parallel to the zygomatic arch, in a rostral to caudal direction.

nerve is blocked by injecting the local anesthetic along the lower orbital rim in a similar fashion (Westhues and Fritsch 1964).

In dogs, regardless of whether the nerve can be palpated, the injection is made over the zygomatic arch where the bone curves ventrally at its caudal aspect.

In the cat, the nerve cannot be palpated so the needle is placed at the caudal border of the zygomatic arc (rostral to the ear canal) and advanced subcutaneously in a ventral to dorsal direction.

Lidocaine (2%) $0.025–0.05\,ml\,kg^{-1}$ with a minimum volume of 0.2 ml is injected when the needle tip is considered to be in the optimal location.

Since the **auriculopalpebral nerve** is a motor nerve and blocking it will prevent blinking, there can be drying of the cornea and the potential for corneal ulceration. Use of eye lubrication is recommended until the block has worn off.

The use of short-acting drugs such as lidocaine is recommended. As always, it is important to aspirate before injecting because this nerve is accompanied by an artery and vein.

This nerve is relatively superficial so it is easy to end up with the needle in the nerve. If there is excessive resistance to injection, the needle should be withdrawn a little to ensure that the drug is not injected into the nerve.

FRONTAL NERVE BLOCK

What is it used for?

- Surgery of the superior eyelid, including laceration repair.
- The **frontal nerve** block can be combined with the **zygomaticotemporal nerve** block* to provide regional anesthesia for rostral craniotomy.

Landmarks:

- Dorsal rim of the orbit.

What equipment and personnel are required?

- Hypodermic needle 25 Ga 16 mm (5/8 in.) or 23 Ga 25 mm (1 in.)
- Syringe of drug(s)
- Sterile gloves

When do I perform the block?

- Prior to surgery, after the hair at the dorsal aspect of the eye is clipped and surgical skin preparation is complete (final skin preparation will be required prior to surgery).

What volume of local anesthetic is used?

- $0.04\,ml\,kg^{-1}$

Goal:

- To safely advance a needle toward the **frontal nerve** and inject a volume of local anesthetic, resulting in blockade of the nerve.

Complexity level:

- Basic

An anatomic study of this block has been published (Kushnir et al. 2018). Those authors reported 32/34 "successful" injections, with success being defined as a length of nerve > 6 mm being stained (Figure 5.5). The two failures were due to intravascular injections.

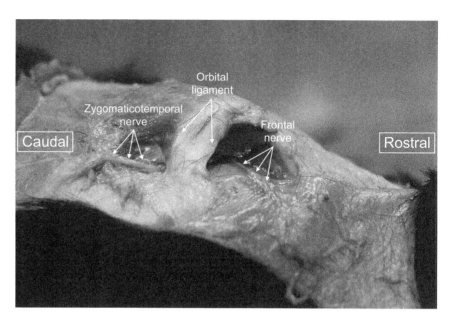

FIGURE 5.5 **Frontal** and **zygomaticotemporal nerves** stained following injection with bupivacaine diluted with methylene blue in a dog cadaver. Source: From Dr. Gal Marwitz and Dr. Yishai Kushnir.

PATIENT SELECTION

INDICATIONS FOR THE BLOCK

Surgery of the superior eyelid, such as laceration repair.

CONTRAINDICATIONS

The usual contraindications apply to this block – it should not be performed if there is a tumor in the vicinity of the injection or if there is an infection, which could make the local anesthetic ineffective.

POTENTIAL SIDE EFFECTS AND COMPLICATIONS

In the cadaver study, failures were due to intravascular injections, therefore, negative pressure to the syringe plunger should be applied before injection (Kushnir et al. 2018).

GENERAL CONSIDERATIONS

CLINICAL ANATOMY

The **frontal nerve** is a branch of the **ophthalmic branch** (V_1) of the **trigeminal nerve** and partially supplies the sensory fibers of the superior eyelid. It passes between the periorbita and the fascia of the extraocular muscles and exits the orbit at the most dorsal part of the orbital rim (zygomatic process of the frontal bone) along a small groove (groove for angularis oculi vein) (Figure 5.1).

EXPECTED DISTRIBUTION OF ANESTHESIA

This technique will block a small area of the middle portion of the superior eyelid. Although the **frontal nerve** innervates the entire superior eyelid, there is overlap on the medial aspect with the **infratrochlear nerve** and on the lateral aspect with the **zygomaticotemporal nerve** such that the only autonomous zone is the middle dorsal area of the eyelid (Figure 5.2).

LOCAL ANESTHETIC: DOSE, VOLUME, AND CONCENTRATION

Kushnir et al. (2018) used 0.04 ml kg^{-1} of 0.5% bupivacaine in their study.

PATIENT PREPARATION AND POSITIONING

The patient should be positioned in sternal or lateral recumbency.

STEP-BY-STEP PERFORMANCE

SURFACE ANATOMY AND LANDMARKS TO BE USED

The nerve exits the orbit through a small indentation (groove) at the most dorsal aspect of the zygomatic process of the frontal bone (which forms the superior portion of the orbital rim). This groove can often be palpated.

NEEDLE INSERTION TECHNIQUE

The puncture site is located at the most dorsal point of the orbital rim where a small notch can be palpated. The needle is inserted ventral to the rim, aiming along the ventral surface of the bone (Figure 5.6).

ADMINISTRATION OF LOCAL ANESTHETIC – WHAT TO LOOK FOR, WHAT TO FEEL FOR, AND DECISION POINTS

Once the needle tip is considered to be at the appropriate location, half the calculated volume can be injected with the other

(a)

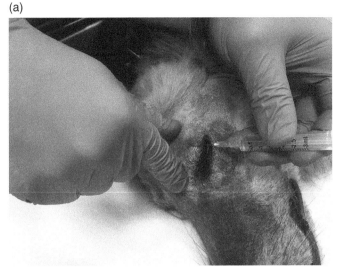

(b)

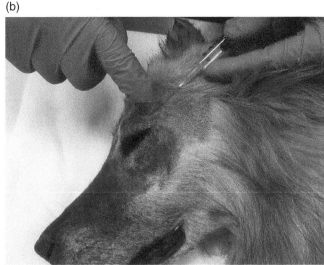

FIGURE 5.6   Administration of **frontal** (a) and **zygomaticotemporal** (b) **nerve** blocks in a dog.

half administered as the needle is withdrawn as described by Kushnir et al. (2018)

COMPLICATIONS AND HOW TO AVOID THEM

Kushnir et al. (2018) reported two failures due to intravascular injections, emphasizing the need for aspiration prior to injection.

COMMON MISTAKES AND HOW TO AVOID THEM

This nerve is relatively superficial so it is easy to end up with the needle in the nerve. If there is excessive resistance to injection the needle should be withdrawn a little to ensure that the drug is not injected into the nerve. Aspiration before injecting is especially important with this block as the nerve runs right next to the angularis oculi vein.

* Zygomaticotemporal nerve block

The **zygomaticotemporal nerve** innervates the lateral commissure of the eyelids but has very little autonomous innervation of the lids themselves. In conjunction with blockade of the **frontal nerve**, the whole of the upper eyelid is desensitized.

The **zygomaticotemporal nerve** is blocked by introducing a needle caudal to the junction of the orbital ligament and the frontal bone, aiming the needle medially and ventrally as if aiming for the nasal planum (Figure 5.6). In an anatomical study, a dose of 0.04 ml kg^{-1} of 0.05% methylene blue diluted with 0.5% bupivacaine was administered with a 25 Ga 1.6 cm (5/8″) needle that had been inserted to its full depth (Kushnir et al. 2018). Half the volume was injected as described above, and then the needle was withdrawn and aimed slightly dorsally, injecting the second half at the full depth of the needle penetration. This gave a high "success" rate (staining>6 mm; Figure 5.5) with 27/28 nerves stained in

non-brachycephalic breeds and 4/6 in brachycephalic breeds, which were not significantly different (Kushnir et al. 2018) (Figure 5.6a, b).

RETROBULBAR ANESTHESIA

BLOCK AT A GLANCE

What is it used for?

- Intraocular surgeries (e.g. phacoemulsification)
- Corneal surgeries (e.g. conjunctival flap)
- Evisceration/enucleation surgeries (note: additional infiltration of the eyelids/periorbital area should be administered).

Landmarks:

- Ventrolateral orbit ("inferior-temporal- palpebral" (ITP) approach) or supra-temporal (ST) in the dog and dorsomedial orbit ("superior-nasal" approach) in the cat (SN).

What equipment and personnel are required?

- Hypodermic or spinal needle 22-Ga, 1.5 in. (3.8 cm) for cats and small dogs or spinal needle 2.5–3.5 in. (6.4–8.9 cm) for larger dogs. The needle is used straight for the ST approach or bent at the midpoint to a curve with about a 20º angle for the ITP or SN techniques.

- Syringe of drug(s)
- Sterile gloves

When do I perform the block?

- Prior to surgery, after the hair around the eye is clipped and skin preparation is complete. Final skin preparation will be required prior to surgery.

What volume of local anesthetic is used?

- 1–3 ml (depending on dog size), 1 ml (adult cats).

Goal:

- To safely advance a needle behind the globe into the extraocular muscle cone and inject a volume of local anesthetic.

Complexity level:

- Intermediate

Clinical pearl:

- This block by itself does not provide sufficient intraoperative analgesia for enucleations.

WHAT DO WE ALREADY KNOW?
DOGS

Retrobulbar anesthesia (RBA) for ophthalmic surgeries in dogs was reported over half a century ago (Westhues and Fritsch 1964). However, at the time, it was not commonly used in small animals because general anesthesia and the use of neuromuscular blockers were preferred (Startup 1969; Severin 1995).

A study investigating three techniques for ophthalmic regional anesthesia in dogs concluded that the ITP approach to RBA, performed via the ventrolateral orbit, resulted in the best injectate distribution and in pupil dilation (mydriasis) (Accola et al. 2006). Although sensory effects were not reported in the Accola et al. study, this technique became popular and has been reported in clinical studies. RBA with 0.5% bupivacaine in comparison to a saline control was reported to provide postoperative analgesia following enucleation in dogs (Myrna et al. 2010). Nine of 11 control dogs required rescue analgesia in the postoperative period in comparison to 2 of 11 dogs in the bupivacaine group. Another study reported administration of RBA for cataract surgery in 10 dogs (10–15 kg) under xylazine–ketamine–diazepam anesthesia (Hazra et al. 2008); however, the technique was different than the one described by Accola et al. (2006). In that study, the needle was inserted at the lateral angle of the eye and advanced toward the opposite mandible, until it touched the medial orbital wall, where 2% lidocaine (2 mL) was deposited behind the globe. Central eye position was obtained in all 10 dogs and globe exposure was excellent except in 1 dog in which the nictitating membrane had completely obstructed the cornea and had to be retracted. An experimental study comparing akinesia and mydriatic effects of RBA (via the ITP approach) and another ophthalmic regional anesthesia technique (sub-Tenon's anesthesia [STA]), reported that only 5 out of 10 eyes of beagle dogs were blocked successfully following 2 ml of lidocaine 2%. An additional injection of 1 mL lidocaine 2% was required in the nonsuccessful eyes to provide akinesia (Ahn et al. 2013b).

Recently, several studies reassessed the success of RBA via the ITP approach. One study reported that in dog cadavers administered 1–2 ml injectate (bupivacaine : contrast agent 1 : 1) according to body weight, only 6 of 15 (40%) injections were successfully deposited intraconally, as assessed by computed tomography (CT) (Shilo-Benjamini et al. 2017a). A second study assessed RBA administration of 2 ml 0.5% bupivacaine : iopamidol (4 : 1) in six dogs (Figure 5.7). Injections were performed under sedation with dexmedetomidine and clinical effects were assessed following reversal with atipamezole (Shilo-Benjamini et al. 2019a). Injectate was observed intraconally on CT in only 2 of 6 (33%) injected orbits. Sensory block, including abolished corneal sensitivity and decreased periorbital sensation, was noted only in dogs with intraconal distribution.

A different approach to RBA via the superior temporal region ("supra-temporal" technique, ST) has been reported. The needle is inserted into the caudal orbit at the notch located above the zygomatic arch, caudal to the orbital ligament. The needle is directed ventromedially and 1–2 ml of a local anesthetic is injected (Severin 1995). This supra-temporal approach was compared to the ITP technique in ten dog cadavers (Chiavaccini et al. 2017). A 22 Ga, 3.81 cm (1.5 inch) spinal needle was used to deposit 0.1 ml kg^{-1} of local anesthetic–contrast agent mixture following perforation of the extraocular muscle cone. There was intraconal distribution in 19/20 injections assessed via CT and the only animal with complete extraconal spread was from the supra-temporal approach. It has also been compared to ITP using ultrasound guided ST in 21 dogs undergoing subconjunctival enucleation. The ST dogs did not receive any intraoperative fentanyl (vs 5/10 for the ITP) but the postoperative pain scores were not different (Briley et al. 2023). In a further retrospective study using ultrasound guided ST only 1/14 dogs required intraoperative fentanyl with the rest of the dogs receiving no opioids throughout their clinical management (Citarella et al. 2023).

A study assessed the relationship between dog size, skull conformation, periorbital length, and their effect on RBA administration. Thirty dog cadaver heads divided equally between skull conformation types (brachy-, dolicho-, and mesaticephalic) were measured. Significant positive correlations were found between the length of the periorbita and body weight and between the length of the periorbita and the cranial length (from the external occipital protuberance at the back of the skull to the median plane between the lower eyelid margins). A mathematical model was applied to estimate the periorbital length based on body weight and

(a)   (b)

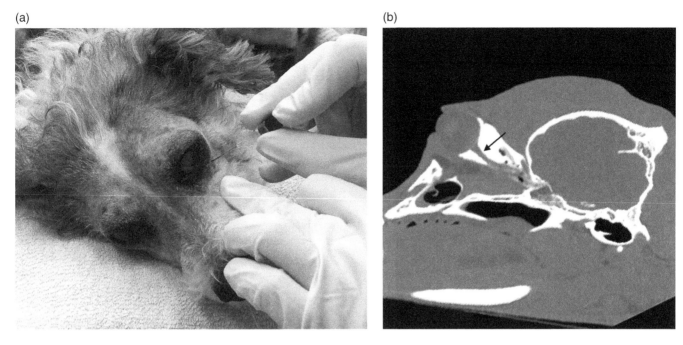

FIGURE 5.7   Administration of retrobulbar block with the inferior-temporal-palpebral approach in a dog (a). A sagittal oblique plane of computed tomography image presenting injectate distribution intraconally following RBA injection in a dog (b). The arrow demonstrates the **optic nerve** in long axis.

cranial length, defined as the distance from the most caudal point of the skull, referred to as the "*inion*," to a point connecting the medial canthi on the midline, referred to as the "*nasion*." No significant difference in this measurement was observed between the different skull types. Retrobulbar injection was performed in 10 dog cadavers using a 1 : 1 0.5% bupivacaine: iopamidol mixture, dosed at 0.1 ml cm^{-1} of the cranial length measured. Intraconal distribution assessed via CT was successful in all injections. The authors concluded that cranial length measurement is suitable for calculating the anesthetic volume required for RBA in dogs, although the clinical effects of using this volume calculation have not been assessed in live animals to date (Klaumann et al. 2018).

A recent study assessed the extraocular muscle cone volume of 188 dogs (376 orbits) using CT imaging. Cone volume was calculated according to: "*r*," the radius-half of the cone base diameter in centimeters, and "*h*," the height of the cone in centimeters, within the formula: $(\pi \cdot r^2 \cdot h)/3$. Skull morphology classified based on the cranial index ([skull width/skull length]·100; dolichocephalic approximately 39, mesocephalic approximately 52, and brachycephalic approximately 81) significantly affected cone volume, with mesocephalic dogs displaying a smaller volume (1.8 ml) than brachycephalic (2.5 ml) and dolichocephalic dogs (2.5 ml). It was found that mean cone volume was significantly greater in large dogs (>22 kg; 2.8 ml) than in medium (8–22 kg; 1.9 ml) and small dogs (≤8 kg; 0.9 ml). Sex also affected cone volume, being larger in males than in females with the same skull morphology (2.2 *versus* 1.6 ml). The final model to estimate cone volume in

mL included body weight and skull morphology, with the basic formula for mesocephalic dogs being 0.7 + (0.06 × weight in kg) and using this formula with addition of 0.37 in dolichocephalic and 0.57 in brachycephalic dogs (Greco et al. 2021). It is important to note that the extraocular muscle cone volume measured in this study is occupied with tissue, such as vessels, nerves, and fat; therefore, the volume of local anesthetic injected is not going to equal this volume. Further studies are required to confirm the clinical effectiveness of the proposed formula.

A retrospective study investigated the effects of RBA on the occurrence of oculocardiac reflex in 145 dogs undergoing enucleation. Overall, the oculocardiac reflex occurred in seven cases (4.8%) of which six dogs did not receive an RBA. The authors concluded that RBA may help prevent the oculocardiac reflex from occurring in dogs during enucleation (Vezina-Audette et al. 2019). A prospective, controlled, randomized, masked clinical study in dogs reported that preoperative RBA (ITP approach; $n = 11$) using 0.1 ml kg^{-1} bupivacaine 0.5% provided superior antinociception postoperatively in comparison to postoperative splash block ($n = 11$) with the same bupivacaine dose. Furthermore, significantly more dogs (4/11) in the splash block group required treatment for hypotension (versus 1/11 in the RBA group), although no difference in isoflurane requirement was noted between groups (Zibura et al. 2020). A retrospective study compared dogs administered RBA ($n = 97$) with dogs not administered regional anesthesia (control; $n = 70$) undergoing enucleation. There was no difference in the inhalant vaporizer settings intraoperatively, nor in additional perioperative analgesics administered between groups; 16 (16.5%) dogs in the RBA *versus* six (8.9%) dogs in the control group (Bartholomew et al. 2020). However, this was a retrospective study with no prespecified controls for intraoperative or postoperative analgesia. A recent prospective, randomized, masked placebo-controlled clinical trial in dogs compared RBA administration (ITP approach) either with ropivacaine 0.75% (0.1 ml kg⁻¹; $n = 12$) or an equivalent volume of 0.9% saline ($n = 12$). Intraoperatively there was no difference with regard to end-tidal isoflurane concentration, heart rate, or rescue analgesia administration. Mean arterial pressure was significantly higher in the ropivacaine-administered group during suture placement (skin closure). Postoperatively, pain scores using a numerical rating scale did not differ between groups, while visual analog scores were significantly higher in the saline-administered group at extubation, but not at the following evaluation times. No difference was reported for postoperative rescue analgesia administration, although time to rescue administration was significantly shorter in the saline-administered group (Scott et al. 2021). The authors did not test for block success; therefore, it is unknown how many animals had adequate regional anesthesia. Additionally, the study was underpowered to detect a difference in pain scores.

Ultrasound guidance has been used in people for ophthalmic regional anesthesia, allowing for imaging of key structures such as the globe, orbit, muscle cone, and **optic nerve**, which increases safety of needle-based anesthetic techniques by avoidance of intraocular, intraneural, intrathecal, or intravascular injections (Gayer and Palte 2016). Orbital structures are shallow; therefore, higher frequency transducers produce optimal resolution for ophthalmic regional anesthesia (i.e. 8–20 MHz). Both linear and curved-array transducers are used in people (Gayer and Palte 2016). Although ultrasound guidance has many advantages, it should be recognized that the eye is a delicate organ, and excessive sonic exposure may induce injury to globe structures. Therefore, the use of ocular-rated ultrasound devices or an "orbital" mode in new-generation bedside ultrasound devices, which reduce Mechanical and Thermal Index output is recommended (Palte et al. 2012; Gayer and Palte 2016). In people, real-time observation of intraconal spread of the local anesthetic is correlated with regional anesthesia success (Luyet et al. 2012). Ultrasound guidance for intraconal RBA has been reported in dogs for the ST technique and in cats (Shilo-Benjamini et al. 2014, Briley et al. 2023, Citarella et al. 2023).

CATS

In cats, the use of the ITP approach that is commonly used in dogs results in deposition of the injectate ventrally, outside the cone, and outside the orbit. For this reason, Shilo-Benjamini and colleagues studied a "superior-nasal" technique (Figure 5.8). Using this approach, the authors reported intraconal distribution of the 1 ml bupivacaine: contrast agent (1 : 1) in 5 of 7 (71%) cat cadaver eyes that were assessed using CT (Shilo-Benjamini et al. 2013). However, in experimental cats, this approach using 0.5% bupivacaine (0.75 ml) and iopamidol (0.25 ml) achieved intraconal distribution and clinical effects in only 3 of 6 (50%) eyes, despite the use of ultrasound to guide the needle intraconally (Shilo-Benjamini et al. 2014). Clinically, RBA has only been reported in two cats prior to enucleation. The first case report described administration of the ITP approach using 2 ml lidocaine/bupivacaine (1 : 1 volume ratio), which resulted in apnea and increased heart rate and blood pressure. At the end of surgery, it was difficult to wean the cat off the ventilator, and when the cat finally recovered it demonstrated neurological signs for approximately three hours. Therefore, brainstem anesthesia due to intrathecal injection of the local anesthetics was suspected (Oliver and Bradbrook 2013). The second case report described administration of the superior-nasal approach using 1 mL bupivacaine 0.25%. According to the cat's responses to surgical manipulations, it was speculated by the authors that the RBA was not deposited intraconally and that the desired local analgesia was not provided (Shilo-Benjamini et al. 2016).

PATIENT SELECTION
INDICATIONS FOR THE BLOCK

- RBA is indicated for any corneal or intraorbital surgery.

- Additionally, it can be used for evisceration or enucleation procedures in combination with local anesthetic infiltration of the eyelids and periorbital area.

CONTRAINDICATIONS

Several conditions may not be appropriate for needle-based ophthalmic injections:

- *Orbital neoplasia* – needle-based regional anesthesia in close proximity to neoplasia may increase the likelihood of spreading tumor cells. In cases of suspected orbital neoplasia, preoperative needle-based regional anesthesia should be avoided.

- *Orbital infection* – in severe eye infections, tissue pH becomes acidic. This will decrease the efficacy of the local anesthetic and absorption may increase, potentially leading to systemic toxicity (Giuliano and Walsh 2013; Chow et al. 2015).

- *Proptosis (globe prolapse)* – globe prolapse is not considered a contraindication, however, from the authors' experience, the effectiveness of preoperative needle-based techniques in this condition is dubious. The reason for this observation may be a result of the abnormal anatomy and the already disrupted tissues.

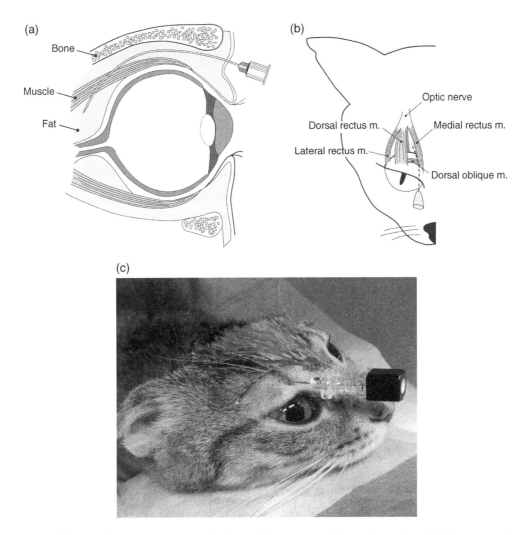

FIGURE 5.8 Diagrams of RBA administration in cats: sagittal view (a); dorsal view (b); administration of RBA in an experimental cat (c). Source: Shilo-Benjamini et al. (2013)/reproduced with permission from Elsevier.

POTENTIAL SIDE EFFECTS AND COMPLICATIONS

Complications are usually divided into ocular or systemic (Chang et al. 1984; Jaichandran 2013; Alhassan et al. 2015):

POTENTIAL OCULAR COMPLICATIONS:

- Corneal abrasion
- Chemosis
- Ecchymosis
- Retrobulbar hemorrhage
- Globe perforation
- **Optic nerve** damage
- Extraocular muscle damage

POTENTIAL SYSTEMIC COMPLICATIONS:

- Manifestation of the oculocardiac reflex
- Local anesthetic toxicity
- Intravascular anesthetic injection
- Intrathecal injection (i.e. into the optic sheath), resulting in seizures, brainstem anesthesia, and cardiorespiratory arrest

GENERAL CONSIDERATIONS
CLINICAL ANATOMY

The extraocular muscles form a cone behind the eye, referred to as the "extraocular muscle cone," and orbital structures or drug application is often described in relation to the cone (i.e. "*intraconal*" – inside the cone, or "*extraconal*" – outside the cone) (Giuliano and Walsh 2013; Samuelson 2013). RBA is commonly considered to be an "*intraconal*" technique, although a couple of veterinary studies reported "extraconal, retrobulbar" techniques (see above) (Hazra et al. 2008; Viscasillas et al. 2019).

EXPECTED DISTRIBUTION OF ANESTHESIA

Local anesthetics that are deposited inside the extraocular muscle cone (intraconally) will distribute around the **optic nerve** and other nerves passing nearby. A successful RBA injection will produce significant dilation of the pupil (>10 mm), centralization of the globe, and loss of corneal sensation.

It is important to note that RBA by itself does not provide complete anesthesia of the eyelids and other periorbital tissues because some of the branches of the **ophthalmic** and **maxillary nerves** pass extraconally. Therefore, it has been recommended that RBA should be accompanied by eyelid/conjunctival infiltration for enucleation or evisceration surgeries (Giuliano 2008; Shilo-Benjamini 2019).

LOCAL ANESTHETIC: DOSE, VOLUME, AND CONCENTRATION

Any local anesthetic can be used. Depending on the duration required, lidocaine could be used for shorter, less invasive procedures (such as cataract surgery) while bupivacaine, ropivacaine, or levobupivacaine can be used for longer, more invasive surgeries or those that would be expected to have some degree of postoperative pain (such as enucleation). However, even for short procedures, there may be some advantage to the use of longer-acting drugs to provide postoperative analgesia.

The volume of local anesthetic used in dogs varies between studies and there is currently no widely agreed-upon volume that is recommended for use (Table 5.2).

In adult cats, intraconal injection of 1 mL of local anesthetic produces excellent distribution around the **optic nerve** and loss of corneal sensitivity (Shilo-Benjamini et al. 2014).

PATIENT PREPARATION AND POSITIONING

The patient should be positioned in sternal or lateral recumbency. Standard aseptic preparation of the periorbital area is recommended before injection.

Table 5.2 Reported local anesthetic volumes used for RBA in dogs.

RBA reported local anesthetic volume	References
2 mL (in Beagles or dogs 10–15 kg)	Accola et al. (2006) and Hazra et al. (2008)
2 mL for body weight ≤15 kg	Myrna et al. (2010) and Ploog et al. (2014)
3 mL for body weight >15 kg	
1 mL for body weight ≤10 kg	Shilo-Benjamini et al. (2017a)
2 mL for body weight >10 kg	
0.1 mL cm^{-1} cranial length (defined as the distance between the inion and the nasion)	Klaumann et al. (2018)

STEP-BY-STEP PERFORMANCE

SURFACE ANATOMY AND LANDMARKS TO BE USED

The orbital bony rim is the main anatomical landmark and should be able to be palpated easily.

USE OF ULTRASOUND

Ultrasound guidance for intraconal RBA has been reported in dogs using the ST approach. This has produced excellent success rates of 96% across two studies using a 5-8 MHz probe (Briley et al. 2023, Citarella et al. 2023). In cats, it has been reported using a blended 5–8 MHz microconvex transducer placed at the dorsal aspect of the orbit (transpalpebral approach; Figure 5.9). However, in that study, the use of ultrasound did not increase RBA block success and the authors hypothesized that success rate was low (50%) due to difficulty in identifying the position of the tip of the curved needle used in that study (Shilo-Benjamini et al. 2014).

NEEDLE INSERTION TECHNIQUE

In both dogs and cats, the needle should be bent into a gentle curve with about a 20° angle. In dogs, the needle should be inserted at the junction between the middle third and the lateral third of the inferior eyelid (ventrolateral; inferiortemporal; Figure 5.7) in close proximity to the wall of the orbit. The needle is then advanced towards the back of the orbit in a medial (nasal) direction.

In cats, the needle is inserted through the superior eyelid at the junction between the dorsal and medial aspects of the orbit (Figure 5.8). This junction can be felt easily by palpating the dorsomedial (superior-nasal) orbital bone. The needle is then advanced towards the back of the orbit with a slight lateral orientation.

When the needle comes in contact with the outer surface of the extraocular muscle cone, the globe may appear to rotate in the direction of the needle as the needle is advanced through this muscle/fascia layer. A "pop" or "click" sensation may be appreciated in dogs as the needle penetrates the fascia of the muscular cone. This is often accompanied by rotation of the globe back to its normal position.

ADMINISTRATION OF LOCAL ANESTHETIC – WHAT TO LOOK FOR, WHAT TO FEEL FOR, AND DECISION POINTS

- It is important to aspirate prior to injection to avoid injecting into a blood vessel or into the cerebrospinal fluid of the **optic nerve** sheath.

- During administration of the local anesthetic, the globe may start bulging as the local anesthetic is distributed intraconally.

- If resistance is noted during injection, the needle should be redirected as this could be due to injection into the **optic nerve** sheath.

(a)

(b)

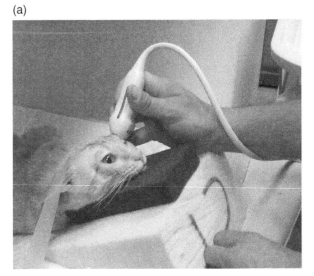
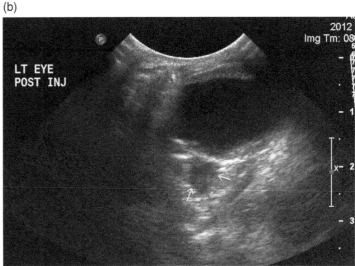

FIGURE 5.9   Ultrasound-guided approach to retrobulbar block in cats. Note the transducer is positioned at the superior eyelid using a transpalpebral approach (a). Ultrasound image following an intraconal RBA injection (b). The white arrows indicate the distribution of the local anesthetic in the muscular cone.

BLOCK EFFECTS AND PATIENT MANAGEMENT

- Complete loss of, or significantly reduced, corneal sensation and reduced periorbital skin sensation should result from an RBA injection.

- Additionally, successful blocks should result in centralization of the globe (akinesia) and pupillary dilation (mydriasis), which are helpful effects to facilitate certain intraocular or corneal surgeries.

- Ophthalmic regional anesthesia results in reduced tear production so the cornea should be treated with lubricants for the duration of the nerve block.

COMPLICATIONS AND HOW TO AVOID THEM

Complication rate of RBA in veterinary medicine is unknown (Shilo-Benjamini 2019), but manifestation of the oculocardiac reflex has been described in horses (Oel et al. 2014) and suspected brainstem anesthesia has been reported in a cat following injection of a local anesthetic using the ITP approach (Oliver and Bradbrook 2013).

Monitoring of a patient's vital signs during and following administration of RBA is very important in order to recognize an inadvertent intravascular or intrathecal injection as soon as it occurs and to be able to administer supportive patient care immediately.

Exophthalmos and conjunctival edema have been reported as minor transient complications in dogs (Shilo-Benjamini et al. 2019a) and cats (Shilo-Benjamini et al. 2014). Uveitis was reported in two eyes of 10 dogs undergoing cataract surgery administered 2 ml of lidocaine

2% (Hazra et al. 2008) and in two eyes out of six experimental dogs administered 2 ml of bupivacaine 0.5% combined with a contrast agent (iopamidol), of which one eye developed a corneal ulcer (Shilo-Benjamini et al. 2019a).

A recent single-center retrospective study in dogs undergoing enucleation assessed complications following RBA ($n = 97$) compared with dogs not administered regional anesthesia (control; $n = 70$). No major adverse events following RBA were related specifically to regional anesthesia. Incidence of hemorrhage was the same (23% in RBA versus 20% in the control group). One of the dogs administered RBA had severe hemorrhage requiring a packed red blood cell transfusion, which may or may not have been associated with amyloidosis that was diagnosed a year following surgery. Other postoperative complications following RBA included hyperalgesia with flank biting ($n = 1$), a postoperative methicillin-resistant *Staphylococcus intermedius* infection ($n = 1$) and fever, urinary incontinence, severe lethargy, and elevated liver enzymes two days after discharge ($n = 1$) (Bartholomew et al. 2020).

COMMON MISTAKES AND HOW TO AVOID THEM

At the doses recommended for RBA, it is not uncommon for extraconal injection of a local anesthetic solution to result in block failure. It may be difficult to appreciate whether the tip of the needle is inside the muscular cone without advanced imaging. If a "popping" sensation occurs (more easily detected in dogs than in cats), then it is more likely that the needle tip is located intraconally. To date, there is no reported technique that will ensure intraconal needle placement.

PERIBULBAR ANESTHESIA

BLOCK AT A GLANCE

What is it used for?

- Intraocular surgeries (e.g. phacoemulsification)
- Evisceration/enucleation surgeries

Landmarks:

- Dogs: ventrolateral orbit (ITP technique) or medial canthus.
- Cats: dorsomedial orbit ("superior-nasal" technique).

What equipment and personnel are required?

- Hypodermic needle.
  - In dogs <15 kg: 25-Ga 1.6 cm (5/8 in.) needle.
  - In dogs 15–40 kg: 22–23-Ga 2.5 cm (1 in.) needle.
  - In dogs >40 kg, a longer needle may be required (22--Ga 3.8 cm [1.5 in.]), but there are no published studies investigating the length of needle required in giant breed dogs.
  - In cats: 25 Ga 1.6 cm (5/8 in.) needle.
- Syringe of drug(s)
- Sterile gloves

When do I perform the block?

- Prior to surgery, after the hair around the eye is clipped and skin preparation is complete. Final skin preparation will be required prior to surgery.

What volume of local anesthetic is used?

- Dogs: Bupivacaine 0.25–0.5% or ropivacaine 0.5–1% 0.3 ml kg^{-1} or 2.33 BW$^{0.33}$ mL (BW = body weight in kg).
- Cats: Bupivacaine or ropivacaine 0.25% 3.5–4 ml per adult cat.
- Drug may require dilution with saline 0.9% to avoid reaching a toxic dose, while still meeting the required volume.

Goal:

- To safely advance a needle outside the extraocular muscle cone and inject a volume of local anesthetic.

Complexity level:

- Basic to intermediate

Clinical pearl:

- This block provides excellent intraoperative analgesia for enucleations.

WHAT DO WE ALREADY KNOW?
DOGS

Several techniques for delivery of peribulbar anesthesia (PBA) have been suggested for use in dogs. A single-injection technique was evaluated in 15 experimental dogs, with or without ultrasound guidance (Wagatsuma et al. 2014). A 22-Ga, 2.5 cm needle was inserted at the ventrolateral eyelid and 0.3 ml kg^{-1} of ropivacaine 1% was injected. Both akinesia and decreased corneal sensitivity were achieved with this technique. Another study reported the use of a single-injection at the medial canthus or a double-injection at the dorsomedial and ventrolateral regions in dog cadavers (Figure 5.10) (Shilo-Benjamini et al. 2017a). A 25-Ga 1.6 cm needle was used and the volume of injectate (bupivacaine : contrast agent 1 : 1) was calculated according to the allometric equation: $2.33 \times BW^{0.33}$ ml (BW = body weight in kg). Partial to complete injectate distribution at the base of the cone and intraconally was evident in 75–88% and 31–57% of the eyes, respectively. Dogs over 20 kg were less likely to have intraconal distribution, which was hypothesized to result from using short needles for all sizes of dogs. The injection at the medial canthus was accompanied by penetration of the third eyelid in 3 out of 16 injections (19%) so it was not used in a subsequent study in experimental dogs (Shilo-Benjamini et al. 2019a). The double-injection PBA technique was further applied in six experimental dogs with a mean body weight of 21 kg using 22-Ga 2.5 cm hypodermic needles and injecting 5 ml of 0.5% bupivacaine/iopamidol (4 : 1) divided equally between the dorsomedial and ventrolateral regions. Injections produced significantly lower periocular skin sensitivity for 2–3 hours and lower corneal sensitivity for 4 hours (complete loss of corneal sensitivity was observed for 4.7 ± 4.1 [range 1–11 hours]) in comparison to control eyes (Shilo-Benjamini et al. 2019a).

CATS

In cat cadavers, administration of a single injection dorsomedially was deemed to provide better injectate distribution than using two injections (i.e. dorsomedially and ventrolaterally), as assessed by CT (Shilo-Benjamini et al. 2013). In that study, a 25-Ga, 1.6 cm needle was inserted in close proximity to the orbital wall, advanced to its full length (Figure 5.11), and 4 ml of bupivacaine/iopamidol (1 : 1) was injected. A significant amount of injectate was observed intraconally in 7/7 eyes injected dorsomedially, of which in 6/7 eyes the injectate surrounded the **optic nerve** 360°. This technique was further assessed in six experimental cats, using 3 ml of injectate (1.5 ml bupivacaine 0.5%, 1 ml saline 0.9%, and 0.5 ml iopamidol). All PBA injections resulted in intraconal distribution (assessed by CT) and produced significantly lower corneal and skin sensation relative to control eyes for three hours (Shilo-Benjamini et al. 2014). Clinically, a case report comparing administration of PBA to RBA in a cat undergoing bilateral enucleation suggested that PBA produced better intra-and postoperative analgesia than the RBA technique (Shilo-Benjamini et al. 2016). In 20 cats

(a)
(b)

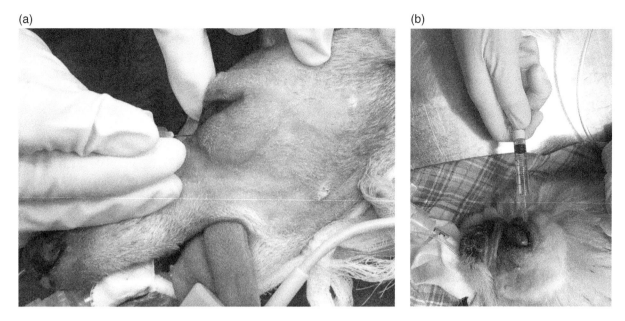

FIGURE 5.10   Administration of PBA single-injection at the medial canthus (a) or a double-injection at the dorsomedial and ventrolateral regions (b) in dogs prior to enucleation surgery.

(a)
(b)

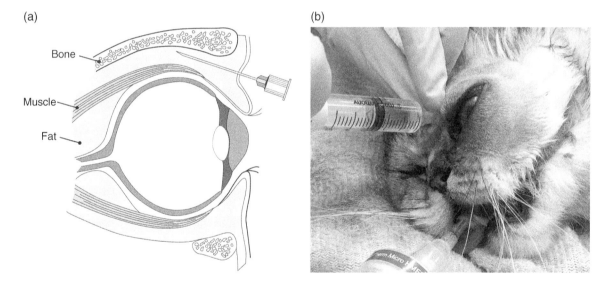

Bone

Muscle

Fat

FIGURE 5.11   Administration of PBA: (a) diagram (sagittal view) and (b) in a cat prior to enucleation. Source: Shilo-Benjamini et al. (2013)/ reproduced with permission from Elsevier.

no block failures were reported using PBA with bupivacaine ± cisatracurium. The addition of the latter shortened the onset of akinesia and increased mydriasis in 10 cats undergoing corneal or lens surgery (Costa et al. 2023).

PATIENT SELECTION

INDICATIONS FOR THE BLOCK

- PBA is primarily indicated for evisceration/enucleation surgery as it provides a wide local anesthetic distribution including the eyelids and periorbital tissues.

- Additionally, it can be used for intraocular surgery (e.g. phacoemulsification).

CONTRAINDICATIONS

Several conditions may not be appropriate for needle-based ophthalmic injections:

- ***Orbital neoplasia*** – needle-based regional anesthesia in close proximity to neoplasia may increase the likelihood of spreading tumor cells. In cases of suspected orbital neoplasia, preoperative needle-based regional anesthesia should be avoided.

- *Orbital infection* – in severe eye infections, tissue pH becomes acidic. This will decrease the efficacy of the local anesthetic and absorption may increase, potentially leading to systemic toxicity (Giuliano and Walsh 2013; Chow et al. 2015).

- *Proptosis (globe prolapse)* – globe prolapse is not considered a contraindication, however, from the authors' experience, the effectiveness of preoperative needle-based techniques in this condition is dubious. The reason for this observation may be a result of the abnormal anatomy and the already disrupted tissues.

- *Glaucoma or descemetocele (corneal thinning where only Descemet's membrane remains)*: glaucoma or descemetocele are not considered contraindications, however, because a transient (but clinically important) increase in intraocular pressure has been reported in cats following PBA (Shilo-Benjamini et al. 2014), this technique should be avoided in patients where a salvage globe procedure, such as conjunctival flap, is planned (Shilo-Benjamini 2019).

POTENTIAL SIDE EFFECTS AND COMPLICATIONS

- Exophthalmos
- Chemosis
- Ecchymosis
- Corneal ulceration can develop due to corneal desiccation from decreased eyelid closure and reduced tear production
- Increased intraocular pressure (IOP) in cats

GENERAL CONSIDERATIONS
CLINICAL ANATOMY

The muscle sheaths are made of thick connective tissue enclosing the extraocular muscles (Samuelson 2013). This sheath seems to be permeable to local anesthetics, as it has been reported in people (Ripart et al. 2001) and cats (Shilo-Benjamini et al. 2014). Adipose tissue occupies the space between orbital fascia sheaths and acts to protect the globe (Samuelson 2013). In people, the spread of a local anesthetic through the adipose tissue of the orbit following peribulbar block was reported to be unpredictable, although increasing the volume injected will increase block success (Nouvellon et al. 2010).

EXPECTED DISTRIBUTION OF ANESTHESIA

The local anesthetic is expected to diffuse from outside the extraocular cone into the cone, as well as to the eyelids and periorbital region. A successful block will produce significant dilation of the pupil (>10 mm), centralization of the globe, and loss of, or significantly reduced, corneal and periocular sensation.

LOCAL ANESTHETIC: DOSE, VOLUME, AND CONCENTRATION

The choice of local anesthetic should depend on the duration of effect required and drug availability. Any local anesthetic can be calculated to its maximum recommended dose and then diluted with 0.9% saline to reach the desired volume.

DOGS

Volumes reported in dogs vary between studies. In one study, a volume of 0.3 ml kg^{-1} was used (Wagatsuma et al. 2014). In a different study, an allometric calculation was used: $2.33 \times BW^{0.33}$ ml (BW = body weight in kg) because orbit size does not increase linearly with body weight (Shilo-Benjamini et al. 2017a). Globe size may vary among dog breeds, but globe diameter is usually 20–22 mm across breeds (Samuelson 2013). Therefore, it should be emphasized that when PBA is administered in tiny-breed dogs or in giant-breed dogs, a basic calculation of X ml kg^{-1} will most likely be either inadequate or excessive, respectively (Table 5.3). The authors recommend that the use of 3–6 ml should be used with the lower dose in small dogs and a maximum dose of 6 mL in large dogs. Table 5.3 shows the calculation of doses from the two published studies, and it is obvious that these may be inadequate or excessive in cases of body weight extremes. A new calculation that fits with the above recommendation is provided in the third column.

A recent study assessing ultrasound-guided PBA used a different approach for volume calculation (Foster et al. 2021). The approach was based on the relationship between cranial length (defined as the distance between the inion and the nasion) and the retrobulbar space as investigated by CT, which was reported to be 0.1 ml cm^{-1} of cranial length (Klaumann et al. 2018). Foster et al. (2021) extrapolated from this calculation and, because the volume of the peribulbar

Table 5.3 Calculations of the reported local anesthetic volumes (in ml) used for PBA in dogs.

Body weight (BW; in kg)	0.3 ml kg^{-1} (Wagatsuma et al. 2014)	$2.33 \times BW^{0.33}$ ml (Shilo-Benjamini et al. 2017a)	$3 \times BW^{0.17}$
2	0.6	2.9	3.4
5	1.5	4.0	3.9
10	3	5.0	4.4
15	4.5	5.7	4.8
20	6	6.3	5.0
30	9	7.2	5.3
40	12	7.9	5.6
50	15	8.5	5.8
60	18	9.0	6.0

space should be greater than the retrobulbar space, the authors used 0.2 ml cm^{-1} of cranial length.

CATS

Cats have a globe diameter of approximately 21 mm, which may be slightly greater than dogs with a similar body weight (Samuelson 2013). A study in adult cat cadavers reported excellent intraconal and extraconal distribution using a volume of 4 ml (Shilo-Benjamini et al. 2013). In a clinical investigation in adult cats, using a volume of 3 ml (bupivacaine 0.25%) there was a less-optimal distribution in some of the eyes. Median corneal and skin sensation were significantly lower than control eyes for three hours, although the duration of effect was variable among cats (Shilo-Benjamini et al. 2014).

The volume required to produce adequate intraconal distribution may be above the maximal recommended dose of the local anesthetic for either species. A study with bupivacaine 0.25% in cats after a peribulbar block reported that a dose of 2 mg kg^{-1} (0.8 ml kg^{-1}) resulted in bupivacaine peak plasma concentrations that were lower (approximately half) than the plasma concentrations reported to produce bradyarrhythmias or seizure activity (Shilo-Benjamini et al. 2017b). Furthermore, the concentrations were very low (approximately one-sixth) in comparison to the plasma concentrations that have been reported to produce hypotension.

Therefore, based on the above studies and the authors' personal experience, the use of 3.5–4 ml in adult cats is recommended to produce good distribution of the local anesthetic into the muscular cone. However, in a study using levobupivacaine at 1.25 mg kg^{-1}, a total volume of 1 mL/eye was sufficient for corneal or lens surgery (Costa et al. 2023). In cachectic cats, the maximum recommended dose of the local anesthetic chosen (i.e. as mg kg^{-1}) should be diluted up to that volume. In kittens, however, since the orbit is not at its final size, the authors use the maximum recommended dose of the local anesthetic (as mg kg^{-1}) diluted to a final volume of approximately 1 ml kg^{-1} (e.g. in a 1.5 kg kitten, 2 mg kg^{-1} bupivacaine 0.5% will be used; 3 mg = 0.6 ml, which will be diluted with 0.9 ml saline to a total volume of 1.5 ml).

PATIENT PREPARATION AND POSITIONING

The patient can be positioned in sternal or lateral recumbency. Standard aseptic preparation of the periorbital area is recommended before injection.

STEP-BY-STEP PERFORMANCE

SURFACE ANATOMY AND LANDMARKS TO BE USED

The bony rim of the orbit is the primary landmark and should be palpated easily.

USE OF ULTRASOUND

Ultrasound-guided technique using a transpalpebral approach with an ophthalmic 15 MHz transducer (Accutome B-Scan Plus) was compared to a blind technique in 15 dogs (Wagatsuma et al. 2014). Complete needle visualization via ultrasound was achieved in only half of the injected eyes (8/15). There were no differences between eyes with regard to block success, although the intraocular pressure (IOP) was significantly higher following the performance of the blind technique (23.3 versus 18.6 mmHg).

Several recent studies have investigated ultrasound-guided peribulbar injection techniques, aiming to inject in close proximity to the orbital fissure where **cranial nerves** III, IV, V (ophthalmic branch), and VI emerge. A posterior extraconal approach was assessed bilaterally in 12 dog cadavers by Viscasillas et al. (2019). A 5–8 MHz microconvex ultrasound transducer was positioned transversely, caudal to the orbital ligament, and tilted caudally to view the orbital fissure (Figure 5.12). An intra-arterial catheter was placed in and sutured to the infraorbital artery. This was flushed with saline in order to visualize the maxillary artery with the ultrasound and provide a source of reference since the nerves themselves were unable to be visualized sonographically. The needle was advanced using an in-plane technique between the ultrasound transducer and the lateral aspect of the frontal bone until the sphenoid complex was reached. A mixture of contrast agent and methylene blue (0.5 ml) was injected in close proximity to the orbital fissure and spread was evaluated using CT and dissection, respectively. A total of 15/24 (63%) injections were considered successful with no difference between left and right sides. No complications such as intracranial spread of contrast, or intraocular or intravascular injection were found in this study (Viscasillas et al. 2019).

Another study evaluated a similar approach in 10 dog cadavers using a 5–8 MHz microconvex transducer positioned caudal to the orbital ligament in a longitudinal plane. An in-plane technique was used with the needle inserted caudal to the orbital ligament above the zygomatic arch and guided to the edge of the myofascial cone, midway along the length from globe to pterygoid bone, and methylene blue dye was injected in five dogs (10 eyes), while methylene blue and contrast agent were injected in the remaining five dogs (10 eyes). Injection volume was 0.2 ml cm^{-1} of cranial length. Contrast distribution in the peribulbar space via CT was evident in 9/10 injections (90%), and a mixed peribulbar/retrobulbar distribution was identified in 1/10 (10%) injection. Contrast was present at the rostral alar foramen in 4/10 (40%), at the orbital fissure in 5/10 (50%), and at the oval foramen in 1/10 (10%) injections. On orbital dissection, peribulbar spread of dye was noted in 19/20 (95%) injections (Foster et al. 2021).

A different study investigated a subzygomatic approach to PBA, where a microconvex transducer was positioned on the surface of the cornea (Mahler et al. 2020). The peribulbar compartment was identified as the interface between the

(a)

(b)

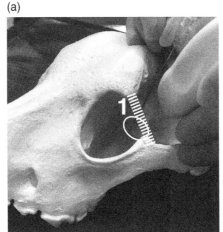
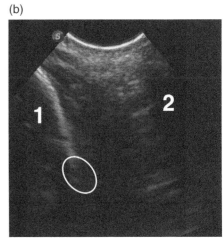

FIGURE 5.12 Administration of an extraconal block with ultrasound-guided posterior approach in the dog. (a) A dog skull showing the position of the probe and needle: the transducer is positioned in a transverse position caudal to the orbital ligament (dotted line). (b) An ultrasound image presenting sonoanatomy of this approach: lateral aspect of the frontal bone (1), coronoid process of the mandible (2), and sphenoid complex (circle). Source: Viscasillas et al. (2019)/Elsevier.

hyperechoic periorbita medially and the hypoechoic *m. masseter* laterally. The needle was introduced through the *m. masseter*, ventral to the zygomatic arch, caudal to the maxilla, and cranial to the vertical ramus of the mandible, in a medial direction. After passing the zygomatic arch, the needle was oriented in a caudodorsal direction and further advanced. Then, using an out-of-plane oblique approach, the tip of the needle was ultrasonographically identified and positioned within the peribulbar compartment, where the injectate was administered. Following successful administration of 1 mL of dye in four orbits, this technique was assessed further in seven orbits using 0.1 ml kg^{-1} of contrast agent, with injectate distribution assessed by CT. The contrast had peribulbar distribution in 6/7 orbits (86%), with migration to the orbital fissure, rostral alar foramen, and mandibular foramen, while in 1/7 orbits distribution occurred in the *m. masseter*. It should be noted that positioning the ultrasound transducer at the cornea, as performed in the study by Mahler et al. (2020), may result in increased heat and injury to globe structures. Therefore, it is recommended that for this approach, only ocular-rated ultrasound devices should be used (Palte et al. 2012; Gayer and Palte 2016).

A potential major complication documented by several studies is a high incidence of intracranial injectate distribution. In one of these studies where the needle was inserted above the zygomatic arch, intracranial spread of contrast was noted following 5/10 (50%) injections via the alar canal, the orbital fissure, or both (Foster et al. 2021). In the second study where the subzygomatic approach was used, in all successful cases, intracranial distribution was observed through the rostral alar foramen, with an incidence of 6/6 (100%) (Mahler et al. 2020).

The studies by Viscasillas et al. (2019), Mahler et al. (2020) and Foster et al. (2021) used cadavers and, to the authors' knowledge, none of the abovereported techniques have been evaluated in live animals. Additionally, none of

these studies compared the use of ultrasound guidance with a strictly anatomical approach to document potential benefits of using an ultrasound-guided technique.

In the authors' opinions, the use of ultrasound guidance for PBA is not necessary. Using the techniques described below, the needle will be kept away from important structures inside the orbit, and success of the block depends mainly on distribution of the local anesthetic, not where it is initially deposited.

NEEDLE INSERTION TECHNIQUE

In dogs, the needle can be inserted at several possible locations: the lateral third of the inferior eyelid, the medial canthus, the dorsomedial junction of the orbit (through the superior eyelid), and the ventrolateral orbit (through the inferior eyelid) (Figure 5.10).

In cats, the needle is inserted through the superior eyelid at the junction between the dorsal and medial aspects of the orbit (Figure 5.11). This junction can be felt easily upon palpation of the orbital bone.

In both dogs and cats, after the needle is inserted, it is advanced in close proximity to the orbital wall toward the back of the orbit.

ADMINISTRATION OF LOCAL ANESTHETIC – WHAT TO LOOK FOR, WHAT TO FEEL FOR, AND DECISION POINTS

Negative aspiration on the syringe should be confirmed prior to drug administration. Injection of the local anesthetic should be performed slowly, which allows the relatively large volume being injected (compared to a retrobulbar technique) to diffuse caudally and around the globe. Exophthalmos and chemosis may be noted postinjection.

BLOCK EFFECTS (SENSORY, MOTOR, ETC.) AND PATIENT MANAGEMENT

Sensory effects include complete loss of, or significantly reduced, corneal sensation and significantly reduced periorbital skin sensation. Motor effects include pupil centralization and dilation, which are important components required during intraocular or corneal surgeries.

Ophthalmic regional anesthesia will result in reduced tear production so the cornea should be protected with lubricants for as long as the block lasts.

COMPLICATIONS AND HOW TO AVOID THEM

Complications include exophthalmos, chemosis, and ecchymosis (due to rostral spread of the relatively large volume of local anesthetic and damage to small blood vessels) (Figure 5.13). These minor complications do not typically interfere with surgery and usually resolve spontaneously within a few hours (Shilo-Benjamini et al. 2014; Wagatsuma et al. 2014; Alhassan et al. 2015; Shilo-Benjamini et al. 2016).

Punctate superficial ulcers were reported following bilateral peribulbar block with 0.3 mL kg[1] of ropivacaine 1% in both eyes of 2 of 15 dogs (Wagatsuma et al. 2014). Uveitis and a corneal ulcer were reported following PBA injections in one out of six dogs administered bupivacaine 0.5% combined with a contrast agent (iopamidol) (Shilo-Benjamini et al. 2019a). Corneal ulceration can develop following PBA due to decreased eyelid closure and reduced tear production therefore eye lubrication is advisable.

A transient, but clinically important increase in IOP was observed in cats following PBA (Shilo-Benjamini et al. 2014). Increases in IOP are not a concern if enucleation is planned, but in animals with glaucoma or with globes at risk of rupture, this block should be used with caution or not used at all (Shilo-Benjamini et al. 2014; Allgoewer 2018).

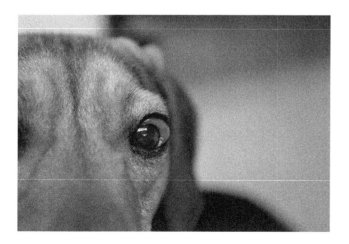

FIGURE 5.13 Exophthalmos, chemosis, and ecchymosis in a dog following PBA. These short-lived minor complications occur due to rostral spread of the large volume injected and damage to minor blood vessels.

Needle-based complications, such as globe perforation (Riad and Akbar 2012) or retrobulbar hemorrhage (Alhassan et al. 2015) have been reported in people following peribulbar block but have not been described in the veterinary literature.

If a medial canthus injection is performed in dogs, the needle may accidentally penetrate the third eyelid which will result in a failure of the block and a swollen third eyelid. Slow injection is likely to reveal this mistake and the needle can be repositioned (Shilo-Benjamini et al. 2017a).

COMMON MISTAKES AND HOW TO AVOID THEM

A needle that is too short may result in less distribution of the injectate caudally and reduced block success or reduced duration of effect. Therefore, the needle should be of appropriate length in relation to the size of the orbit.

Because of the relatively large volume of local anesthetic that is required for PBA (relative to RBA), the needle may be repulsed during injection, resulting in reduced distribution of the local anesthetic caudally. To avoid this, the needle should be held securely in place during injection.

If a double-injection technique is being performed, it is advisable to place both needles before any injections are made, otherwise, insertion of the second needle is made more difficult by the exophthalmos that is produced following the first injection (Shilo-Benjamini et al. 2019a).

SUB-TENON'S CAPSULE ANESTHESIA

BLOCK AT A GLANCE

What is it used for?

- Intraocular surgeries (e.g. phacoemulsification)
- Corneal surgeries (e.g. conjunctival flap)

Landmarks:

- A 4–5 mm snip incision is made into the dorsomedial or dorsolateral portion of the bulbar conjunctiva, approximately 5 mm away from the limbus using conjunctival scissors.

What equipment and personnel are required?

- Curved mosquito hemostat
- Colibri forceps or 0.5 mm rat tooth thumb forceps
- Westcott conjunctival scissors or other ophthalmic scissors
- cm (1 in.), 19 Ga STA cannula
- Syringe of drug(s)
- Sterile gloves

When do I perform the block?

- This block is performed by the surgeon immediately prior to surgery, after aseptic orbital and periorbital preparation, and after draping the surgical site.

What volume of local anesthetic is used?

- Lidocaine 2%, 2 ml per adult dog or bupivacaine 0.25–0.5%, 1-2 ml in dogs under 5 kg, 2-3 ml in dogs over 5-25 kg and 3-5 ml in dogs >25 kg.

Goal:

- Insert a cannula into Tenon's (episcleral) capsule and inject a small volume of local anesthetic.

Complexity level:

- Intermediate

Clinical pearl:

- The tip of the cannula should be advanced **past** the globe's equator.

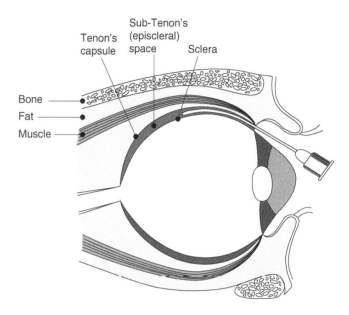

FIGURE 5.14 Diagram of STA administration (sagittal view). Source: Shilo-Benjamini 2019/reproduced with permission from Elsevier.

WHAT DO WE ALREADY KNOW?

STA is a cannula-based injection technique that has been shown to be a simple, safe, and effective alternative to needle-based retro- or peribulbar anesthetic techniques in people (Jaichandran 2013; Palte 2015). To perform this technique, a specialized, blunt cannula is inserted surgically under sterile conditions along the curvature of the sclera into Tenon's capsule, and a local anesthetic is injected. To do so, a small incision is made in the conjunctiva and Tenon's capsule, several millimeters from the limbus. The local anesthetic diffuses from this location and blocks the **short ciliary nerves** that are merged with the **long ciliary nerves**, resulting in dilation of the pupil and analgesia, respectively.

In dogs, an incision is made in the dorsomedial portion of the bulbar conjunctiva, 5 mm from the limbus, and a 19-Ga STA cannula is inserted (Figure 5.14). In people, a variety of needles and cannulas have been described but none seem to provide great advantages over the others (Kumar et al. 2004; Riad et al. 2012). Following injection, the conjunctival incision is not closed but is allowed to heal by second intention.

The effects of sub-Tenon's blocks using 2 mL of lidocaine 2% in experimental dogs were reported to provide consistent akinesia and mydriasis (pupil diameter >10 mm) (Ahn et al. 2013c). Akinesia and mydriasis onset and duration were approximately 5 and 90 minutes, respectively (Ahn et al. 2013b).

Sub-Tenon's blocks using 2 ml lidocaine 2% were evaluated in seven dogs undergoing phacoemulsification. The blocks were effective for providing akinesia and mydriasis during phacoemulsification and isoflurane requirements were significantly lower in the blocked group when compared to the control group that received systemic atracurium to achieve a central eye for surgery (Ahn et al. 2013a).

The sub-Tenon's technique was reported to be an effective alternative to systemic neuromuscular blockade in 12 dogs requiring bilateral cataract surgery. Administration of 2–3 ml bupivacaine (0.25–0.5%; according to body weight) on the first operated eye was compared to 0.01 mg kg^{-1} pancuronium administered intravenously during the second operated eye (Bayley and Read 2018). In a larger study with 133 eyes in 99 dogs a number of eyes did not achieve akinesia (23/133) and the intraoperative and postoperative complication rates were higher compared with NMB alone (Bayley et al. 2023).

PATIENT SELECTION
INDICATIONS FOR THE BLOCK

- Intraocular surgeries (e.g. phacoemulsification)
- Corneal surgeries (e.g. conjunctival flap)

CONTRAINDICATIONS

- Previous STA injections
- Infection at the injection site
- Globe perforation or trauma
- Ocular pemphigoid (because of adhesions at the injection site) (Kumar et al. 2011; Guise 2012). Ocular pemphigoid has not been reported in companion animals however, in cats, herpes virus may cause a similar phenomenon of adhesions (symblepharon).

POTENTIAL SIDE EFFECTS AND COMPLICATIONS

- Chemosis
- Ecchymosis
- Corneal ulcer (could be the result of corneal desiccation)

GENERAL CONSIDERATIONS
CLINICAL ANATOMY

Tenon's capsule (also referred to as the vagina bulbi or bulbar sheath) is a thick connective tissue enclosing the globe and sclera from the outside and it is one of the three important fascial structures of the orbit (Murphy and Pollock 1993). The space created between the connective tissue and the sclera is filled with loose connective tissue and is referred to as Tenon's (episcleral) space (Samuelson 2013).

EXPECTED DISTRIBUTION OF ANESTHESIA

The local anesthetic is expected to diffuse throughout Tenon's space and may diffuse caudally into the intraconal space with increasing volumes of injectate. Successful STA will produce significant dilation of the pupil (>10 mm), centralization of the globe, and loss of corneal sensation.

LOCAL ANESTHETIC: DOSE, VOLUME, AND CONCENTRATION

- 2 ml lidocaine 2% (Ahn et al. 2013a, b, c).
- 2–3 ml bupivacaine 0.25–0.5% (2 ml in dogs under 5 kg and 3 ml in dogs over 5 kg) (Bayley and Read 2018).
- The size of the globe does not vary greatly between dogs and cats and there is little increase in size as the weight of the animal increases. Globe diameter is approximately 20–22 mm. There are no reports of STA in cats, but a volume of 2 ml can probably be used in cats as well. However, the maximum recommended dose of the drug used should be calculated.

PATIENT PREPARATION AND POSITIONING

The patient can be positioned in sternal or lateral recumbency (both have been reported in dogs). Standard preparation of the eye (conjunctiva and cornea) is required before making an incision in the conjunctiva. Some authors clip the cilia as part of the patient's preparation.

STEP-BY-STEP PERFORMANCE
SURFACE ANATOMY AND LANDMARKS TO BE USED

The dorsal portion of the bulbar conjunctiva should be identified and assessed for abnormalities. An incision will be made approximately 5 mm from the limbus (medial or lateral areas have been reported in dogs).

USE OF ULTRASOUND

Ultrasound guidance for this block has not been reported in veterinary medicine. In people, following STA administration, an ultrasonic observation of "T-sign" was indicative of distribution of the local anesthetic circumferentially around the posterior pole of the eye and correlated with successful block (Guise 2012; Palte 2015).

CANNULA INSERTION TECHNIQUE

- Certain equipment is required in order to make the incision: an eyelid speculum, curved mosquito hemostat, 0.5 mm rat tooth thumb forceps or Colibri forceps, and curved Westcott conjunctival scissors.
- A drop of a topical ophthalmic local anesthetic can be administered prior to making the incision.
- First, the conjunctiva is raised with a hemostat or forceps. This is followed by making a 4–5 mm snip incision using scissors at the dorsomedial or dorsolateral portion of the bulbar conjunctiva, 3–5 mm from the limbus.
- Tenon's capsule is grasped with forceps and blunt dissection using conjunctival scissors (while keeping the scissors closed) is performed posteriorly, staying on the "longitudinal" line of the globe, creating a small tunnel.
- A 2.5 cm (1 in.), 19-Ga STA cannula is inserted through the incision into the tunnel and is advanced past the globe's equator.
- The local anesthetic is injected slowly, facilitating caudal distribution of the injected solution.
- The cannula is removed, and the tunnel and incision are left to heal by second intention (i.e. not sutured) (Ahn et al. 2013c; Bayley and Read 2018).

ADMINISTRATION OF LOCAL ANESTHETIC – WHAT TO LOOK FOR, WHAT TO FEEL FOR, AND DECISION POINTS

After performing the incision, administration of 0.1 ml of the local anesthetic solution into the capsule can help to differentiate between Tenon's capsule and the underlying sclera, by spreading them apart (Bayley and Read 2018).

During injection, the cannula can be redirected slightly from side to side in order to allow injection of local anesthetic in different directions, enhancing diffusion of the local anesthetic behind the eye.

BLOCK EFFECTS (SENSORY, MOTOR, ETC.) AND PATIENT MANAGEMENT

Sensory effects include complete loss of, or significantly reduced, corneal sensation. Motor effects include pupil centralization (akinesia) and dilation (mydriasis), which are important components required during intraocular or corneal surgeries.

COMPLICATIONS AND HOW TO AVOID THEM

Chemosis and ecchymosis have been reported in dogs following STA (Ahn et al. 2013c; Bayley and Read 2018). Postoperatively, a corneal ulcer was reported in 1/12 eyes following STA in dogs, which resolved with medical treatment after a week (Bayley and Read 2018). Ulceration could be the result of corneal desiccation, and therefore globe lubrication should continue for as long as the block is anticipated to last.

Although fewer complications are reported with STA when compared to needle-based techniques such as retro- or PBA, retrobulbar hemorrhage, globe perforation, and central spread of local anesthetics leading to brainstem anesthesia and death, have been reported in people (Kumar et al. 2011; Jaichandran 2013; Palte 2015). Further studies on small animals are needed.

COMMON MISTAKES AND HOW TO AVOID THEM

- In order to minimize the local anesthetic from draining back out of the tunnel, it is important to keep the tunnel as narrow as possible by keeping the blades closed during dissection.

- The local anesthetic should be injected slowly. If the injection rate is too rapid, it can cause pain and may result in chemosis.

- The local anesthetic volume should be kept low, and probably should not exceed 3 mL (the maximum volume reported in dogs to date). In people, when increased volumes are used, it results in increased IOP and may make it more difficult to access the anterior chamber surgically.

- Make sure that the conjunctiva does not get swollen during injection (this significant chemosis means that the spread of local anesthetic is migrating anteriorly rather than posteriorly). If it does, the cannula should be pushed from a rostral to a caudal direction (i.e. further posteriorly).

- If it is difficult to inject, the cannula may be too far into the capsule and may be obstructed. In this case, the cannula should be withdrawn slightly, and injection reattempted (Guise 2012; Ahn et al. 2013c; Bayley and Read 2018).

- Ocular massage following injection should be avoided, as this was reported to result in substantial increase in IOP and bleeding into the anterior chamber (Guise 2012).

TOPICAL ORBITAL ANESTHESIA TECHNIQUES

WHAT DO WE ALREADY KNOW?

Topical infiltration techniques may be used following enucleation surgery in dogs, replacing RBA or PBA in cases where there may be contraindications or reluctance to use needle-based techniques (Ploog et al. 2014; Chow et al. 2015; Shilo-Benjamini 2019).

These techniques are simple, inexpensive, and can be performed easily by nonspecialist veterinarians. These postoperative techniques can also be useful in cases where RBA or PBA are contraindicated, such as if ophthalmic neoplasia is present, or in cases of severe infections of the globe and periorbital tissues (Giuliano and Walsh 2013; Chow et al. 2015). In the authors' experience, proptosis is another indication to consider using a postoperative topical technique because needle-based techniques such as RBA and PBA have decreased accuracy in these patients. The reason for this may be the disrupted anatomy of the globe, adnexa, and traumatized tissues, affecting local anesthetic distribution in these cases.

SPLASH BLOCK

Installation of bupivacaine 0.5% ($0.1\,\text{ml}\,\text{kg}^{-1}$) into the orbit after having removed the globe and establishing hemostasis has been reported (Chow et al. 2015). In that report, a 22-Ga, hypodermic needle was used to splash the local anesthetic into the empty orbit (Figure 5.15) and the local anesthetic was left in place for 30 seconds by lifting the skin surrounding the orbit, following which skin sutures were placed. Those authors compared the splash block to RBA and reported that there were no differences in postoperative pain between groups. Limitations of that study included the use of several pain assessors (interobserver variability was not evaluated), questionable RBA success, and the use of a questionable pain scoring scale. No complications were reported to occur in any of the dogs; however, only 16 dogs were included in the splash block group.

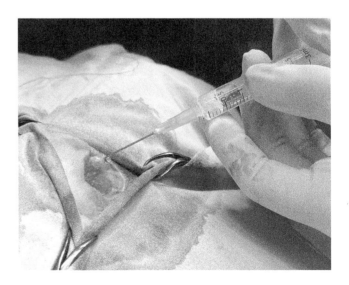

FIGURE 5.15   Splash block is administered in a cat following enucleation and before suture placement.

LOCAL ANESTHETIC-INFUSED HEMOSTATIC SPONGES

Evaluation of absorbable gelatin sponge (Gelfoam®) infused with lidocaine (1–1.5 ml) and bupivacaine (1–1.5 ml) placed into the orbit intraoperatively following globe extraction has been reported (Ploog et al. 2014). Postoperative analgesia provided by the infused Gelfoam® was comparable to the same drugs administered via preoperative RBA, although, uneven groups (8 versus 11), questionable RBA success, and use of a questionable pain scoring scale were limitations of this study. Another study evaluated intraorbital placement of Gelfoam® infused with 2 mg kg⁻¹ ropivacaine 1% compared with an equivalent volume of saline following enucleation in dogs (10 dogs in each group) (Shilo-Benjamini et al. 2019b) (Figure 5.16). At extubation, the median pain score was significantly higher in the saline control group (8 versus 3) and significantly more dogs were administered rescue analgesia compared to the ropivacaine group (7 versus 1). In addition, significantly more dogs in the saline control group were reported by the owners to have "crying" or "attention-seeking" behaviors on the first day following enucleation (7 versus 1). Both studies reported no complications to Gelfoam® insertion, however, the small number of dogs studied in these reports (8 and 10, respectively) does not completely rule out complications that might occur following this technique.

From the authors' experience, the Gelfoam® should be soaked in the local anesthetic for several minutes (until the local is absorbed into the Gelfoam®) before it is placed in the orbit.

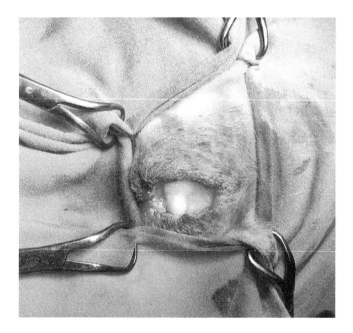

FIGURE 5.16 Absorbable gelatin sponge (Gelfoam®) infused with local anesthetics inserted into the orbit in a dog following enucleation.

INFILTRATION OF THE EYELIDS

Infiltration of the eyelids with a local anesthetic is indicated for a variety of procedures, including canthoplasty, entropion or ectropion repair, wedge resection, laceration repair, eyelid reconstructive procedures, or as an adjunct to RBA. It may also help to decrease postsurgical entropion by causing slight eversion of the eyelids (Giuliano and Walsh 2013).

Long-acting local anesthetics such as bupivacaine or ropivacaine are recommended for postoperative pain control due to their prolonged duration of effect. The use of bupivacaine liposome injectable suspension (Nocita®) for infiltration of tissues following ophthalmic surgery has potential to result in prolonged analgesia (up to 72 hours) however there are no published studies to support this use at present. Addition of epinephrine to a local anesthetic to further increase its duration of action is possible but must be weighed against the possible decrease in local tissue blood flow.

EQUIPMENT

- Hypodermic needle 25 or 27-Ga.
- Syringe of drug(s)
- Gloves

TECHNIQUE

Depending on the procedure, infiltration of the eyelids can be performed before surgery, to provide better intraoperative analgesia and decrease general anesthetic dose, or after surgery in order to not distort lid conformation and damage surgical repair of some reconstructive procedures.

The local anesthetic is injected into the skin and subcutaneous tissues using a small gauge needle (Figure 5.17). The needle should be inserted at the incision line (if performed before surgery) or adjacent to the incision (if performed after surgery). Depending on the size of the patient and the length of the needle being used, the needle can be inserted up to the hub, and the local anesthetic is injected as the needle is slowly withdrawn. Typically, two or more injection sites will be necessary to adequately infiltrate the entire eyelid.

CLINICAL TIPS

- To avoid local anesthetic leaking from the infiltrated tissues, use the smallest gauge needle possible.

- Infiltration of a large volume will result in significant eyelid swelling and may distort lid conformation. For this reason, some authors infiltrate the eyelids only after surgery (e.g. entropion or ectropion repair). Another way to avoid lid distortion is to use a small volume of a more concentrated local anesthetic.

- If it is desirable to decrease the amount of bleeding during surgery, a local anesthetic with epinephrine can be administered.

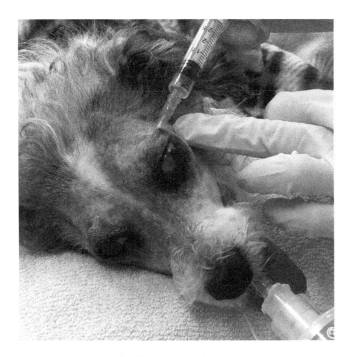

FIGURE 5.17   Eyelid infiltration in a dog.

• In dogs with entropion, a strong spastic component may be exacerbated by surgical manipulation of the eyelids. Infiltration of local anesthetic to slightly evert the eyelids may reduce the need for additional sutures (Giuliano 2008).

INTRACAMERAL ANESTHESIA

WHAT DO WE ALREADY KNOW?

Injection of a local anesthetic into the anterior chamber, "intracameral anesthesia" (ICA), has been used as an alternative to mydriatic drug administration when those drugs (e.g. sympathomimetics and anticholinergics) are contraindicated or to provide pain management for intraocular surgeries (Gerding et al. 2004; Park et al. 2009a; Park et al. 2010). This technique is reported to be safe and effective for providing additional analgesia in people undergoing cataract surgery when compared to administration of topical anesthesia alone (Ezra et al. 2008). However, exposure of the corneal endothelium to local anesthetics at typically used concentrations may result in apoptosis and pathology. Exposure of the anterior chamber to lidocaine at ≤1% appears to result in minimal changes, however, 0.5% bupivacaine and 1% ropivacaine both cause clinically significant corneal thickening and opacification (Eggeling et al. 2000; Iradier et al. 2000; Guzey et al. 2002; Yang et al. 2002; Cakmak et al. 2005; Chuang et al. 2007). A study in dogs indicated no lasting effects of ICA following administration of 1% or 2% lidocaine (Gerding et al. 2004).

DOGS

The technique in dogs is performed at a location slightly lateral to the 12 o'clock position of the limbus. Using an operating microscope, a 30-Ga needle is introduced through the limbus into the anterior chamber and 0.1–0.3 ml of aqueous humor is aspirated into a syringe. Following aspiration, a second 30-Ga needle is inserted slightly lateral to the first needle, and an equivalent volume of 1–2% lidocaine is injected into the anterior chamber (Park et al. 2009a; Park et al. 2010).

Several studies have reported the use of ICA with lidocaine in dogs. One study tested the effects of 0.1 mL 1–2% lidocaine in one eye of 16 dogs in comparison to 0.1 ml of balanced salt solution injected into the contralateral eye (control). In that study, a 25-Ga needle was used. No significant differences were found in morphological features, including corneal thickness, endothelial cell density, or intraocular pressure when comparing baseline values with those over seven days following the injections (Gerding et al. 2004).

Another study evaluated the volume of lidocaine for ICA required to produce mydriasis (defined as mean pupil diameter >10 mm) in dogs (Park et al. 2009a). Volumes of 0.1, 0.2, and 0.3 ml of lidocaine 1% or 2% in comparison to saline injection were tested. Lidocaine 2% decreased onset and increased duration of mydriasis in comparison to the 1% solution and 0.2–0.3 ml decreased the onset (one to five minutes) and increased duration of effect (approximately 120 minutes).

A third study evaluated the intraoperative and postoperative analgesia produced following ICA with either 0.3 ml lidocaine 2% or 0.3 ml of balanced salt solution for phacoemulsification in dogs. During surgery, the requirement for isoflurane was significantly lower in dogs administered lidocaine in comparison to dogs administered a balanced salt solution. Following surgery, dogs that were administered lidocaine had a significantly increased interval to the time for rescue analgesia (approximately 5 hours) in comparison to dogs in the control group (approximately 1.5 hours) (Park et al. 2010).

CATS

The mydriatic effects of ICA with 0.2 or 0.3 ml lidocaine 2% were compared with 0.2 ml epinephrine (0.1 mg ml^{-1}), a balanced salt solution, and topical administration of one drop of 0.5% tropicamide in 50 adult cats (Amorim et al. 2019). Epinephrine provided the shortest onset, longest duration (approximately 200 minutes), and greatest pupil dilation (10–13 mm) in comparison to all other treatments. Lidocaine 0.2 ml and 0.3 ml provided pupil dilation of 8–10 and 9–11 mm, with a median duration of 65 and 160 minutes, respectively.

PATIENT SELECTION

INDICATIONS FOR THE BLOCK

Intraocular surgeries, such as cataracts, intraocular lens implantation, and vitreoretinal surgery to expose the lens and posterior segments. In dogs, ICA was reported as useful during phacoemulsification (Park et al. 2010).

CONTRAINDICATIONS

Any infection or trauma to the globe.

POTENTIAL SIDE EFFECTS AND COMPLICATIONS

No obvious gross or microscopic changes to the corneal endothelium were identified following ICA with preservative-free lidocaine in dogs (Gerding et al. 2004). However, the use of preservative-free 0.5% bupivacaine, 0.75% levobupivacaine, 1% ropivacaine, and 2% lidocaine was reported to result in corneal pathologies in rabbits, although these changes were temporary and resolved within seven days of the injections (Guzey et al. 2002; Borazan et al. 2009). No adverse effects were reported in dogs or cats, even when the concentration and volume of lidocaine were increased from what is recommended in people (Park et al. 2009a, 2010; Amorim et al. 2019). A meta-analysis study suggested no differences in adverse effects when topical anesthesia was used with or without intracameral anesthesia in people (Ezra et al. 2008).

GENERAL CONSIDERATION

CLINICAL ANATOMY

Anterior chamber, cornea, and limbus.

EXPECTED DISTRIBUTION OF ANESTHESIA

The local anesthetic is expected to diffuse throughout the anterior chamber. It is hypothesized that diffusion of the local anesthetic around the iris and the ciliary body affects the small nerve fibers located within these structures (Park et al. 2010). A successful injection will produce significant dilation of the pupil (>10 mm) and intraocular analgesia.

LOCAL ANESTHETIC: DOSE, VOLUME, AND CONCENTRATION

0.2–0.3 ml lidocaine 2%

PATIENT PREPARATION AND POSITIONING

- The patient can be positioned in sternal or lateral recumbency.
- Aseptic preparation of the eye is required before injection.

STEP-BY-STEP PERFORMANCE

SURFACE ANATOMY AND LANDMARKS TO BE USED

The dorsal portion of the limbus.

NEEDLE INSERTION TECHNIQUE

Using an operating microscope for magnification to help guide needle placement, a 30-Ga needle is inserted slightly lateral to the 12 o'clock position of the limbus into the anterior chamber, and 0.2–0.3 ml of aqueous humor is aspirated. Then, a second 30-Ga needle is inserted slightly lateral to the first needle, and an equivalent volume of the local anesthetic is injected into the anterior chamber.

BLOCK EFFECTS (SENSORY, MOTOR, ETC.) AND PATIENT MANAGEMENT

Sensory effects include complete loss or significantly reduced corneal sensation. Motor effects include pupil centralization and dilation, which are important components required during intraocular or corneal surgeries.

COMPLICATIONS AND HOW TO AVOID THEM

Although ICA in dogs was not associated with any gross or microscopic corneal changes, a transient visual loss in a man following ICA for cataract surgery was reported. It was hypothesized that a posterior capsule rupture was present, which led to retinal toxicity (Eshraghi et al. 2015). In that case, vision gradually returned to normal over the three days following injection. Therefore, in cases where a capsule rupture is suspected, ICA should probably be avoided.

REFERENCES

Accola PJ, Bentley E, Smith LJ et al. (2006) Development of a retrobulbar injection technique for ocular surgery and analgesia in dogs. J Am Vet Med Assoc 229, 220–225.

Ahn J, Jeong M, Lee E et al. (2013a) Effects of peribulbar anesthesia (sub-Tenon injection of a local anesthetic) on akinesia of extraocular muscles, mydriasis, and intraoperative and postoperative analgesia in dogs undergoing phacoemulsification. Am J Vet Res 74, 1126–1132.

Ahn J, Jeong M, Park Y et al. (2013b) Comparison of systemic atracurium, retrobulbar lidocaine, and sub-Tenon's lidocaine injections in akinesia and mydriasis in dogs. Vet Ophthalmol 16, 440–445.

Ahn JS, Jeong MB, Park YW et al. (2013c) A sub-Tenon's capsule injection of lidocaine induces extraocular muscle akinesia and mydriasis in dogs. Vet J 196, 103–108.

Alhassan MB, Kyari F, Ejere HO (2015) Peribulbar versus retrobulbar anaesthesia for cataract surgery. Cochrane Database Syst Rev, CD004083.

Allgoewer I (2018) Principles of ophthalmic surgery; anesthesia of the ophthalmic patient. In: Slatter's Fundamentals of Veterinary Ophthalmology, 6th edition. Maggs D, Miller P, Ofri R (eds.) Elsevier, USA. pp. 89–100.

Amorim TM, Dower NMB, Stocco MB et al. (2019) Effects of intracameral injection of epinephrine and 2% lidocaine on pupil diameter, intraocular pressure, and cardiovascular parameters in healthy cats. Vet Ophthalmol 22, 276–283.

Ansari H, Weinberg L, Spencer N (2013) Toxic epitheliopathy from a single application of preservative free oxybuprocaine (0.4%) in a patient with Sjogren's syndrome. BMJ Case Rep 2013. doi: 10.1136/bcr-2013-010487.

Bardocci A, Lofoco G, Perdicaro S et al. (2003) Lidocaine 2% gel versus lidocaine 4% unpreserved drops for topical anesthesia in cataract surgery: a randomized controlled trial. Ophthalmology 110, 144–149.

Bartholomew KJ, Smith LJ, Bentley E et al. (2020) Retrospective analysis of complications associated with retrobulbar bupivacaine in dogs undergoing enucleation surgery. Vet Anaesth Analg 47, 588–594.

Bayley KD, Gates MC, Anastassiadis Z et al. (2023) The use of sub-Tenon'sanesthesia versus a low-dose neuromuscular blockade for canine cataract surgery: A comparative study of 224 eyes. Vet Ophthalmology, 1-13. doi:10.1111/vop.13111

Bayley KD, Read RA (2018) Sub-Tenon's anesthesia for canine cataract surgery. Vet Ophthalmol 21, 601–611.

Binder DR, Herring IP (2006) Duration of corneal anesthesia following topical administration of 0.5% proparacaine hydrochloride solution in clinically normal cats. Am J Vet Res 67, 1780–1782.

Borazan M, Karalezli A, Akova YA et al. (2008) Comparative clinical trial of topical anaesthetic agents for cataract surgery with phacoemulsification: lidocaine 2% drops, levobupivacaine 0.75% drops, and ropivacaine 1% drops. Eye (Lond) 22, 425–429.

Borazan M, Karalezli A, Oto S et al. (2009) Induction of apoptosis of rabbit corneal endothelial cells by preservative-free lidocaine hydrochloride 2%, ropivacaine 1%, or levobupivacaine 0.75%. J Cataract Refract Surg 35, 753–758.

Britton B, Hervey R, Kasten K et al. (1976) Intraocular irritation evaluation of benzalkonium chloride in rabbits. Ophthalmic Surg 7, 46–55.

Cakmak SS, Olmez G, Nergiz Y et al. (2005) The effects of intracameral ropivacaine on the corneal endothelium. Jpn J Ophthalmol 49, 267–268.

Chang JL, Gonzalez-Abola E, Larson CE et al. (1984) Brain stem anesthesia following retrobulbar block. Anesthesiology 61, 789–790.

Chiavaccini L, Micieli F, Meomartino L et al. (2017) A novel supra-temporal approach to retrobulbar anaesthesia in dogs: preliminary study in cadavers. Vet J 223, 68–70.

Chow DW, Wong MY, Westermeyer HD (2015) Comparison of two bupivacaine delivery methods to control postoperative pain after enucleation in dogs. Vet Ophthalmol 18, 422–428.

Chuang LH, Yeung L, Ku WC et al. (2007) Safety and efficacy of topical anesthesia combined with a lower concentration of intracameral lidocaine in phacoemulsification: paired human eye study. J Cataract Refract Surg 33, 293–296.

Citarella G, Cornoa D, Parsons E et al. (2023) The outcomes of an opioid-free anaesthetic plan in fourteen dogs undergoing enucleation using an ultrasound-guided supra-temporal retrobulbar block: A retrospective case series. Animals 13, 2059. https://doi.org/10.3390/ani13132059

Costa GL, Leonardi F, Interlandi C et al. (2023) Levobupivacaine combined with cisatracurium in peribulbar anaesthesia in cats undergoing corneal and lens surgery. Animals 13, 170. https://doi.org/10.3390/ani13010170

Costa D, Pena MT, Rios J et al. (2014) Evaluation of corneal anaesthesia after the application of topical 2 per cent lidocaine, 0.5 per cent bupivacaine and 1 per cent ropivacaine in dogs. Vet Rec 174, 478.

Dannaker CJ, Maibach HI, Austin E (2001) Allergic contact dermatitis to proparacaine with subsequent cross-sensitization to tetracaine from ophthalmic preparations. Am J Contact Dermat 12, 177–179.

Dass BA, Soong HK, Lee B (1988) Effects of proparacaine on actin cytoskeleton of corneal epithelium. J Ocul Pharmacol 4, 187–194.

Deb K, Subramaniam R, Dehran M et al. (2001) Safety and efficacy of peribulbar block as adjunct to general anaesthesia for paediatric ophthalmic surgery. Paediatr Anaesth 11, 161–167.

Douet JY, Michel J, Regnier A (2013) Degree and duration of corneal anesthesia after topical application of 0.4% oxybuprocaine hydrochloride ophthalmic solution in ophthalmically normal dogs. Am J Vet Res 74, 1321–1326.

Eggeling P, Pleyer U, Hartmann C et al. (2000) Corneal endothelial toxicity of different lidocaine concentrations. J Cataract Refract Surg 26, 1403–1408.

Eshraghi B, Katoozpour R, Anvari P (2015) Transient complete visual loss after intracameral anesthetic injection in cataract surgery. J Curr Ophthalmol 27, 129–131.

Ezra DG, Nambiar A, Allan BD (2008) Supplementary intracameral lidocaine for phacoemulsification under topical anesthesia. A meta-analysis of randomized controlled trials. Ophthalmology 115, 455–487.

Fayon M, Gauthier M, Blanc VF et al. (1995) Intraoperative cardiac arrest due to the oculocardiac reflex and subsequent death in a child with occult Epstein-Barr virus myocarditis. Anesthesiology 83, 622–624.

Fentiman KE, Rankin AJ, Meekins JM et al. (2018) Effects of topical ophthalmic application of 0.5% proparacaine hydrochloride on aerobic bacterial culture results for naturally occurring infected corneal ulcers in dogs. J Am Vet Med Assoc 253, 1140–1145.

Foster A, Medina-Serra R, Sanchis-Mora S et al. (2021) In-plane ultrasound-guided peribulbar block in the dog: an anatomical cadaver study. Vet Anaesth Analg 48, 272–276.

Fuchsjager-Mayrl G, Zehetmayer M, Plass H et al. (2002) Alkalinization increases penetration of lidocaine across the human cornea. J Cataract Refract Surg 28, 692–696.

Gayer S, Palte HD (2016) Ultrasound-guided ophthalmic regional anesthesia. Curr Opin Anaesthesiol 29, 655–661.

Gerding PA, Jr., Turner TL, Hamor RE et al. (2004) Effects of intracameral injection of preservative-free lidocaine on the anterior segment of the eyes in dogs. Am J Vet Res 65, 1325–1330.

Ghali AM, El Btarny AM (2010) The effect on outcome of peribulbar anaesthesia in conjunction with general anesthesia for vitreoretinal surgery. Anaesthesia 65, 249–253.

Giudici V, Baeza S, Douet JY et al. (2015) Corneal anesthesia following application of 0.4% oxybuprocaine hydrochloride ophthalmic solution to normal feline eyes. Vet Ophthalmol 18, 141–146.

Giuliano E, Walsh K (2013) The eye. In: Small Animal Regional Anesthesia and Analgesia, 1st edition. Campoy L, Read M (eds.) Wiley, USA. pp. 103–118.

Giuliano EA (2008) Regional anesthesia as an adjunct for eyelid surgery in dogs. Top Companion Anim Med 23, 51–56.

Greco A, Costanza D, Senatore A et al. (2021) A computed tomography-based method for the assessment of canine retrobulbar cone volume for ophthalmic anaesthesia. Vet Anaesth Analg 48, 759–766.

Guise P (2012) Sub-Tenon's anesthesia: an update. Local Reg Anesth 5, 35–46.

Gupta N, Kumar R, Kumar S et al. (2007) A prospective randomised double blind study to evaluate the effect of peribulbar block or topical application of local anaesthesia combined with general anesthesia on intra-operative and postoperative complications during paediatric strabismus surgery. Anaesthesia 62, 1110–1113.

Guzey M, Satici A, Dogan Z et al. (2002) The effects of bupivacaine and lidocaine on the corneal endothelium when applied into the anterior chamber at the concentrations supplied commercially. Ophthalmologica 216, 113–117.

Hazra S, De D, Roy B et al. (2008) Use of ketamine, xylazine, and diazepam anesthesia with retrobulbar block for phacoemulsification in dogs. Vet Ophthalmol 11, 255–259.

Herring IP, Bobofchak MA, Landry MP et al. (2005) Duration of effect and effect of multiple doses of topical ophthalmic 0.5% proparacaine hydrochloride in clinically normal dogs. Am J Vet Res 66, 77–80.

Iradier MT, Fernandez C, Bohorquez P et al. (2000) Intraocular lidocaine in phacoemulsification: an endothelium and blood-aqueous barrier permeability study. Ophthalmology 107, 896–900; discussion 900-891.

Irving W, Annear M, Whittaker C et al. (2023) Effect of dexmedetomidine added to retrobulbar blockade with lignocaine and bupivacaine in dogs undergoing enucleation surgery. Veterinary Ophthalmology, 1–10.

Jaichandran V (2013) Ophthalmic regional anaesthesia: A review and update. Indian J Anaesth 57, 7–13.

Khatatbeh AE, Qubain WN (2012) The effectiveness of lidocaine vs tetracaine as topical anesthetic agents for the removal of corneal stitches. Int J Biol Med Res 3, 1512–1515.

Klaumann PR, Moreno JCD, Montiani-Ferreira F (2018) A morphometric study of the canine skull and periorbita and its implications for regional ocular anesthesia. Vet Ophthalmol 21, 19–26.

Koch SA, Rubin LF (1969) Ocular sensitivity of dogs to topical tetracaine HCl. J Am Vet Med Assoc 154, 15–16.

Kumar CM, Dodds C, McLure H et al. (2004) A comparison of three sub-Tenon's cannulae. Eye (Lond) 18, 873–876.

Kumar CM, Eid H, Dodds C (2011) Sub-Tenon's anaesthesia: complications and their prevention. Eye (Lond) 25, 694–703.

Kushnir Y, Marwitz GS, Shilo-Benjamini Y et al. (2018) Description of a regional anaesthesia technique for the dorsal cranium in the dog: a cadaveric study. Vet Anaesth Analg 45, 684–694.

Liu JC, Steinemann TL, McDonald MB et al. (1993) Topical bupivacaine and proparacaine: a comparison of toxicity, onset of action, and duration of action. Cornea 12, 228–232.

Luyet C, Eng KT, Kertes PJ et al. (2012) Real-time evaluation of diffusion of the local anesthetic solution during peribulbar block using ultrasound imaging and clinical correlates of diffusion. Reg Anesth Pain Med 37, 455–459.

Mahler S, Betti E, Guintard C (2020) Evaluation of injectate distribution after ultrasound-guided peribulbar injections in canine cadavers. Vet Anaesth Analg 47, 720–723.

McLeod GA (2004) Density of spinal anaesthetic solutions of bupivacaine, levobupivacaine, and ropivacaine with and without dextrose. Br J Anaesth 92, 547–551.

Morel J, Pascal J, Charier D et al. (2006) Preoperative peribulbar block in patients undergoing retinal detachment surgery under general anesthesia: a randomized double-blind study. Anesth Analg 102, 1082–1087.

Murphy C, Pollock R (1993) The eye. In: Miller's Anatomy of the Dog, 3rd edition. Evans H (ed.) Saunders, USA. pp. 1009–10057.

Myrna KE, Bentley E, Smith LJ (2010) Effectiveness of injection of local anesthetic into the retrobulbar space for postoperative analgesia following eye enucleation in dogs. J Am Vet Med Assoc 237, 174–177.

Nouvellon E, Cuvillon P, Ripart J et al. (2010) Anaesthesia for cataract surgery. Drugs Aging 27, 21–38.

Novack GD (2011) Drop size: an issue wrapped in a non-issue wrapped in an issue. Ocul Surf 9, 185–188.

Oduntan O, Ruskell G (1992) The source of sensory fibres of the inferior conjunctiva of monkeys. Graefes Arch Clin Exp Ophthalmol 230, 258–263.

Oel C, Gerhards H, Gehlen H (2014) Effect of retrobulbar nerve block on heart rate variability during enucleation in horses under general anesthesia. Vet Ophthalmol 17, 170–174.

Oliver JA, Bradbrook CA (2013) Suspected brainstem anesthesia following retrobulbar block in a cat. Vet Ophthalmol 16, 225–228.

Palte HD (2015) Ophthalmic regional blocks: management, challenges, and solutions. Local Reg Anesth 8, 57–70.

Palte HD, Gayer S, Arrieta E et al. (2012) Are ultrasound-guided ophthalmic blocks injurious to the eye? A comparative rabbit model study of two ultrasound devices evaluating intraorbital thermal and structural changes. Anesth Analg 115, 194–201.

Park SA, Kim NR, Park YW et al. (2009a) Evaluation of the mydriatic effect of intracameral lidocaine hydrochloride injection in eyes of clinically normal dogs. Am J Vet Res 70, 1521–1525.

Park SA, Lee I, Lee YL et al. (2009b) Combination auriculopalpebral nerve block and local anesthesia for placement of a nictitating membrane-to-superotemporal bulbar conjunctiva flap in dogs. J Am Anim Hosp Assoc 45, 164–167.

Park SA, Park YW, Son WG et al. (2010) Evaluation of the analgesic effect of intracameral lidocaine hydrochloride injection on intraoperative and postoperative pain in healthy dogs undergoing phacoemulsification. Am J Vet Res 71, 216–222.

Patel M, Fraunfelder FW (2013) Toxicity of topical ophthalmic anesthetics. Expert Opin Drug Metab Toxicol 9, 983–988.

Pelosini L, Treffene S, Hollick EJ (2009) Antibacterial activity of preservative-free topical anesthetic drops in current use in ophthalmology departments. Cornea 28, 58–61.

Ploog CL, Swinger RL, Spade J et al. (2014) Use of lidocaine-bupivacaine-infused absorbable gelatin hemostatic sponges versus lidocaine-bupivacaine retrobulbar injections for postoperative analgesia following eye enucleation in dogs. J Am Vet Med Assoc 244, 57–62.

Pucket JD, Allbaugh RA, Rankin AJ et al. (2013) Comparison of efficacy and duration of effect on corneal sensitivity among anesthetic agents following ocular administration in clinically normal horses. Am J Vet Res 74, 459–464.

Reaux-Le Goazigo A, Poras H, Ben-Dhaou C et al. (2019) Dual enkephalinase inhibitor PL265: a novel topical treatment to alleviate corneal pain and inflammation. Pain 160, 307–321.

Regnier A, Berton I, Concordet D et al. (2018) Effect of topical application of 2% lidocaine gel on corneal sensitivity of clinically normal equine eyes. Vet Anaesth Analg 45, 158–164.

Riad W, Ahmad N, Kumar CM (2012) Comparison of metal and flexible sub-Tenon cannulas. J Cataract Refract Surg 38, 1398–1402.

Riad W, Akbar F (2012) Ophthalmic regional blockade complication rate: a single center audit of 33,363 ophthalmic operations. J Clin Anesth 24, 193–195.

Ripart J, Lefrant JY, de La Coussaye JE et al. (2001) Peribulbar versus retrobulbar anesthesia for ophthalmic surgery: an anatomical comparison of extraconal and intraconal injections. Anesthesiology 94, 56–62.

Ripart J, Lefrant JY, Vivien B et al. (2000) Ophthalmic regional anesthesia: medial canthus episcleral (sub-tenon) anesthesia is more efficient than peribulbar anesthesia: A double-blind randomized study. Anesthesiology 92, 1278–1285.

Ripart J, Metge L, Prat-Pradal D et al. (1998) Medial canthus single-injection episcleral (sub-tenon anesthesia): computed tomography imaging. Anesth Analg 87, 42–45.

Samuelson D (2013) Ophthalmic anatomy. In: Veterinary Ophthalmology, 5th edition. Gelatt K, Gilger B, Kern T (eds.) Wiley-Blackwell, USA. pp. 39–170.

Scott EM, Vallone LV, Olson NL et al. (2021) Analgesic effects of a retrobulbar block with 0.75% ropivacaine in dogs undergoing enucleation. Vet Anaesth Analg 48, 749–758.

Severin G (1995) Chemical restraint and anesthesia. In: Severin's Veterinary Ophthalmology notes, 3rd edition. Severin G (ed.) DesignPointe Communication Inc, USA. pp. 100–105.

Shah H, Reichel E, Busbee B (2010) A novel lidocaine hydrochloride ophthalmic gel for topical ocular anesthesia. Local Reg Anesth 3, 57–63.

Shende D, Sadhasivam S, Madan R (2000) Effects of peribulbar bupivacaine as an adjunct to general anaesthesia on peri-operative outcome following retinal detachment surgery. Anaesthesia 55, 970–975.

Shilo-Benjamini Y (2019) A review of ophthalmic local and regional anesthesia in dogs and cats. Vet Anaesth Analg 46, 14–27.

Shilo-Benjamini Y, Kahane N, Ofri R (2016) Pain management with peribulbar anesthesia versus retrobulbar anesthesia in a cat undergoing bilateral enucleation. Isr J Vet Med 71, 37–40.

Shilo-Benjamini Y, Pascoe PJ, Maggs DJ et al. (2019a) Retrobulbar vs peribulbar regional anesthesia techniques using bupivacaine in dogs. Vet Ophthalmol 22, 183–191.

Shilo-Benjamini Y, Pascoe PJ, Maggs DJ et al. (2013) Retrobulbar and peribulbar regional techniques in cats: a preliminary study in cadavers. Vet Anaesth Analg 40, 623–631.

Shilo-Benjamini Y, Pascoe PJ, Maggs DJ et al. (2014) Comparison of peribulbar and retrobulbar regional anesthesia with bupivacaine in cats. Am J Vet Res 75, 1029–1039.

Shilo-Benjamini Y, Pascoe PJ, Wisner ER et al. (2017a) A comparison of retrobulbar and two peribulbar regional anesthetic techniques in dog cadavers. Vet Anaesth Analg 44, 925–932.

Shilo-Benjamini Y, Pypendop BH, Newbold G et al. (2017b) Plasma bupivacaine concentrations following orbital injections in cats. Vet Anaesth Analg 44, 178–182.

Shilo-Benjamini Y, Slav SA, Kahane N et al. (2019b) Analgesic effects of intraorbital insertion of an absorbable gelatin hemostatic sponge soaked with 1% ropivacaine solution following enucleation in dogs. J Am Vet Med Assoc 255, 1255–1262.

Short CE, Rebhun WC (1980) Complications caused by the oculocardiac reflex during anesthesia in a foal. J Am Vet Med Assoc 176, 630–631.

Stadler S, Dennler M, Hetzel U et al. (2017) Sub-Tenon's injection in equine cadaver eyes: MRI visualization of anesthetic fluid distribution and comparison of two different volumes. Vet Ophthalmol 20, 488–495.

Startup F (1969) Anesthesia for ophthalmic surgery. In: Diseases of the Canine Eye. Startup F (ed.) Bailliere Tindall and Cassell, London. pp. 70–76.

Stiles J, Honda CN, Krohne SG et al. (2003) Effect of topical administration of 1% morphine sulfate solution on signs of pain and corneal wound healing in dogs. Am J Vet Res 64, 813–818.

Sun R, Hamilton RC, Gimbel HV (1999) Comparison of 4 topical anesthetic agents for effect and corneal toxicity in rabbits. J Cataract Refract Surg 25, 1232–1236.

Thomson SM, Oliver JA, Gould DJ et al. (2013) Preliminary investigations into the analgesic effects of topical ocular 1% morphine solution in dogs and cats. Vet Anaesth Analg 40, 632–640.

Trolle-Lassen C (1958) Investigations into the sensitivity of the human eye to hypo- and hypertonic solutions as well as solutions with unphysiological hydrogen ion concentrations. Pharm Weekbl 93, 148–155.

Tsegaw A, Tsegaw A, Abula T et al. (2017) Bacterial contamination of multi-dose eye drops at Ophthalmology Department, University of Gondar, Northwest Ethiopia. Middle East Afr J Ophthalmol 24, 81–86.

Venturi F, Blocker T, Dees DD et al. (2017) Corneal anesthetic effect and ocular tolerance of 3.5% lidocaine gel in comparison with 0.5% aqueous proparacaine and 0.5% viscous tetracaine in normal canines. Vet Ophthalmol 20, 405–410.

Vezina-Audette R (2020) Anesthesia case of the month. J Am Vet Med Assoc 256, 176–178.

Vezina-Audette R, Steagall PVM, Gianotti G (2019) Prevalence of and covariates associated with the oculocardiac reflex occurring in dogs during enucleation. J Am Vet Med Assoc 255, 454–458.

Viscasillas J, Everson R, Mapletoft EK et al. (2019) Ultrasound-guided posterior extraconal block in the dog: anatomical study in cadavers. Vet Anaesth Analg 46, 246–250.

Wagatsuma JT, Deschk M, Floriano BP et al. (2014) Comparison of anesthetic efficacy and adverse effects associated with peribulbar injection of ropivacaine performed with and without ultrasound guidance in dogs. Am J Vet Res 75, 1040–1048.

Waldman N, Densie IK, Herbison P (2014) Topical tetracaine used for 24 hours is safe and rated highly effective by patients for the treatment of pain caused by corneal abrasions: a double-blind, randomized clinical trial. Acad Emerg Med 21, 374–382.

Weaver CS, Rusyniak DE, Brizendine EJ et al. (2003) A prospective, randomized, double-blind comparison of buffered versus plain tetracaine in reducing the pain of topical ophthalmic anesthesia. Ann Emerg Med 41, 827–831.

Westhues M, Fritsch R (1964) Regional anaesthesia of head and limbs. In: Animal Anaesthesia: Local Anaesthesia. Lippincott, USA. pp. 76–139.

Williams DL (2005) Analysis of tear uptake by the Schirmer tear test strip in the canine eye. Vet Ophthalmol 8, 325–330.

Yang H, Zheng D, Zhang Z (2002) Effect of intracameral lidocaine anesthesia on the anterior segment of rabbit eyes. Yan Ke Xue Bao 18, 54–58, 62.

Zibura AE, Posner LP, Ru H et al. (2020) A preoperative bupivacaine retrobulbar block offers superior antinociception compared with an intraoperative splash block in dogs undergoing enucleation. Vet Ophthalmol 23, 225–233.

Ultrasound-Guided Blocks for the Ear

Luis Campoy and Jaime Viscasillas

CHAPTER 6

BLOCK AT A GLANCE

What is it used for?

- To supplement anesthesia and analgesia for procedures involving the ear and ear canal such as total or partial ear canal ablation, polyp removal, and ear flushing.

Landmarks/transducer position:

Great Auricular Nerve Block – The primary landmarks are the wing of the atlas and the maxillary vein. The transducer should be positioned in a dorsoventral orientation over the lateral aspect of the neck, ventral to the wing of the atlas, and parallel to the caudal border of the mandibular ramus.

Auriculotemporal Nerve Block – The primary landmarks are the temporomandibular joint (TMJ), the zygomatic process of the temporal bone, and the external acoustic meatus. The transducer should be positioned over the temporal area at the base of the ear, following the ventral edge of the zygomatic process of the temporal bone with a slight tilt toward the external meatus and the marker oriented rostrally.

What equipment and personnel are required?

- 21G 100 mm or 22G 50 mm (depending on dog's size) blunt atraumatic needle
- Syringe of drug(s)
- Ultrasound machine
- High frequency (15–6 MHz) linear array transducer +/− protective sleeve
- Gloves
- Coupling agent (e.g. alcohol)
- +/− Assistant to perform the injection

When do I perform the block?

- Prior to the procedure, after the area is clipped and surgical skin preparation is complete.

What volume of local anesthetic is used?

- **Great auricular nerve block** – $0.1\,\mathrm{ml\,kg^{-1}}$
- **Auriculotemporal nerve block** – $0.05\,\mathrm{ml\,kg^{-1}}$

Goal:

- **Great auricular nerve block** – The local anesthetic should spread caudal to the tympanic bulla and ventral to the wing of the atlas.
- **Auriculotemporal nerve block** – The local anesthetic should spread rostral to the vertical ear canal.

Complexity level:

- Advanced

Clinical pearls:

- Ipsilateral facial nerve paralysis and/or Horner's syndrome may be observed.

WHAT DO WE ALREADY KNOW?

Published literature on local anesthetic techniques for otologic surgical procedures, such as total ear canal ablations or lateral bulla osteotomies for the treatment of otitis media, is scarce (Radlinsky et al. 2005; Wolfe et al. 2006). Buback et al. (1996) evaluated three different methods of providing analgesia for total ear canal ablation and lateral bulla osteotomy in dogs. Their study compared three analgesic protocols, with 10 subjects per group. One group (1) received systemic opioids alone, a second group (2) received systemic opioids combined with a local anesthetic (bupivacaine 0.5%) splash block, and a third group (3) received systemic opioids combined with pre-operative bupivacaine 0.5% nerve blocks (**great auricular** and **auriculotemporal nerve** blocks performed blindly using anatomical landmarks). Pain scores were not significantly different between groups, however, mean pain scores were less than 3 (on a scale of 1–5) for all groups at all observed time points. Rough recoveries were noted in 30%, 0%, and 20% for groups 1, 2, and 3, respectively. In all three groups, 94% of dogs were moderately to heavily sedated at the time of extubation. Sixty percent of dogs in group 3 remained moderately to heavily sedated two hours post extubation and 23% of the dogs

Small Animal Regional Anesthesia and Analgesia, Second Edition. Edited by Matt Read, Luis Campoy, and Berit Fischer.
© 2024 John Wiley & Sons, Inc. Published 2024 by John Wiley & Sons, Inc.

required additional analgesia (oxymorphone) or tranquilization post-surgery (one dog in group 1, two dogs in group 2, and four dogs in group 3). More recently, Stathopoulou et al. (2018) reported successful nerve staining of the **great auricular** and **auriculotemporal nerves** in dog and fox cadavers in 24 out of 24 and 22 out of 24 injections following bilateral blocks, respectively. The investigators reported concurrent staining of the **facial nerve** following three injections. The technique to perform this block in the dog is also described in Otero and Portela (2019).

A study examining the feasibility and efficacy of ultrasound-guided blocks of the **great auricular** and **auriculotemporal nerves** in veterinary species does not currently exist; however, they have been described in humans. Thallaj et al. (2010) reported an observational volunteer study with human subjects that described the feasibility of imaging the great auricular nerve and blocking it. The **great auricular nerve** was successfully imaged and blocked in all volunteers; however, the authors found heterogeneity in the distribution pattern of the sensory blockade with only the tail of the helix, antitragus, lubula, and mandibular angle always being consistently blocked (Thallaj et al. 2010).

Flores and Herring (2016) reported a series of two cases describing the successful use of an ultrasound-guided **great auricular nerve** block performed in the emergency room for the treatment of an ear laceration and drainage of an abscess. Liu et al. (2020) published a randomized controlled trial evaluating perioperative analgesia provided by blockade of the **great auricular nerve** in people undergoing middle ear microsurgery. Those authors found that patients who received blocks had significantly greater analgesia for the first 24 hours than those who did not receive blocks. Hemodynamic changes associated with sympathetic stimulation described as increases in heart rate and blood pressure were also significantly less in patients who had received **great auricular nerve** blocks (Liu et al. 2020).

PATIENT SELECTION
INDICATIONS FOR THE BLOCK

- Otologic surgical procedures such as incision and drainage of abscesses or cysts, laceration repair of the external ear, foreign body removal, polyp removal, total or partial ear canal ablation, and ventral or lateral bulla osteotomy.

CONTRAINDICATIONS

- Inability to identify the target structures ultrasonographically.
- Skin infection at any of the intended puncture sites.
- Preexisting peripheral nerve disease.
- Patient is too small relative to the transducer size.

POTENTIAL SIDE EFFECTS AND COMPLICATIONS

- Ipsilateral **facial nerve** palsy/paralysis can result from the surgical procedure itself or may be related to the unintended rostral migration of the local anesthetic following an **auriculotemporal nerve** block, affecting the **facial nerve** or a branch such as the **auriculopalpebral nerve**. If this occurs, the patient will exhibit **facial nerve** deficits or even more selective deficits, such as **auriculopalpebral nerve** deficits, manifesting in an inability to blink. In these instances, eye lubrication and corneal protection should be provided, as necessary.

- **Lingual nerve** palsy may result from unintended migration of the local anesthetic solution to the **lingual nerve** following performance of an **auriculotemporal nerve** block.

- Hematoma formation (and possibly intravascular injection) are additional potential complications, specifically from the maxillary vein during the **great auricular nerve** block and caudal auricular and superficial temporal arteries while performing the **auriculotemporal nerve** block. A negative aspiration test should always be verified prior to injection of the local anesthetic solution.

GENERAL CONSIDERATIONS
CLINICAL ANATOMY

Sensory innervation to the ear, the ear canal, and the tympanic membrane are supplied by the **great auricular nerve** (originating from the cervical plexus, **second cervical spinal nerve** – C_2), the **auriculotemporal nerve** (a branch of the **trigeminal nerve**, **mandibular nerve** – V_3), and the **greater** and **lesser occipital nerves** (**cervical plexus, second cervical spinal nerve** – C_2). The **auricular branch** of the **facial nerve** (CN VII) and the **auricular branch** of the **vagus nerve** (CN X) may contribute additional sensory contributions to this area of the body.

The **great auricular nerve** emerges between the ventral edge of the *m. omotransversarius* and the dorsal border of the *m. sternocephalicus*. It subsequently runs superficial to the *m. omotransversarius* along the caudodorsal aspect of the parotid salivary gland and dorsal to the mandibular salivary gland. It then runs toward the base of the pinna before innervating the apex of the pinna after dividing into **anterior** and **posterior branches**.

The **auriculotemporal nerve** is the most proximal branch of the **mandibular nerve** (CN V_3). After it branches off from the **mandibular nerve** at the foramen ovale, the **auriculotemporal nerve** turns medial and caudal to the retroarticular process of the temporal bone, taking a dorsal path toward the ear. In the region caudal to the condylar process of the mandible (ventral to the acoustic meatus), the nerve is in close proximity with the superficial branches of the facial nerve, the glossopharyngeal nerve, and the superficial temporal artery. After emerging onto the face, the nerve divides into a plexus spreading over the temporal region (Figures 6.1 and 6.2).

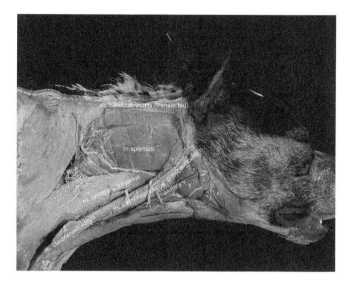

FIGURE 6.1   Dissection of the right cervical area of a dog. The **great auricular nerve** is branching out of the cervical plexus and runs toward the base of the right ear on the surface of the *m. sternocephalicus*, dorsal to the maxillary vein. 1, mandibular salivary gland and 2, parotid salivary gland. Source: With permission from Virtual Canine Anatomy, Colorado State University.

EXPECTED DISTRIBUTION OF ANESTHESIA

Sensory innervation to the ear (pinna), ear canal, and tympanic membrane is highly complex, with areas of overlap between multiple different nerve domains. The **great auricular nerve** innervates most of the cutaneous latero-caudal (convex) surface of the ear, as well as the lateral aspect of the pinna. There is some overlapping with the **greater occipital nerve** (mostly on the rostral concave surface). The **transverse cervical nerve** (a branch of C$_2$) provides sensory innervation to a region of skin ventral to the ear.

The **auriculotemporal nerve** is sensory to the skin of the external acoustic meatus (ear canal) near the tympanic membrane. The **rostral auricular nerves** (branches of the **auriculotemporal nerve**) supply the skin over the lateral aspect of the tragus, a small portion of the medioventral part of the pinna's rostral (concave) surface, the medial border of the pinna, the skin over the ventral aspect of the temporal region, ventrally over the zygomatic arch, and an area of skin extending dorsal and ventral from the zygomatic arch.

The **lesser occipital nerve** innervates the dorsal aspect of the temporal area, and the medial border, the caudal (convex) surface, and the apex of the pinna. There is some overlap with the **auricular branches** of the **facial nerve**.

The ear canal is innervated by the **auricular branch** of the **vagus nerve** (CN X), **auricular branch** of the **facial nerve** (CN VII), and the **trigeminal nerve** (CN V).

The external surface of the tympanic membrane is innervated by the **auriculotemporal nerve** and the **auricular branch** of the **vagus nerve**, whereas the internal

(a)

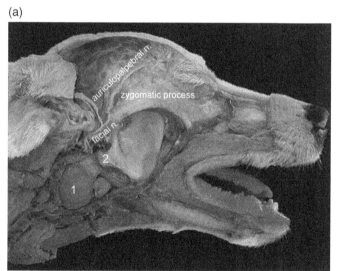

(b)

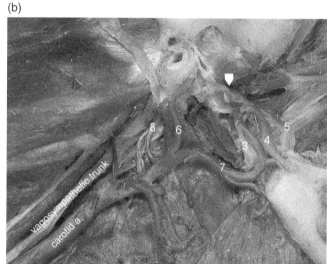

FIGURE 6.2   (a) Dissection of the right side of the head and neck of a dog showing the **facial nerve** rostral to the ear canal and the **auriculopalpebral nerve** branching off. 1, mandibular salivary gland and 2, angular process of mandible. (b) Close-up view of the right retromandibular area of a dog. The mandibular ramus and temporomandibular joint (TMJ) have been partially removed to expose the **auriculotemporal nerve** (arrowhead) branching off of the **mandibular nerve**. The nerve is found between the TMJ and the ear canal; 3, **mylohyoid nerve**; 4, **inferior alveolar nerve**; 5, **lingual nerve**; 6, superficial temporal artery; 7, maxillary artery; and 8, **glossopharyngeal nerve**. Source: With permission from Virtual Canine Anatomy, Colorado State University.

surface of the tympanic membrane is innervated by the **glossopharyngeal nerve** (CN IX).

LOCAL ANESTHETIC: DOSE, VOLUME, AND CONCENTRATION

Any local anesthetic (e.g. bupivacaine, ropivacaine, and levobupivacaine) can be used to perform the blocks, with or without the coadministration of an adjuvant (e.g. dexmedetomidine, dexamethasone, and buprenorphine). For the great auricular nerve block, 0.1 ml kg^{-1} is used. For the auriculotemporal nerve block, 0.05 ml kg^{-1} is used.

PATIENT PREPARATION AND POSITIONING

The animal should be positioned in lateral recumbency with the side to be blocked uppermost. An area around the base of the ear, the temporal region, the mastoid process, the lateral aspect of the occipital area, and the proximal cervical region (following the projection of the *m. omotransversarius*) should be clipped free of hair, and standard surgical preparation of the skin should be performed.

STEP-BY-STEP PERFORMANCE

SURFACE ANATOMY AND LANDMARKS TO BE USED

For the **great auricular nerve** block, the ultrasound transducer should be positioned in a dorsoventral orientation over the lateral aspect of the neck, ventral to the wing of the atlas and over the mandibular salivary gland, with the marker oriented ventrally (Figure 6.3). The **great auricular nerve** can be found lateroventral to the wing of the atlas, dorsal to the maxillary vein and the mandibular salivary gland, on the surface of the *m. sternocephalicus* (Figure 6.4).

For the **auriculotemporal nerve** block, the ultrasound transducer should be oriented following the direction of the zygomatic process of the temporal bone, caudal to the condylar process, and ventral to the external ear canal with a slight tilt so the external ear canal can be imaged (Figure 6.3). The **auriculotemporal nerve** can be found in the parotid region, rostral and slightly ventral to the external ear canal (Figure 6.4).

ULTRASOUND ANATOMY

The **great auricular nerve** can be identified immediately dorsal to the maxillary vein and the mandibular salivary gland, deep to the *m. platysma*, ventral to the *mm. splenius* and *omotransversarius*, and running over the surface of the *m. sternocephalicus*. This area of interest is very superficial so the use of a standoff pad may be necessary to optimize the image.

The **auriculotemporal nerve** can be identified rostral and slightly ventral to the external ear canal, caudal to the condylar process and the parotid gland.

NEEDLE INSERTION TECHNIQUE

For the **great auricular nerve** block, the needle should be introduced in-plane in a dorsoventral direction and advanced until the needle tip is in the plane between *m. platysma* and *m. cleidocervicalis*, dorsal to the maxillary vein and the mandibular salivary gland. The **great auricular nerve** is on the surface of the *m. sternocephalicus*.

For the **auriculotemporal nerve** block, an out-of-plane needle approach is recommended. The needle should be advanced towards the condylar process of the mandible, ensuring a rostral position with respect to the external ear canal. This is a highly vascular area; care and appropriate needle path planning should be used.

(a)

(b)

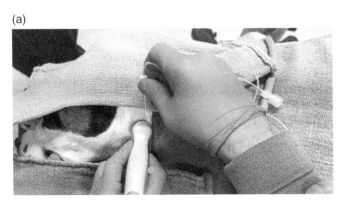
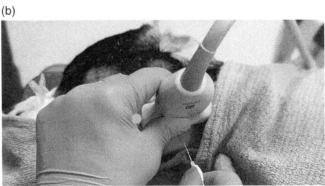

FIGURE 6.3   (a) Left **great auricular nerve** block is being performed in a dog positioned in right lateral recumbency. The ultrasound transducer is positioned over the cranial cervical area, just ventral to the wing of the atlas using a dorsoventral orientation. The marker (green circle) is oriented ventrally. The needle is being advanced in-plane in a ventral direction. (b) Left **auriculotemporal nerve** block is being performed in a dog positioned in right lateral recumbency. The ultrasound transducer is positioned over the temporal area, immediately ventral to the ear canal, with a discrete tilt so as to include the ear canal in the ultrasound image. The marker (green circle) is oriented rostrally. The needle is being advanced out-of-plane, rostral to the ear canal.

(a)

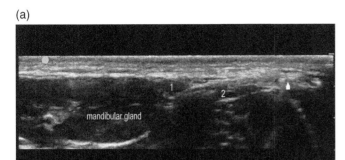

(b)

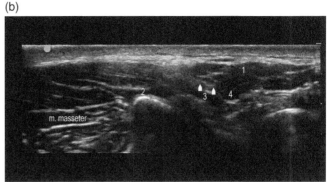

FIGURE 6.4 (a) Ultrasonographic image relevant to the **great auricular nerve** block. The marker (green circle) is oriented ventrally. Note the position of the mandibular salivary gland and the maxillary vein (1). The great auricular nerve (arrowhead) runs on the surface of the **m. sternocephalicus** (2). (b) Ultrasonographic image relevant to the **auriculotemporal nerve** block. The marker (green circle) is oriented rostrally. Observe the position of the parotid salivary gland in its very dorsal aspect (1), the condylar process (2), and the maxillary vein (in its long axis) (3). The **facial** and **auriculotemporal nerves** (arrowheads) are very close to each other (the more ventral the transducer is placed, the greater the separation between these two nerves) and are located immediately rostral to the ear canal (4).

EXPECTED MOTOR RESPONSES FROM NERVE STIMULATION

When performing an **auriculotemporal nerve** block, a motor response from stimulation of the **facial nerve** may be observed (motion of the pinna).

ADMINISTRATION OF LOCAL ANESTHETIC – WHAT TO LOOK FOR, WHAT TO FEEL FOR, AND DECISION POINTS

For the **great auricular nerve** block, the local anesthetic (0.1 ml kg^{-1}) should be injected in the muscular plane between the **mm. platysma** and **cleidocervicalis/sternocephalicus**, dorsal to the maxillary vein and mandibular salivary gland. For the **auriculotemporal nerve** block, position the needle tip slightly ventral and rostral to the ear canal. Due to the high vascularity of the area, a negative aspiration test must be verified before the injection. A smaller volume (0.05 ml kg^{-1}) is recommended to minimize migration and blockade of the **facial nerve**.

BLOCK EFFECTS AND PATIENT MANAGEMENT

This block will primarily affect the sensory innervation of the pinna, ear canal, and tympanic membrane. However, nerve deficits associated with unintentional local anesthetic migration may be observed. Patients must remain under observation should clinically recognizable side effects occur (see below).

COMPLICATIONS AND HOW TO AVOID THEM

Accidental migration of the local anesthetic toward the **hypoglossal, glossopharyngeal, vagosympathetic trunk, mandibular nerve branches**, and **auriculotemporal nerves** may occur and, therefore, subsequent complications may manifest.

Deviation of the tongue (**hypoglossal nerve** palsy), loss of gag reflex, inability to cough (**glossopharyngeal nerve** palsy), Horner's syndrome (**vagosympathetic trunk** palsy), partial loss of lingual sensory function, and possible inability to blink (**auriculopalpebral nerve** palsy) may be observed. There are no reports of using this technique in clinical patients to date so the incidence of complications and side effects is not currently known.

COMMON MISTAKES AND HOW TO AVOID THEM

When performing an ultrasound-guided **auriculotemporal nerve** block in combination with electrolocation, if motor responses such as blinking (**auriculopalpebral nerve**) or chewing (motor supply to the **m. digastricus**) are elicited, it may indicate that the needle is located too far caudal. The needle should be repositioned in a more rostral location. Alternatively, if only blinking is observed, it may be that the needle is stimulating the **auriculopalpebral nerve** only, in which case, the needle may be in a too rostral location.

HOW TO TALK TO CLIENTS/PROFESSIONAL COLLEAGUES

- For an experienced clinician, performance of both blocks should take less than 10 minutes.

- Additional pain management in the postoperative period may include icing of the affected area and administration of oral analgesics (e.g. NSAIDs and pregabalin) for five to seven days.

- Patients should remain under close observation and the ipsilateral eye should be lubricated regularly if complications such as **auriculopalpebral nerve** palsy occur.

REFERENCES

Buback JL, Boothe HW, Carroll GL et al. (1996) Comparison of three methods for relief of pain after ear canal ablation in dogs. Vet Surg 25, 380–385.

Flores S, Herring AA (2016) Ultrasound-guided greater auricular nerve block for emergency department ear laceration and ear abscess drainage. J Emerg Med 50, 651–655.

Liu J, Yuan K, Zhou H et al. (2020) A randomized controlled trial evaluating the hemodynamic impact of ultrasound-guided great auricular nerve block in middle ear microsurgery. BMC Anesthesiol 20, 234.

Otero P, Portela D (2019) Nerve blocks of the auricular region. In: Manual of Small Animal Regional Anesthesia, 2nd edition. Inter-Medica, Buenos Aires. pp. 367–374

Radlinsky MG, Mason DE, Roush JK et al. (2005) Use of a continuous, local infusion of bupivacaine for postoperative analgesia in dogs undergoing total ear canal ablation. J Am Vet Med Assoc 227, 414–419.

Stathopoulou TR, Pinelas R, Haar GT, Cornelis I, Viscasillas J (2018) Description of a new approach for great auricular and auriculotemporal nerve blocks: A cadaveric study in foxes and dogs. Vet Med Sci 4, 91–97.

Thallaj A, Marhofer P, Moriggl B et al. (2010) Great auricular nerve blockade using high resolution ultrasound: a volunteer study. Anaesthesia 65, 836–840.

Wolfe TM, Bateman SW, Cole LK et al. (2006) Evaluation of a local anesthetic delivery system for the postoperative analgesic management of canine total ear canal ablation – a randomized, controlled, double-blinded study. Vet Anaesth Analg 33, 328–339.

Ultrasound-Guided Brachial Plexus Block (Subscalene Approach)

Pablo E. Otero

BLOCK AT A GLANCE

What is it used for?

- This block is used to provide regional anesthesia and analgesia for surgeries of the thoracic limb distal to, and including, the shoulder joint (e.g. shoulder arthroscopy, arthrotomy, humeral fracture repair, etc.).

Landmarks/transducer position

- The ultrasound transducer is positioned on the lateral aspect of the neck, parallel to the long axis of the **m. scalenus**, cranial to the first rib, and proximal to the costochondral junction.

What equipment and personnel are required?

- 21G or 22G short-bevel insulated needle:
  - 50 mm (2 in.) for cats and dogs smaller than 5 kg
  - 75 mm (3 in.) for dogs weighing 5–30 kg
  - 100 mm (4 in.) for dogs weighing more than 30 kg
- Syringe of drug(s)
- Ultrasound machine
- High frequency (e.g. 15–6 MHz) linear array transducer +/− protective sleeve
- Gloves
- Coupling agent (e.g. alcohol)
- +/− Nerve stimulator
- +/− Assistant to help perform the injection

When do I perform the block?

- Prior to surgery, after the patient has been clipped and skin preparation is complete. Final skin preparation before surgery is still required.

What volume of local anesthetic is used?

- 0.4 ml kg⁻¹ total volume, divided into two aliquots (0.1 and 0.3 ml kg⁻¹ for administration cranial and caudal to the ventral branches of the seventh cervical nerve (C7), respectively).

Goal:

- During injection, the local anesthetic should be observed spreading around the nerve roots of C6, C7, C8, and T1 within the subscalene space deep into the deep fascia of the neck.

Complexity level:

- Advanced

Clinical pearls:

- This block will cause motor paralysis of the ipsilateral diaphragm due to concurrent **phrenic nerve** blockade. Therefore, performing this block bilaterally is not advised.
- **Recurrent laryngeal nerve** blockade with subsequent laryngeal hemiplegia may occur as a side effect.
- Patients may require bandaging of the blocked limb and assistance with ambulation (e.g. use of a sling or harness) to avoid injury until motor function is regained.

WHAT DO WE ALREADY KNOW?

Otero et al. (2017) described the ultrasound anatomy of the subscalene space and compared the distribution of two volumes of dye (0.3 and 0.4 ml kg⁻¹) in canine cadavers. They found that C7, C8, and T1 could be completely stained using either volume of dye, whereas, C6 was successfully stained only in the higher-volume group. The **phrenic nerve** was completely stained in all cases. No intrapleural, mediastinal, or epidural distribution was reported. This approach was also described by Otero et al. (2019).

Another study evaluated diaphragmatic function using M-mode ultrasonography following subscalene brachial plexus blocks in dogs undergoing thoracic limb surgery. Twenty minutes after injection of bupivacaine 0.5% (0.3 ml kg⁻¹), a significant reduction in the caudal displacement of the ipsilateral diaphragm was observed (Fuensalida et al. 2017). Those authors used the lack of cardiovascular response to surgery in the dogs as evidence of acceptable sensory blockade and suggested that the decrease in diaphragm displacement could be correlated with successful injections.

In a case report, Horner's syndrome occurred following a brachial plexus block using the subscalene approach (Chohan 2019). That author speculated that bupivacaine injected near the first rib could have spread and disrupted the sympathetic output from the cervicothoracic (stellate) and middle cervical ganglia and result in this temporary, but undesirable side effect.

PATIENT SELECTION
INDICATIONS FOR THE BLOCK

This block can be used to provide anesthesia and analgesia for a wide range of surgical procedures involving the thoracic limb. It is preferentially used for procedures involving the proximal third of the thoracic limb, such as humeral fractures, shoulder surgery (e.g. arthroscopy, arthrotomy), and forelimb amputation. When used for amputations, it is important to note that the brachial plexus block does not desensitize the muscles of the dorsal region (e.g. the **mm. trapezius** and **rhomboideus**) or the dermatomes of the caudal scapular and tricipital regions. These areas are innervated by cutaneous branches of the dorsal and ventral branches of the thoracic nerves (i.e. T2–T4), and supplemental analgesia will be required.

CONTRAINDICATIONS

- Skin infection or other lesions at the intended needle puncture site.
- Inability to identify the relevant anatomy during ultrasound scanning.

POTENTIAL SIDE EFFECTS AND COMPLICATIONS

- Diaphragmatic hemiparalysis – As stated above, utilizing this approach to block the brachial plexus will block the ipsilateral **phrenic nerve**. In animals with preexisting respiratory disease, this may further impair ventilatory function and caution should be exercised.
- Temporary laryngeal hemiplegia – The **recurrent laryngeal nerve** lies deep to the common carotid artery in the angle between the **m. longus colli** and the trachea (Evans and de Lahunta 2013). Inadvertent puncture of the prevertebral fascia can result in local anesthetic spread into this area and blockade of the **recurrent laryngeal nerve**.
- Horner's syndrome – The presence of the vagosympathetic trunk within the carotid sheath and the cervicothoracic and middle cervical ganglia lying in close association with the **m. longus colli** may result in the development of an ipsilateral Horner's syndrome following puncture of the prevertebral fascia and/or spread of the local anesthetic.
- There is potential to cause vascular trauma (resulting in hemorrhage and hematoma formation) due to the close proximity of the needle's trajectory to the jugular vein, the carotid artery, and the axillary artery. If an injection is made following intravascular puncture, subsequent local anesthetic toxicity is possible.
- Block failure – Spread of local anesthetic outside the deep fascia of the neck and into the **m. scalenus** prevents the local anesthetic from spreading adequately within the neurovascular bundle and blockade of the brachial plexus roots will fail.
- Iatrogenic nerve injury – Avoid injection of the local anesthetic if the muscular response is obtained with less than 0.3 mA or if resistance is perceived during injection.
- Pneumothorax and cardiac arrhythmias – Care should be taken not to advance the needle further than the cranial edge of the first rib to avoid inadvertent pleural and/or cardiac puncture.
- Cervical epidural distribution of the local anesthetic.

GENERAL CONSIDERATIONS
CLINICAL ANATOMY

The brachial plexus is a network of nerves formed by the ventral roots of the C6, C7, C8, and T1 spinal nerves. Occasionally, the brachial plexus receives contributions from C5 and T2. As the ventral roots of the spinal nerves leave the spinal cord through their respective intervertebral foramina, they divide into cranial, medial, and caudal branches, which then become the different nerves that supply the thoracic limb.

In the dog, the **m. scalenus** is comprised of dorsal and medial muscle bellies that extend from the transverse processes of C4 through C7 and insert on the dorsal and lateral aspects of the first eight ribs (Evans and de Lahunta 2013). Between the medial aspect of the **m. scalenus** and the lateral aspect of the **m. longus colli**, the ventral branches of the C6, C7, C8, and T1 spinal nerves are aligned in the same intermuscular plane (Figure 7.1). They lie in areolar tissue and are surrounded by the deep fascia of the neck.

The **phrenic nerve** arises from the ventral branches of the C5, C6, and C7 spinal nerves. It runs medial to the brachial plexus and in the same interfascial compartment (Figure 7.1b). Therefore, blockade of the brachial plexus at this level may induce dysfunction of the ipsilateral diaphragm.

(a)

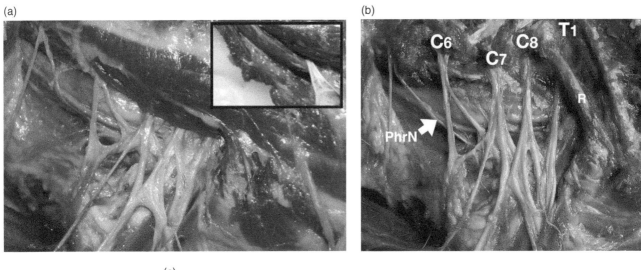

(b)

(c)

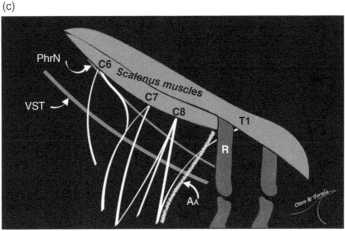

FIGURE 7.1   (a) Anatomy of the lateral aspect of the left brachial plexus in a dog. The dissection shows the relationship between the ventral branches of the brachial plexus and the bellies of the ***mm. scalenus*** and ***longus colli***. The insert shows the root of C6 between the ***mm. scalenus*** and ***longus colli***. (b) The ventral branches of the left brachial plexus after removing the lateral muscles. (c) Schematic illustration of (a). AA, axillary artery; C6, C7, C8, and T1, ventral branches of the corresponding spinal nerves; PhrN, **phrenic nerve**; R, first rib; and VST, vagosympathetic trunk.

EXPECTED DISTRIBUTION OF ANESTHESIA

- The brachial plexus contains the fibers that are responsible for the innervation of the entire thoracic limb except for the skin over the tricipital region of the brachium (caudomedial aspect), which is innervated by a branch of T2, the **intercostobrachial nerve**.

- Blockade of the C6, C7, C8, and T1 nerve roots will provide sensory anesthesia to the shoulder joint, brachium, antebrachium, and manus.

LOCAL ANESTHETIC: DOSE, VOLUME, AND CONCENTRATION

Long-acting local anesthetics are recommended (e.g. bupivacaine, ropivacaine, or levobupivacaine). High concentrations (0.5%) will promote more complete sensory and motor

blockade, whereas lower concentrations (≤0.2%) will provide acceptable blockade of the sensory fibers but result in a shorter duration of motor blockade (Ford et al. 1984). Portela et al. (2018) recommended using 0.4 ml kg^{-1}, divided into equal aliquots to be administered at each nerve branch, however, this author recommends using only two aliquots – 0.1 ml kg^{-1} to be injected cranial to C7, and 0.3 ml kg^{-1} to be injected caudal to C7, respectively.

PATIENT PREPARATION AND POSITIONING

The patient should be positioned in lateral recumbency with the limb to be blocked positioned uppermost and in a neutral position (Figure 7.2). To further facilitate the procedure, consider placing a small cushion or towel under the opposite/ dependent shoulder. This allows the patient's neck to be extended and the operative limb to be displaced caudally,

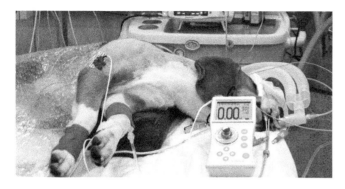

FIGURE 7.2 A dog has been positioned for a subscalene approach to the right brachial plexus. Note that a cushion has been placed under the dog's left shoulder, allowing for the more caudal displacement of the right thoracic limb, facilitating the procedure.

making ultrasound imaging more consistent and needle advancement easier.

The hair overlying the shoulder joint, brachium, and lateral aspect of the cervical and craniothoracic spine extending from C4 to T2 should be clipped and aseptically prepared.

STEP-BY-STEP PERFORMANCE
SURFACE ANATOMY AND LANDMARKS TO BE USED

The ultrasound transducer should initially be positioned parallel to the long axis of the **m. scalenus**, cranial to the first rib, and immediately dorsal to its costochondral junction (Figure 7.3). The transducer should then be moved caudally (while displacing the scapula) until the first rib comes into the field of view, and dorsally until the ventral branches of the spinal nerves can be observed medial to the belly of the **m. scalenus**, deep to the deep fascia of the neck.

Small movements of the transducer may be required to optimize the image of the nerve branches and the deep fascia of the neck and to identify the axillary artery, which is located caudal and medial to the T1 root.

ULTRASOUND ANATOMY

The neurovascular bundle containing the brachial plexus roots (C6, C7, C8, and T1) is visualized surrounded by the deep fascia of the neck in the center of the ultrasound screen and viewed on its long axis at a depth of approximately 2.5–3.5 cm depth in a midsize dog (Figure 7.4). The axillary artery should be observed medial to the C8–T1 nerve complex (Figure 7.5). It is important to visualize the cranial border of the first rib and the intermittent incursion of the pleura in the field of view during inspiration to minimize accidental pleural puncture.

NEEDLE INSERTION TECHNIQUE

The needle should be advanced in-plane through the deep fascia of the neck using a cranial-to-caudal trajectory, aiming towards the caudal aspect of C7 nerve root (Figure 7.3). After negative aspiration, a test dose may be administered to observe the dispersion of spread within the interfascial plane, indicating correct positioning of the needle.

EXPECTED MOTOR RESPONSES FROM NERVE STIMULATION

When the block is assisted by a nerve stimulator, the motor responses observed will depend on the nerve root stimulated:

- **C6** – Adduction and extension of the shoulder, advancement of limb.

- **C7** – Flexion of the elbow and the shoulder.

- **C8, T1** – Extension of elbow, carpus, and digits. Flexion of the carpus and digits.

(a)

(b)

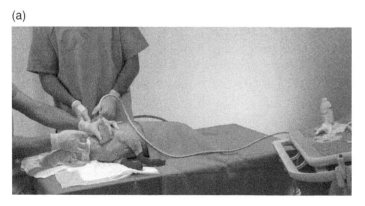
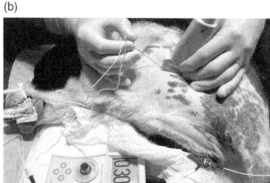

FIGURE 7.3 (a) Positioning for an ultrasound-guided subscalene approach to the left brachial plexus of a canine cadaver. The subject has been positioned in right lateral recumbency with the left thoracic limb uppermost. The transducer has been placed on the lateral aspect of the neck and the needle is being introduced in-plane along the axis of the operator's view towards the ultrasound monitor. (b) Alternative form of positioning, with the anesthetist standing behind the patient and the ultrasound machine positioned across the patient in the near field (not shown).

(a)

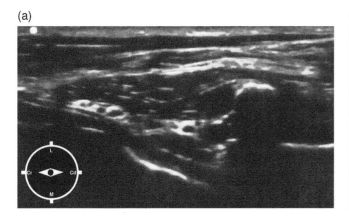

(b)

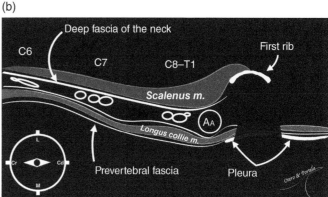

FIGURE 7.4   (a) Longitudinal (long-axis) ultrasound image of the caudal area of the canine neck, immediately cranial to the first rib. (b) Schematic illustration of (a). AA, axillary artery. Source: With permission from Drs. Pablo Otero (Chapter Contributor) and Diego Portela.

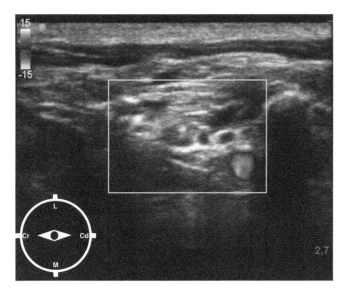

FIGURE 7.5   Color flow Doppler ultrasound image showing the axillary artery medial to the ventral branches of the brachial plexus. The nerves are located cranial to the first rib, along the ventral aspect of the *m. scalenus*.

ADMINISTRATION OF LOCAL ANESTHETIC – WHAT TO LOOK FOR, WHAT TO FEEL FOR, AND DECISION POINTS

Once the needle is in its final location, 0.3 ml kg⁻¹ of the calculated volume should be injected. During injection, the interfascial plane containing the brachial plexus roots will distend and the injected solution will distribute around the nerve roots (Figure 7.6). This hydrodissection will result in the deep fascia of the neck and the prevertebral fascia moving laterally and medially away from the target nerves, respectively. After the injection of the first aliquot, the needle should be withdrawn and redirected, toward the cranial aspect of the C7 nerve root. Once negative aspiration has been confirmed,

the remainder of the calculated volume may be injected (0.1 ml kg⁻¹). During its introduction, the needle should not be advanced beyond the root of C8.

The needle should not be advanced further than the cranial border of the first rib to minimize the risk of pleural puncture and thus possible pneumothorax. Puncture of the prevertebral fascia which lies deep to the **m. longus colli** should also be avoided. If puncture of this fascia occurs, it may create the potential for communication between the injection site and the tracheal and carotid sheath, where the **recurrent laryngeal nerve** and the vagosympathetic trunk are located. Injection of the local anesthetic solution may, therefore, induce blockade of these structures (see Complications below).

BLOCK EFFECTS (SENSORY, MOTOR, ETC.) AND PATIENT MANAGEMENT

This block will completely desensitize the entire thoracic limb, from the shoulder to the digits, with the exception of the skin over the tricipital region that is innervated by the cutaneous branches of the **intercostobrachialis nerve**.

Blockade of the **phrenic nerve** should be expected; however, unilateral blockade of the diaphragm should not significantly impair the ability of a healthy animal to ventilate appropriately. Nonetheless, ventilatory function should be monitored until diaphragmatic function returns to normal.

Because of concurrent motor blockade and subsequent paralysis of the limb, monitoring of the patient postoperatively should include adequate monitoring for skin abrasions or ulcers on the dorsal aspect of the manus that may occur from knuckling.

COMPLICATIONS AND HOW TO AVOID THEM

Inadvertent puncture of the axillary artery or the pleura is possible if the needle is advanced through the caudal margin of the nerve bundle. As such, continuous observation of the

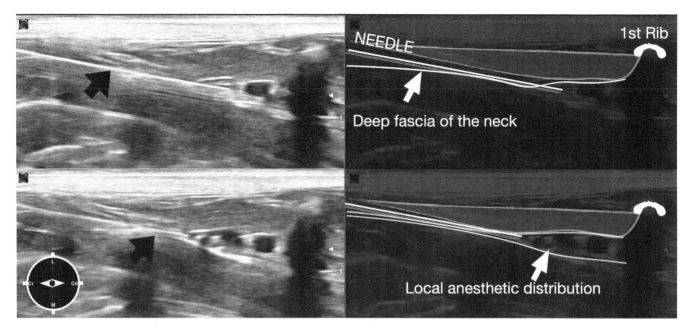

FIGURE 7.6   Ultrasound-guided subscalene brachial plexus block in a dog. The needle can be visualized in-plane (black arrowhead). After puncturing the lateral aspect of the interfascial plane, the needle tip is caudal to the C7 nerve root. The local anesthetic can be visualized surrounding the nerve roots as an anechoic area medial to the deep fascia of the neck.

needle tip position is crucial to optimizing patient safety and the potential for success of this block. To prevent intravascular injection, negative aspiration of the syringe should be confirmed prior to drug administration and the injectate should be directly observed spreading around the nerve roots.

Temporary laryngeal hemiplegia is possible following the performance of this block. Although the **recurrent laryngeal nerve** is found in a different interfascial plane than the one containing the brachial plexus, the two compartments are very close to each other. As a result, puncture of the prevertebral fascia (the medial aspect of the interfascial space that contains the brachial plexus roots) would favor the accumulation of anesthetic in the vicinity of the recurrent laryngeal nerve. For this reason, the anesthetist must be cautious when inserting the needle and stop its advancement immediately after piercing the lateral surface of the deep fascia of the neck (the lateral aspect of the target interfascial space). Taking these precautions may also prevent inadvertent blockade of the vagosympathetic trunk and its associated sympathetic ganglia, which could result in development of Horner's syndrome.

COMMON MISTAKES AND HOW TO AVOID THEM

A common mistake is to incorrectly position the tip of the needle in the *m. scalenus* (i.e. outside the interfascial plane), resulting in administration of the local anesthetic away from

the nerve roots and subsequent failure of the block. A test injection should be performed under ultrasound visualization to ensure correct needle positioning before the full volume of local anesthetic is administered.

HOW TO TALK TO CLIENTS/PROFESSIONAL COLLEAGUES

When planning to include the subscalene approach to block the brachial plexus as part of perioperative pain management, it is important to appreciate how long it might take to perform this block. The subscalene approach is an advanced technique and might require a longer execution time compared to other blocks. Another important aspect to discuss with surgeons is postoperative analgesic expectations. This block provides excellent postoperative analgesia, commonly lasting up to eight hours when long-acting local anesthetics are used. Despite this, rescue analgesia should always be available and promptly administered based on the use of a pain scoring system.

Owners and staff should be aware of the concomitant **phrenic nerve** block and the possible consequences (e.g. additional postoperative care and extended discharge). In addition, the possible adverse effects of the technique should be clarified – such as laryngeal paralysis or Horner's syndrome – which, although they resolve spontaneously in a few hours, could require additional care.

Chohan AS (2019) Anesthesia case of the month. J Am Vet Med 255, 1016–1018.

Evans HE, de Lahunta A (2013) The autonomic nervous system. In: Miller's Anatomy of the Dog, 4th edition. Evans HE, de Lahunta A (eds.) Saunders Elsevier, USA. pp. 575–588.

Ford DJ, Raj PP, Singh P et al (1984) Differential peripheral nerve block by local anesthetics in the cat. Anesthesiology 60, 28–33.

Fuensalida S, Ceballos M, Verdier N et al. (2017) Sonographic evaluation of diaphragm function during a subscalenic brachial plexus block in dogs: technique and clinical applications. Proceedings Manchester AVA Spring Meeting April 2017. Vet Anesth Analg 44, 983–988.

Otero PE, Fuensalida SE, Briganti A et al. (2017) Ultrasound-guided subscalenic brachial plexus block in dogs: a cadaveric study. Proceeding Proceedings Manchester AVA Spring Meeting April 2017. Vet Anesth Analg 44, 983–988.

Otero PE, Fuensalida SE, Verdier N et al. (2019) Peripheral nerve blocks of the thoracic limb. In: Manual of Small Animal Regional Anesthesia, 2nd edition. Otero PE, Portela DA (eds.) Inter-Medica, Buenos Aires. pp. 71–77.

Portela DA, Verdier N, Otero PE (2018) Regional anesthetic techniques for the thoracic limb and thorax in small animals: a review of the literature and technique description. Vet J 241, 8–19.

Ultrasound-Guided Brachial Plexus Block (Axillary Approach)

Luis Campoy

CHAPTER 8

BLOCK AT A GLANCE

What is it used for?

- To supplement anesthesia for surgeries distal to and including the shoulder joint.

Landmarks/transducer position:

- The ultrasound transducer should be placed over the **mm. pectorales superficiales** on the axillary region in a parasagittal plane, with the marker oriented caudally.

- The needle puncture site is located dorsal to the cranial edge of the **mm. pectorales superficiales** and lateral to the jugular vein.

What equipment and personnel are required?

- 21G 100 mm (4 in.) (or similar) blunt atraumatic needle

- Syringe of drug(s)

- Ultrasound machine

- High frequency (15–6 MHz) linear array transducer +/− protective sleeve

- Gloves

- Coupling agent (e.g. alcohol)

- Assistant to help position leg and perform the injection

When do I perform the block?

- Prior to surgery, after the area is clipped and skin preparation is complete. Final skin preparation will still be needed prior to surgery.

What volume of local anesthetic is used?

- 0.4 ml kg^{-1}

Goal:

- During injection, the local anesthetic should spread dorsal to the axillary artery to block C8, cranioventral to the artery to block C6 and C7 and, finally, caudal to the axillary vein to block T1.

Complexity level:

- Intermediate to advanced, depending on the size of the patient and ability to visualize the anatomy.

Clinical pearl:

- This block will cause motor blockade of the entire thoracic limb, including the shoulder joint.

WHAT DO WE ALREADY KNOW?

Campoy et al. (2010) first described an ultrasound-guided axillary approach to the brachial plexus in dogs. Their approach targeted the nerve roots of the brachial plexus as they cross the ventral edge of the **m. scalenus** in the axillary region. Since then, different refinements, comparisons, and alternative approaches have been published. Akasaka and Shimizu (2017) compared ultrasound-guided and electrolocation-guided techniques for blocking the brachial plexus at the level of the axilla. They demonstrated that, while the success rates did not differ between groups, the ultrasound-guided technique took less time to perform and had both a shorter onset and longer duration of action when compared to the electrolocation-guided technique. Additionally, the ultrasound technique was able to be tolerated in dogs receiving only sedation. Benigni et al. (2019) had similar findings when comparing an ultrasound-guided brachial plexus block with electrolocation for thoracic limb surgery in dogs. In their study, successful blocks were obtained in 14/16 and 12/16 attempts following ultrasound-guided and electrolocation-guided techniques, respectively, and were not significantly different. Adverse effects included hypotension in three dogs and Horner's syndrome in three dogs; however, the incidence of these complications was not significantly different between groups.

Recently, da Silva et al. (2020) reported a modification to the previously published axillary approach after studying two cadavers and 50 clinical cases. Those authors imaged the

Small Animal Regional Anesthesia and Analgesia, Second Edition. Edited by Matt Read, Luis Campoy, and Berit Fischer.
© 2024 John Wiley & Sons, Inc. Published 2024 by John Wiley & Sons, Inc.

axillary area of dogs positioned in dorsal recumbency with their thoracic limbs flexed in a natural position. Their study aimed to identify the most common locations of the nerves of the brachial plexus in relation to the axillary artery. The authors divided the ultrasound image into four quadrants, with the axillary artery located at the center of the image. If 9 o'clock was caudal and 3 o'clock was cranial, the **musculocutaneous nerve** (C7) was found cranial to the axillary artery in all of the dogs, the **radial nerve** (C8) was found in sector 2 (6–9 o'clock position) in 92% of the dogs, the **median nerve** (T1) was found in sector 1 (9–12 o'clock position) in 92% of the dogs and the **ulnar nerve** (T1) was found in sector 1 (9–12 o'clock position) in 98% of the dogs.

Ultrasound-guided approaches to performing brachial plexus blocks have also been described in cats. Ansón et al. (2015) compared two different techniques for an axillary approach in 12 feline cadavers positioned in dorsal recumbency. In one group, both thoracic limbs were adducted (thoracic limbs flexed and orientated caudally) and in the other, the limb to be blocked was abducted 90° while the contralateral was adducted. In the latter group, the success rate (staining of all nerve roots involved) was 100% (versus 66% in the first group) with no complications observed. In the second group (adducted group) staining of the **phrenic nerve** in three out of six cats and evidence of jugular hematoma in two out of six cats were observed. Following this cadaver study, the same authors evaluated their approach clinically in eight cats. Sensory and motor blockade were assessed after recovery with 6/8 cats demonstrating complete blockade of the limb and the remaining two cats having partial blockade described as being either delayed or attenuated responses to stimulus (Ansón et al. 2017).

PATIENT SELECTION
INDICATIONS FOR THE BLOCK

This block can be used to provide anesthesia and analgesia for surgical procedures involving the shoulder or humerus such as shoulder arthrotomies and humeral fracture repair. For shoulder surgeries, only single infiltration of the C6 area is necessary. Thoracic limb amputations are beyond the scope of this block since some of the anatomical structures involved are not served by the nerves of the brachial plexus.

CONTRAINDICATIONS

- Skin infection or other lesions at the intended puncture site.
- Peripheral nerve disease affecting the thoracic limb.
- Inability to identify the relevant landmarks (e.g. severe trauma in the axillary region).
- Respiratory disease/depression resulting in hypoxia or hypoventilation.
- Bleeding diathesis – The axillary artery and vein are in close proximity to the target nerves of the brachial plexus

and course down the proximal limb following the general direction of the nerve roots. The artery sits immediately ventral to the C8 root, and the vein is usually found cranial to the T1 nerve root. Understanding the location of these vessels relative to the root's brachial plexus is important for minimizing the possibility of needle trauma.

- Allergic reactions to local anesthetics.

POTENTIAL SIDE EFFECTS AND COMPLICATIONS

- The **phrenic nerve** runs along the ventral border of the **m. scalenus** and provides motor innervation to the diaphragm. Ventilatory insufficiency may result from inadvertent blockade of the **phrenic nerve** following ultrasound-guided brachial plexus block at this level since the local anesthetic may affect the ipsilateral **phrenic nerve** as it originates from the C5, C6, and C7 nerve roots. Although unilateral and bilateral diaphragmatic blockade in healthy awake and anesthetized dogs does not appear to significantly compromise respiratory function (De Troyer and Kelly 1982; Katagiri et al. 1994), caution should be used in patients with impaired pulmonary function or reserves. These patients may be at higher risk because diaphragmatic hemiparalysis after unilateral phrenic nerve blockade may have a detrimental effect on the expansion of both lungs (De Troyer et al. 2009), and therefore, a bilateral blockade in patients with compromised respiratory function should be carried out with extreme caution.

- In the axillary space, the axillary vessels run parallel to the nerve roots so inadvertent vascular laceration and subsequent axillary hematoma may result from brachial plexus blockade at this location. The axillary artery is located ventral to the C8 root and the axillary vein is located cranioventral to the T1 root along the caudal aspect of the brachial plexus. Since, the axillary vessels serve as key anatomic landmarks for informing final needle positioning during the execution of this technique, understanding the location of these vessels relative to each of the nerves of the brachial plexus is important for minimizing the possibility of puncturing or lacerating these large vascular structures.

- Local anesthetic systemic toxicity as a result of intravascular administration of the local anesthetic solution.

- Pneumothorax

- Horner's syndrome

GENERAL CONSIDERATIONS
CLINICAL ANATOMY

The primary contributors to the sensory and motor functions of the thoracic limb are the ventral branches of the C6, C7, C8, and T1 spinal nerves (Figure 8.1, Table 8.1). In a very small number of dogs, individual variation may result in additional contributions from the C5 and T2 spinal nerves. The ventral branches of the nerves leave their respective intervertebral foramina and join with adjacent nerves to form the roots of the brachial plexus. The roots enter the axillary area through the ventral border of the ***m. scalenus*** before forming the brachial plexus and its associated peripheral sensory and motor branches that serve the thoracic limb. The brachial plexus supplies almost all the innervation to the structures of the limb, except for a few muscles (***mm. trapezius, omotransversarius, brachiocephalicus, and rhomboideus***) and the skin over the dorsal shoulder region.

The **phrenic nerves** originate bilaterally in this general area, receiving contributions from the ventral branches of the C5, C6, and C7 spinal nerves on each side of the body. The nerve fibers that become the **phrenic nerve** branch off proximal to those that continue ventrally and contribute to the formation of the brachial plexus. The fibers of the **phrenic nerve** course ventral to the ***m. scalenus*** on each side of the body before forming a trunk that passes medial to each brachial plexus before entering the mediastinum between the first and second rib to serve their respective hemidiaphragms.

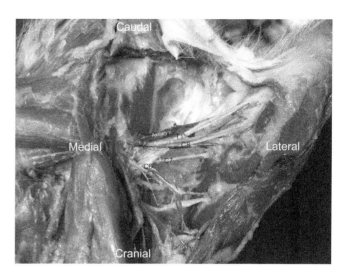

FIGURE 8.1   Dissection of the left axillary area of a dog in dorsal recumbency depicting the axillary vasculature and the roots of the brachial plexus. Note that the ***mm. pectorales*** have been removed on the left side to expose the relevant anatomy. Observe the relationship between the axillary artery and the C8 root.

EXPECTED DISTRIBUTION OF ANESTHESIA

Table 8.1   Sensory and motor distributions of the nerves to the thoracic limb.

Nerve	Spinal nerve contributions	Sensory to	Motor to
Suprascapular nerve	C6, C7	Lateral aspect of shoulder joint	*m. supraspinatus, m. infraspinatus, m. subscapularis,*
Subscapular nerve	C6, C7		*m. subscapularis*
Musculocutaneous nerve	C6, C7	Craniomedial forearm (antebrachium) distal to elbow	*m. coracobrachialis, m. biceps brachii, m. brachialis*
Axillary nerve	C7, C8	Caudal aspect of shoulder joint capsule, craniolateral aspect of the arm (brachium), and part of forearm (antebrachium)	*m. brachiocephalicus, m. teres major, m. teres minor, m. deltoideus.*
Radial nerve	C7, C8, T1	Lateral aspect of elbow joint, dorsal aspect of forearm (antebrachium), and paw	*m. triceps brachii, m. anconeus, m. extensor carpi radialis, m. extensor digitorum., m. extensor carpi ulnaris, mm. supinator communis and lateralis, m. abductor pollicus longus, m. ulnaris lateralis*
Median nerve	C8, T1	Medial aspect of elbow joint, medial and palmar aspects of forearm (antebrachium) and paw	*m. flexor carpi radialis, mm. flexor digitorum superficialis and profundus,* *m. pronator teres, m. pronator quadratus.*
Ulnar nerve	C8, T1	Caudal aspect of elbow joint, caudolateral aspect of forearm (antebrachium) and paw	*m. flexor carpi ulnaris, mm. flexor digitorum superficialis and profundus*

LOCAL ANESTHETIC: DOSE, VOLUME, AND CONCENTRATION

Any local anesthetic (e.g., bupivacaine, ropivacaine, and levobupivacaine) can be used to perform an axillary brachial plexus nerve block, with or without the coadministration of an adjuvant (e.g. dexmedetomidine, dexamethasone, and buprenorphine). The author most commonly uses

bupivacaine 0.5% combined with dexmedetomidine ($1\,\mu g\,ml^{-1}$) at a volume of $0.4\,ml\,kg^{-1}$.

PATIENT PREPARATION AND POSITIONING

For a right-handed anesthetist (i.e. with the needle being held in the dominant hand and the ultrasound transducer being held in the nondominant hand), the patient should be positioned in dorsal recumbency with the head of the patient on the anesthetist's right side and the ultrasound machine positioned on the opposite side of the table. The leg to be blocked should be abducted and extended slightly in order to stretch the nerves and vessels and facilitate the anesthetist obtaining a short axis view of these structures with the ultrasound (Figure 8.2).

STEP-BY-STEP PERFORMANCE

SURFACE ANATOMY AND LANDMARKS TO BE USED

With the leg extended and abducted, the ultrasound transducer should be positioned on the skin of the ventral axillary region (i.e. over the **mm. pectorales superficiales**) in the fossa that is created between the manubrium of the sternum and the supraglenoid tubercle of the scapula. The transducer should be oriented in a parasagittal plane with the marker positioned caudally so that the needle will approach the target area from the right side of the ultrasound screen, as it will approach the nerves *in situ*. The axillary vessels should be visualized in their short axis. Gliding and slightly tilting the transducer medially as well as slightly abducting and extending the limb may help with image optimization.

ULTRASOUND ANATOMY

In the near field, the most prominent superficial structure will be the **mm. pectorales superficiales**, with the **m. pectoralis profundus** dorsal to it (i.e. deep on the image). Dorsal to these muscles within the axillary space, the axillary artery, and the vein should be observed. These vessels serve as important

anatomic landmarks for the procedure and should be centered on the screen so they are in the area of highest resolution. Surrounding the axillary vessels, the roots of the brachial plexus may be visible as four small, round hyperechoic structures (Figure 8.3). The C6 and C7 nerve roots are usually found cranial and ventral to the artery, while the C8 nerve root is usually located dorsal to the axillary artery and the T1 nerve root is located caudal to the axillary vein. The first rib can be observed caudal to the axillary vein.

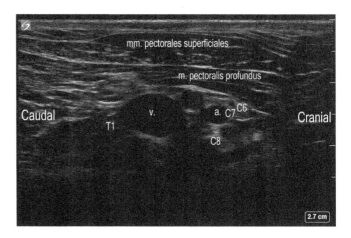

FIGURE 8.3   Optimal ultrasound image for the axillary approach to a brachial plexus block. The marker (blue logo) is oriented caudally. Note the position of the axillary artery (a.) and the axillary vein (v.) relative to the roots of the brachial plexus (C6, C7, C8, and T1).

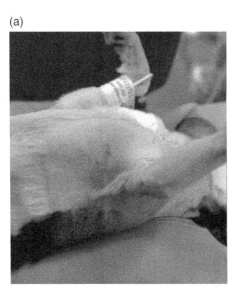

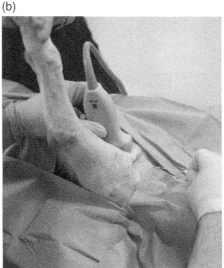

FIGURE 8.2   (a) Dog positioned in dorsal recumbency for brachial plexus block of the left thoracic limb. The leg is extended and slightly abducted to open up the axillary space and stretch the axillary nerves and vessels. (b) The ultrasound transducer is positioned over the axillary region (**mm. pectorales superficiales**) with the marker (blue circle) oriented caudally. The needle is parallel and in-plane with the transducer.

NEEDLE INSERTION TECHNIQUE

After the axillary artery and vein and the target nerve roots of the brachial plexus have been identified, the needle should be inserted in-plane, dorsal to the cranial edge of the **mm. pectorales** and lateral to the jugular vein (Figure 8.4). The needle should initially be advanced in a cranial-to-caudal direction toward the dorsal (deep) aspect of the axillary artery where the root of C8 is located.

EXPECTED MOTOR RESPONSES FROM NERVE STIMULATION

If electrostimulation is used to help identify the different roots of the brachial plexus, stimulation of C6 will result in contraction of the **mm. supra-** and **infraspinatus**, resulting in shoulder rotation, flexion, or extension. Stimulation of C7 will result in contraction of the **m. biceps brachii**, resulting in elbow flexion. Contractions of the **m. triceps brachii** with subsequent elbow extension should be observed when the needle is in close proximity to C8 and stimulation of T1 will result in contractions of the **mm. pronator teres** and **quadratus** with subsequent pronation of the antebrachium.

ADMINISTRATION OF LOCAL ANESTHETIC – WHAT TO LOOK FOR, WHAT TO FEEL FOR, AND DECISION POINTS

Following a negative aspiration test, the local anesthetic should be injected around the C8 nerve root dorsal to the axillary artery. The needle should then be advanced caudally toward the T1 root, using caution to not puncture the axillary vein or enter the chest (the needle should not be advanced caudal to the first rib). Following verification of a negative aspiration test at this new location, a second infiltration of the local anesthetic solution should be injected. Finally, as the needle is being withdrawn from the patient, the area cranioventral to the axillary artery, where the roots of C6 and C7 can be found, should be infiltrated with the reminder of the local anesthetic solution after performing a final aspiration test.

BLOCK EFFECTS AND PATIENT MANAGEMENT

This block will produce absence of motor function in the entire thoracic limb, including the shoulder joint. Patients will likely need assistance upon recovery from anesthesia to help them achieve sternal recumbency, stand, and ambulate. Patients may also need some assistance to remain in sternal recumbency.

COMPLICATIONS AND HOW TO AVOID THEM

If the axillary vessels cannot be identified as two distinct structures, the transducer is most often located too far lateral or too much pressure is being applied to the transducer on the skin (i.e. the vein is being compressed). Gliding the transducer medially and, on some occasions, tilting the transducer one way or the other on the limb may help achieve a true short-axis view of the axillary vessels. Additionally, slight extension and abduction of the limb may also help with visualizing the axillary vessels and the nerve roots.

(a)

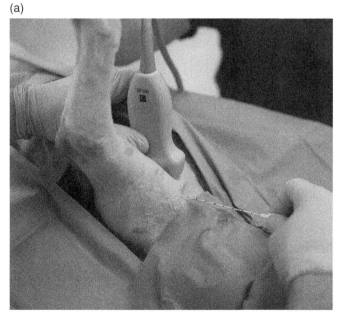

(b)

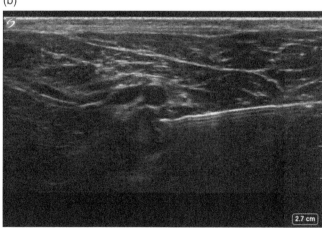

FIGURE 8.4 (a) Left brachial plexus block being performed with the dog positioned in dorsal recumbency. The ultrasound transducer is positioned over the axillary area with the marker (blue circle) oriented caudally. The needle is advanced in-plane with the transducer. (b) Corresponding ultrasound image. The marker (blue logo) is located caudally. Note the needle tip located at the dorsal aspect of the axillary artery where the C8 root can be found. Local anesthetic is being injected and is seen as a hypoechoic pocket.

COMMON MISTAKES AND HOW TO AVOID THEM

Due to the large amount of interstitial tissue and dead space that exists in the axillary area, there is a tendency for the injectate to form large pockets as it is being injected. The needle should be moved and relocated accordingly to ensure appropriate and even distribution of local anesthetic around the targeted nerve roots.

HOW TO TALK TO CLIENTS/PROFESSIONAL COLLEAGUES

- For an experienced anesthetist, the block should take less than five minutes to perform.

- Depending on the local anesthetic that is used, an axillary brachial plexus block will provide analgesia to the affected area for 10–18 hours.

- Additional pain management in the postoperative period should include application of cold compresses to the incision site (e.g. for 15 minutes, 3–4 times a day) and administration of oral analgesics (e.g. NSAIDs and pregabalin) for the following 5–7 days.

- Patients will not be able to use the blocked limb for several hours. Sling-assisted walking for elimination purposes is recommended.

- Complications could include block failure, hematoma, nerve trauma, systemic toxicity, and/or pneumothorax.

REFERENCES

Akasaka M, Shimizu M (2017) Comparison of ultrasound- and electrostimulation-guided nerve blocks of brachial plexus in dogs. Vet Anaesth Analg 44, 625–635.

Ansón A, Laredo FG, Gil F et al. (2017) Evaluation of an ultrasound-guided technique for axillary brachial plexus blockade in cats. J Feline Med Surg 19, 146–152.

Ansón A, Laredo FG, Gil F et al. (2015) Comparison of two techniques for ultrasound-guided axillary brachial plexus blockade in cats. J Feline Med Surg 17, 476–485.

Benigni L, Lafuente P, Viscasillas J (2019) Clinical comparison of two techniques of brachial plexus block for forelimb surgery in dogs. Vet J 244, 23–27.

Campoy L, Bezuidenhout AJ, Gleed RD et al. (2010) Ultrasound-guided approach for axillary brachial plexus, femoral nerve, and sciatic nerve blocks in dogs. Vet Anaesth Analg 37, 144–153.

da Silva LC, Futema F, Cortopassi SR (2020) Ultrasonographic study of a modified axillary approach to block the major branches of the brachial plexus in dogs. Vet Anaesth Analg 47, 82–87.

De Troyer A, Kelly S (1982) Chest wall mechanics in dogs with acute diaphragm paralysis. J Appl Physiol 53, 373–379.

De Troyer A, Leduc D, Cappello M (2009) Bilateral impact on the lung of hemidiaphragmatic paralysis in the dog. Respir Physiol Neurobiol 166, 68–72.

Katagiri M, Young RN, Platt RS et al. (1994) Respiratory muscle compensation for unilateral or bilateral hemidiaphragm paralysis in awake canines. J Appl Physiol 77, 1972–1982.

Ultrasound-Guided Proximal RUMM Block (Axillary Sheath)

CHAPTER 9

Matt Read

What is it used for?

- To supplement anesthesia for conditions distal to the mid-humerus, including humeral condylar fractures, elbow arthroscopy, radius and ulna fractures, radial ostectomies for correction of angular limb deformities, carpal arthrodesis, etc.

Landmarks/transducer position:

- The patient should be positioned in dorsal recumbency with the limb to be blocked rotated externally, or abducted in a neutral position. When it is time to perform the block, it is helpful to have an assistant extend and support the limb.

- The ultrasound transducer should initially be placed on the medial aspect of the humerus over the humeral head.

What equipment and personnel are required?

- 21G 100 mm (or similar) blunt atraumatic needle. A 22G 50 mm needle may be used in toy breeds or cats.

- Syringe of drug(s)

- Ultrasound machine

- High frequency (15–6 MHz) linear array transducer +/− protective sleeve and standoff

- Gloves

- Coupling agent (e.g. alcohol)

- +/− Assistant to help position the patient and perform the injection

When do I perform the block?

- Prior to surgery, after the limb is clipped and skin preparation is complete. Final skin preparation will still be needed prior to surgery.

What volume of local anesthetic is used?

- 0.2–0.4 ml kg^{-1}

Goal:

- During injection, the local anesthetic should be observed spreading within, and distending, the axillary sheath. Compression of the artery and vein may be observed.

Complexity level:

- Basic to intermediate, depending on the size of the patient.

Clinical pearl:

- This block will produce motor paralysis of the elbow and structures distal to it.

WHAT DO WE ALREADY KNOW?

The distal third of the brachium and the structures distal to it are innervated by the **RUMM** (**radial**, **ulnar**, **median**, and **musculocutaneous**) **nerves** that supply the bones, ligaments, muscles, and skin (Otero et al. 2021). Unlike "distal" approaches to performing RUMM blocks that typically involve injecting local anesthetic solutions at two or more sites in the area of the distal third of the brachium, an ultrasound-guided "proximal RUMM" block targets the four primary nerves of the distal thoracic limb at a single site where the RUMM nerves are located together within the axillary sheath.

Although distal approaches can be used to induce more selective sensory blockade, based on how and where on the limb distal RUMM blocks are performed, they may be technically difficult to execute, take more time to perform, involve repositioning the patient and/or multiple needle punctures, and result in patchy anesthesia (Tayari et al. 2019). "Proximal RUMM" block techniques, cover a greater anatomical area than distal RUMM blocks (i.e. including the distal humerus

Small Animal Regional Anesthesia and Analgesia, Second Edition. Edited by Matt Read, Luis Campoy, and Berit Fischer.
© 2024 John Wiley & Sons, Inc. Published 2024 by John Wiley & Sons, Inc.

and elbow), can be carried out in less time, with less needle manipulation, and with greater likelihood of success.

Tayari et al. (2019) were the first to describe and document the use of a proximal RUMM block technique in dogs. They initially performed a cadaver study to describe the regional anatomy of the upper thoracic limb, confirm the existence and describe the ultrasonographic appearance of the "axillary sheath," and document the distribution of a dye solution after it was injected into the sheath and dissipated around the **RUMM nerves**. Next, they performed a clinical study whereby they performed proximal RUMM blocks using ropivacaine 0.5% in medium-sized dogs that presented for a variety of thoracic limb surgical procedures. To use this approach, the ultrasound transducer was placed on the medial aspect of the limb and the needle advanced from a cranial location. Although they did not compare efficacy of the blocks by way of a concurrent control group, they documented low required doses of intraoperative opioids to treat sympathetic responses from surgical stimulation and no need for postoperative rescue analgesia within the first eight hours in 14 of 15 dogs. They also reported no neurological complications over a 30 day follow-up period.

A different approach to performing a proximal RUMM block in a small dog undergoing distal humeral fracture repair was reported by Otero et al. (2021) in a letter to the editor. Those authors described administering bupivacaine 0.5% at a single injection site with the ultrasound transducer on lateral aspect of the limb and the resulting anesthetic stability during surgery that resulted from this intervention. This brief report helped further document the utility and benefits of using a proximal approach to selectively block the major nerves of the distal thoracic limb while avoiding the potential side effects of a brachial plexus approach (e.g. vascular laceration, phrenic nerve involvement, penetration of thorax with needle, Horner's syndrome, etc.).

An ultrasound-guided proximal approach to staining the **RUMM nerves** in cat cadavers has been described (Pratt and Martinez-Taboada 2021). In that study, the ultrasound transducer was positioned laterally on the proximal limb, and cranial and caudal needle approaches to the **RUMM nerves** were compared. Unlike dogs, no axillary sheath was able to be identified in any of the subjects when they were dissected and dye staining was found to be variable, with several injections being made away from the target nerves. Overall, using their criteria for success (>20 mm continuous stain on all nerves), the cranial and caudal approaches were successful in 6/9 and 5/9 injections. Those authors concluded that, although both approaches resulted in promising staining, the considerable variability in dye distribution and presumed absence of an axillary sheath in this species, necessitates further investigation using live models to compare the clinical efficacy between this novel approach and traditional RUMM blocks in cats.

More recently, Iizuka et al. (2023) reported the results of a retrospective study that evaluated the use of proximal RUMM blocks in small-breed dogs that were presented for repair of radius/ulna fractures. Using the technique that was previously described by Tayari et al. (2019), those investigators found that administration of bupivacaine 0.25% or 0.5% significantly reduced the requirement for fentanyl infusions intraoperatively (median = 0.8 μg kg⁻¹ h⁻¹ (IQR = 0–1.9) versus 8.4 ug kg⁻¹ h⁻¹ (7.2–10), RUMM block versus no block, respectively) and that use of the higher concentration of bupivacaine was more reliable for eliminating the need for fentanyl intraoperatively (five of seven dogs received no fentanyl in the 0.5% bupivacaine group versus one of eight dogs in the 0.25% bupivacaine group). Overall, they found that the use of the proximal RUMM block was beneficial in this population of clinical patients, as documented by more stable anesthesia and no reported complications associated with the blocks at the time of performance or at the two-week follow-up.

Based on the still limited number of reports in the literature and lack of controlled, blinded, and randomized studies comparing proximal RUMM blocks to other regional anesthetic techniques of the thoracic limb, further studies are warranted to document the efficacy, safety, and risk associated with the use of this technique in both dogs and cats. However, in the author's clinical experience with this technique, it is highly effective and can be used successfully across a range of canine and feline patients undergoing painful procedures with minimal risk of complications.

PATIENT SELECTION

INDICATIONS FOR THE BLOCK

Surgical procedures that may benefit from use of an ultrasound-guided proximal RUMM block include those involving the distal humerus and elbow (e.g. repair of humeral condylar fractures, elbow arthroscopy, and canine unicompartmental elbow (CUE) arthroplasty) and any other procedure involving anything distal to these anatomical structures (e.g. radius and ulna fractures, radial ostectomies for angular limb deformity correction, stabilization of carpal fractures, carpal arthrodesis, etc.). Whether to perform a proximal RUMM block or one of the other blocks of the thoracic limb will be based on the anatomy involved in the surgical procedure, the desired degree and duration of postoperative motor blockade, patient signalment and size, ease of imaging based on concurrent issues (e.g. bruising, limb swelling from injury), the personal preference and experience of the anesthetist, the equipment available, etc.

CONTRAINDICATIONS

- Skin infection or other issues (e.g. bruising, swelling) at the intended needle puncture site or site of imaging.

- Peripheral nerve disease affecting the thoracic limb.

- Small patient sizes (i.e. small breed dogs, cats, approx. <5 kg), while not contraindicated, can present technical challenges. Use of a small-footprint linear ultrasound transducer (25 mm or "hockey stick") and/or standoff may be necessary.

- Allergic reactions to local anesthetics.

POTENTIAL SIDE EFFECTS AND COMPLICATIONS

- Due to the presence of the axillary artery and vein within the axillary sheath, there is potential for the needle to puncture the artery and/or vein after it penetrates the sheath, resulting in hemorrhage and/or hematoma formation.

- If a vessel is punctured without the operator recognizing the issue and a local anesthetic is administered at an excessive dose, there might be potential for local anesthetic systemic toxicity (LAST).

- Motor function of the elbow will be lost when using this approach to block the **RUMM nerves**. The duration of sensory and motor blockade should be monitored and the patient prevented from injuring itself as a result of dragging and/or scuffing the paw, etc.

GENERAL CONSIDERATIONS
CLINICAL ANATOMY

In the proximal brachium of the dog, the four major nerves (RUMM) that serve the distal thoracic limb are all located within the axillary sheath, a connective covering formed by the deep axillary fascia that wraps around the neurovascular structures (Tayari et al. 2019) (Figure 9.1). At this location in cats, despite evidence that the axillary sheath may not exist (Pratt and Martinez-Taboada 2021), the nerves can be accessed at the same site using a single injection. The axillary artery and vein lie with the nerves within the axillary sheath but in a more caudal position. When using a cranial to caudal approach, the needle will only traverse the **mm. biceps brachii** and/or **coracobrachialis** on its way to the target location cranial to the axillary artery, making this a relatively safe technique in terms of risk of vascular puncture, penetration of the thorax, involvement of the **phrenic nerve** or sympathetic trunk, etc. A caudal to cranial approach will mean the needle must pass the artery and vein on its way to its final position, risking vascular puncture.

(a)

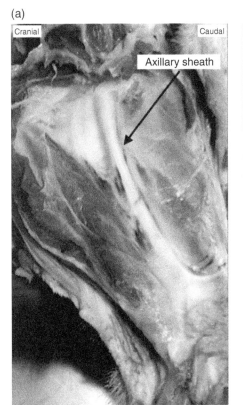

(b)

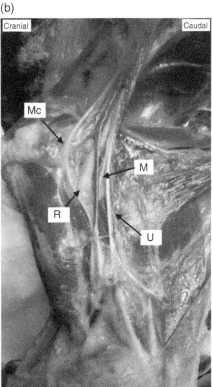

(c)

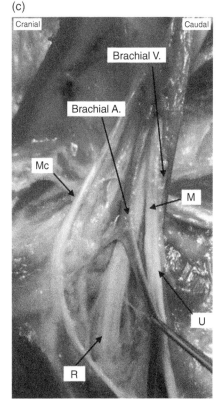

FIGURE 9.1   Visualization of the **radial** (R), **ulnar** (U), **median** (M), and **musculocutaneous** (Mc) **nerves** after removal of the **mm. pectoralis** in a dog cadaver. (a) Axillary sheath containing the nervous vascular bundle. (b) **R, U, M,** and **Mc nerve** exposure after opening the axillary sheath; notice how close the sheath maintains them. The axillary artery and vein continue into the brachial artery and vein. (c) Enlargement of (b); it is possible to see the exact point where the **Mc** splits into two branches. Source: Tayari et al. (2019)/with permission from Elsevier.

EXPECTED DISTRIBUTION OF ANESTHESIA

A successful proximal RUMM block will provide anesthesia for procedures involving structures distal to the mid-humerus.

LOCAL ANESTHETIC: DOSE, VOLUME, AND CONCENTRATION

Any local anesthetic (e.g. bupivacaine, ropivacaine, levobupivacaine) can be used to perform a proximal RUMM block, with or without the coadministration of an adjuvant (e.g. dexmedetomidine, dexamethasone, buprenorphine).

Tayari et al. (2019) used 0.15 ml kg^{-1} ropivacaine 0.5%, administered at three locations: 0.03 ml kg^{-1} to block the **musculocutaneous nerve**, 0.07 ml kg^{-1} to block the **radial nerve**, and 0.05 ml kg^{-1} to block the **ulnar** and **median nerves**. Otero et al. (2021) used 0.15 ml kg^{-1} bupivacaine 0.5% divided between two locations: 0.05 ml kg^{-1} to block the **musculocutaneous nerve** and 0.1 ml kg^{-1} to block the **radial**, **ulnar**, and **median nerves**. Iizuka et al. (2023) used either 0.3 ml kg^{-1} bupivacaine 0.5% or 0.6 ml kg^{-1} bupivacaine 0.25% to block the **RUMM nerves**, with the final volume ultimately being determined by observing the distribution of the drug around the nerves. The author typically prepares 0.2–0.4 ml kg^{-1} ropivacaine 0.5%, depending on the size of the patient (i.e. lower relative volumes for larger patients). Depending on the observed distribution of the local anesthetic during administration, not all of this volume may be used in all patients – once the axillary sheath has been visibly distended by the local anesthetic and the nerves are surrounded, there is little benefit to administering more volume.

PATIENT PREPARATION AND POSITIONING

The patient should be positioned in dorsal recumbency with the front legs abducted and rotated externally, hanging in a natural position (Figure 9.2). The leg to be blocked should be clipped free of hair to the level of the shoulder and standard surgical preparation of the skin over the injection site (i.e. cranial aspect of brachium) should be performed.

The anesthetist should stand on one side of the patient with the ultrasound machine positioned on the opposite side of the patient. For a right-handed anesthetist, the patient's head should be located on the anesthetist's right side, regardless of which leg is being blocked. This will result in the needle approaching the axillary sheath from a cranial-to-caudal direction through the *m. biceps brachii*, minimizing the chances of puncturing the vessels within the sheath. The opposite orientation can be used by a left-handed anesthetist.

When it is time to perform the block, it is helpful to have an assistant hold the patient's paw and extend the limb (Figure 9.2), allowing the anesthetist to apply appropriate pressure with the ultrasound transducer without pushing the limb away. This maneuver is especially helpful for small patients where it can be challenging to apply enough pressure to get good skin contact with the transducer without compressing the vein and losing track of the location of the vessels within the sheath as the needle is being advanced. Extending the limb also stretches the axillary sheath and its associated structures, helping to align the nerves and vessels in the same direction so they all appear in a similar short-axis view.

(a)

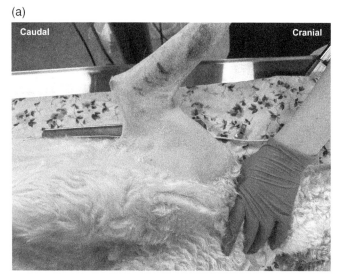

(b)

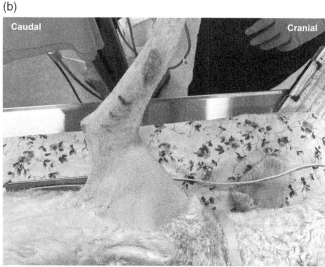

FIGURE 9.2 (a) A dog has been positioned for a proximal RUMM block prior to stabilization of a radius/ulna fracture. (b) An assistant has extended the limb and is available to support it during the procedure.

STEP-BY-STEP PERFORMANCE

SURFACE ANATOMY AND LANDMARKS TO BE USED

The ultrasound transducer should initially be placed on the skin on the medial aspect of the thoracic limb at the level of the humeral head (Figure 9.3). The transducer should be oriented perpendicular to the humerus (i.e. transverse to the long axis of the humerus) with its marker located caudally. For right-handed anesthetists standing with the patient's head to their right side, this will result in the needle approaching the target area with the same orientation on the ultrasound screen as it is moving in the patient.

ULTRASOUND ANATOMY

The axillary artery should initially be used as the primary sonographic landmark and will appear as a circular, pulsing, and anechoic structure (Figure 9.4). Once the artery is identified, the transducer should be manipulated to place the artery in a short-axis view, and the depth and gain controls adjusted to optimize the image and place the artery (and, therefore, the other structures within the axillary sheath) in the center of the ultrasound screen. Keeping the artery in the center of the screen, the transducer should then be slowly moved distally and proximally along the limb until the muscles surrounding the axillary sheath can be identified: the *m. pectoralis profundus* (medial), the *mm. biceps brachii* (craniomedial) and *coracobrachialis* (craniolateral), and the *mm. triceps brachii* (lateral).

The axillary sheath and structures within it usually appear most obvious at a location along the limb where the *mm. biceps brachii* and *coracobrachialis* are seen as discrete, "feather-like" structures. Once the axillary sheath

and its associated structures are identified, scan the area to confirm the presence of the **radial nerve** within the sheath (it eventually leaves the sheath as it courses distally down the limb) and that the **musculocutaneous nerve** has not yet split into its two components (one branch runs cranially to the *m. biceps brachii* and one branch runs distally to the elbow region; Tayari et al. 2019). After the ideal location is found, stop moving the transducer and save this initial image.

The axillary sheath will appear as a thin, hyperechoic line that surrounds the hypoechoic artery, vein, and nerves. The vein will appear as an ovoid, compressible anechoic structure caudal to the artery. Depending on the amount of pressure being applied by the transducer on the limb, the vein may be compressed and may not always be seen, even in larger patients. Make sure to vary the pressure being applied so as to identify the vein's location prior to needle placement or inadvertent puncture of this vessel may occur.

In most cases, the **musculocutaneous nerve** will be identified most cranially, the **radial nerve** will be identified immediately cranial and deep (i.e. more lateral) to the axillary artery, and the **ulnar** and **median nerves** will be located in close proximity to each other between the axillary artery and vein. In some patients (especially smaller ones), the individual nerves may not be able to be visualized as discrete structures within the neurovascular bundle but the hyperechoic line that demarcates the limits of the axillary sheath will still be identifiable.

Color Doppler can be used to differentiate the artery and vein from the nerves. Saving an image in the medical record that shows the location and integrity of the artery and vein prior to needle placement is suggested, especially in small patients where image optimization is more challenging (Figure 9.4c).

NEEDLE INSERTION TECHNIQUE

When performing a proximal RUMM block, all of the structures of interest are typically located superficially beneath the skin (i.e. less than 3 cm), even in large breed dogs. In small breed dogs and cats, these structures are extremely superficial (less than 0.5 cm) so take care to continuously visualize the needle tip as it is being advanced. If it is on too acute an angle, it may inadvertently leave the patient and damage the ultrasound transducer.

The needle will puncture the skin on the cranial aspect of the limb (Figure 9.5). The needle should be advanced in-plane on a caudal trajectory through the *m. biceps brachii* toward the axillary sheath (Figure 9.6). Although other needle approaches can be used, using this needle trajectory avoids the humerus and major vessels within the sheath, making needle advancement easier and safer than if it approaches the sheath from a different direction.

After the needle crosses the *m. biceps brachii*, gentle pressure should be applied to the needle until it penetrates the

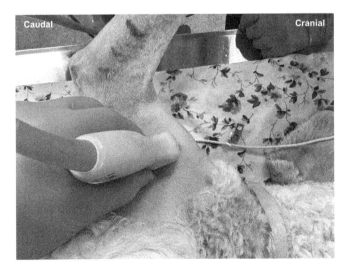

FIGURE 9.3   The ultrasound transducer has been placed perpendicular to limb over the humeral head, allowing for a short-axis view of the structures within the axillary sheath to be obtained.

(a)

(b)

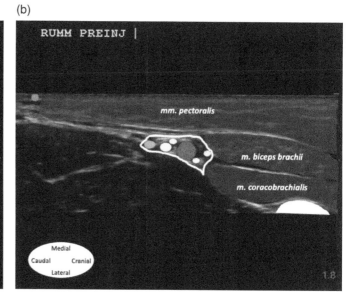

(c)

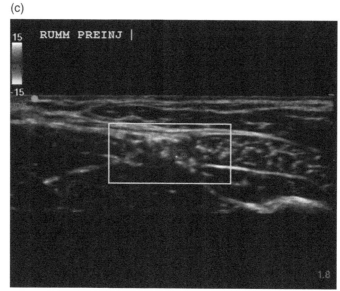

FIGURE 9.4   (a) Pre-block ultrasonographic image of the target area for a proximal RUMM block in a dog. (b) Same image with labels. Note the positions and appearances of the *mm. pectoralis profundus, biceps brachii* and *coracobrachialis*, the humerus, and the location of the nerves and vessels relative to each other within the axillary sheath. (c) Corresponding image demonstrating use of color Doppler to identify the axillary artery.

axillary sheath. At this point, especially in small patients, it can be helpful to angle the needle tip slightly laterally so that when it punctures the sheath, the needle does not advance too far and contact the artery. A palpable "click" or "pop" sensation may be appreciated by the anesthetist as the needle tip penetrates the sheath, which may also be simultaneously visualized occurring on the ultrasound screen.

Unlike the axillary approach to a brachial plexus block, this technique involves the needle being advanced distal to the shoulder joint so there is no risk of intrathoracic needle placement or **phrenic nerve** blockade.

EXPECTED MOTOR RESPONSES FROM NERVE STIMULATION

If nerve stimulation is being used, when the needle tip penetrates the axillary sheath and comes in close proximity to the nerves, motor responses may be observed. Depending on the final position of the needle tip within the axillary sheath and the current intensity, elbow flexion (resulting from **musculocutaneous nerve** stimulation), elbow extension (resulting from **radial nerve** stimulation), or internal rotation of the antebrachium, and/or carpal or digital flexion (resulting from **ulnar** and **median nerve** stimulation) may be observed.

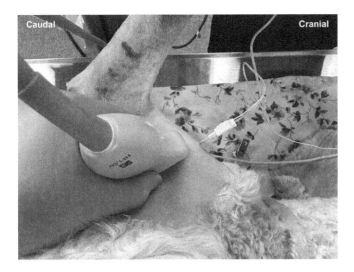

FIGURE 9.5   An insulated needle has been advanced in-plane from the cranial aspect of the limb into the axillary sheath.

ADMINISTRATION OF LOCAL ANESTHETIC – WHAT TO LOOK FOR, WHAT TO FEEL FOR, AND DECISION POINTS

Once the tip of the needle is positioned within the axillary sheath, a negative aspiration test should be performed and a test dose of the local anesthetic solution can be administered. No resistance to injection should be appreciated and distention of the sheath should be observed on the ultrasound screen as the calculated volume of local anesthetic solution is slowly administered. A successful injection will result in the local anesthetic solution being seen to disperse around the structures within the sheath, without appearing within any of the surrounding muscles (Figure 9.7).

Depending on patient size, the needle may need to be repositioned in order to fully block each of the nerves. Tayari et al. (2019) reported blocking each of the nerves individually in dogs that were 20 ± 8 kg (mean $\pm$ SD). Otero et al. (2021) blocked the target nerves at two sites in a 1.5 kg puppy. In the author's experience, since it is not always possible to reposition the needle in small patients without risking patient injury, all of the calculated volume can be administered at a single location without seeming to affect overall success. Instead, slow administration of the injectate is recommended to ensure a more homogeneous dispersion within the axillary sheath.

Saving an image using color Doppler to show the location and integrity of the artery and vein following injection can be useful to further highlight and document distention of the axillary sheath and the final distribution of the local anesthetic solution following injection.

BLOCK EFFECTS AND PATIENT MANAGEMENT

This block will cause sensory and motor blockade of the thoracic limb from the mid-humerus distal. Until the block has worn off, larger patients may require assistance (e.g. use of a sling) when being walked.

COMPLICATIONS AND HOW TO AVOID THEM

- Close monitoring of needle position using ultrasound is crucial to patient safety and success of this block. As described above, since the structures of interest are located superficially, it can be difficult to optimize the ultrasound image and manipulate the needle, especially in small patients (e.g. cats and small dogs).

(a)

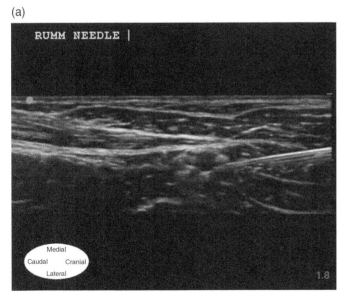

(b)

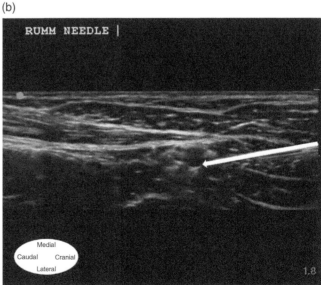

FIGURE 9.6   (a) Ultrasonographic image of proximal RUMM block in a dog. (b) Same image with white arrow representing position of needle. The needle tip has been advanced into its final position inside the axillary sheath.

(a)

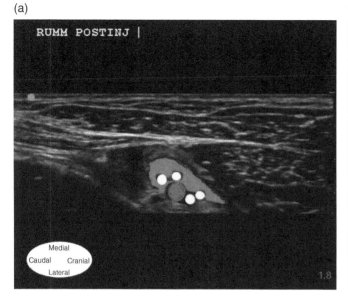

(b)

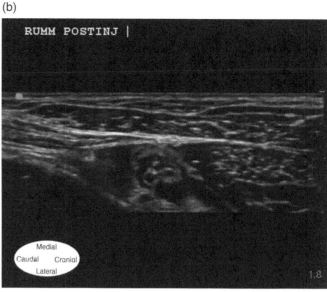

FIGURE 9.7 (a) Postinjection ultrasonographic image following a proximal RUMM block. (b) Same image with labels. Local anesthetic solution (hypoechoic) can be observed spreading around the axillary artery and nerves within the axillary sheath.

- Due to the close proximity of the nerves and vessels within the axillary sheath, it is possible to inadvertently puncture the vessels (especially the vein) if the needle is advanced too far into the sheath. The use of color Doppler and varying the amount of pressure being applied by the transducer on the skin may be helpful for confirming the location of the vessels before advancing the needle into the sheath.

- To avoid potentially damaging the nerves and vessels within the neurovascular bundle, once the needle has penetrated the sheath, it does not need to be advanced or manipulated further.

- Negative blood aspiration should be verified prior to drug administration to minimize the chances of inadvertently performing an intravascular injection.

COMMON MISTAKES AND HOW TO AVOID THEM

A common mistake is injecting outside the axillary sheath into the surrounding muscles (most commonly, in the author's experience, into the **m. biceps brachii** if the axillary sheath has not yet been penetrated). Prior to administering the full calculated volume of local anesthetic solution, the anesthetist should confirm that the needle has successfully penetrated the sheath and is in the correct location by performing a test injection and observing distension of the sheath.

HOW TO TALK TO CLIENTS/PROFESSIONAL COLLEAGUES

- For an experienced anesthetist, a proximal RUMM block should take less than five minutes to perform.

- Depending on the local anesthetic solution that is used, a proximal RUMM block will provide analgesia to the affected area for up to 18–24 hours.

- Additional pain management in the postoperative period should include icing of the incision site (e.g. 15 minutes, 3–4 times a day) and administration of oral analgesics (e.g. NSAIDs and pregabalin) for the following 5–7 days.

- Patients are usually able to walk with support immediately following recovery from anesthesia, can eat four to six hours post recovery, and should be able to void.

- Motor deficits will be observed at the level of the elbow and distal. Since the block is performed at the proximal brachium, shoulder function will be preserved.

REFERENCES

Iizuka T, Anazawa T, Nishimura R et al. (2023) Fentanyl sparing effect of ultrasound-guided proximal radial, ulnar, median, and musculocutaneous nerve (RUMM) block for radial and ulnar fracture repair in dogs: a retrospective case-control study. J Vet Med Sci 85, 49–54.

Otero, PE, Guerrero JA, Verdier N et al. (2021) Use of a lateral ultrasound-guided approach for the proximal radial, ulnar, median and musculocutaneous (RUMM)

block in a small dog undergoing distal humerus fracture repair. Vet Anaesth Analg 48, 815–817.

Pratt SB, Martinez-Taboada F (2021) Lateral ultrasound-guided axillary RUMM block in cats: a pilot cadaveric study. J Fel Med Surg 23, 310–315.

Tayari H, Otero P, Rossetti A et al. (2019) Proximal RUMM block in dogs: preliminary results of cadaveric and clinical studies. Vet Anaesth Analg 46, 384–394.

Ultrasound-Guided (Distal) RUMM Block

Matt Read and Luis Campoy

CHAPTER 10

BLOCK AT A GLANCE

What is it used for?

- To supplement anesthesia for conditions distal to the elbow, including repair of radius and ulna fractures, ostectomy/osteotomy for angular limb deformity correction, carpal arthrodesis, etc.

Landmarks/transducer position:

- The patient should be positioned in lateral recumbency with the limb to be blocked positioned uppermost in a natural, extended position.

- The ultrasound transducer should be placed perpendicular to the long axis of the humerus on the lateral aspect of the limb over the *m. triceps brachii*, approximately halfway between the mid-humerus and the lateral epicondyle.

What equipment and personnel are required?

- 21G 100 mm (or similar) blunt atraumatic needle. A 20G 50 mm needle may be used in toy breeds or cats.

- Syringe of drug(s)

- Ultrasound machine

- High frequency (15–6 MHz) linear array transducer +/− protective sleeve

- Gloves

- Coupling agent (e.g. alcohol)

- +/−Assistant to perform the injection

When do I perform the block?

- Prior to surgery, after the area is clipped and surgical skin preparation is complete. Final skin preparation will still be needed prior to surgery.

What volume of local anesthetic is used?

- $0.3–0.4\,\mathrm{ml\,kg^{-1}}$

Goal:

- During the initial injection, the local anesthetic should be observed spreading around the **radial nerve**.

- A second injection is performed after the needle is redirected towards the *fascia brachialis* and penetration of the fascial sheath containing the **ulnar**, **median**, and **musculocutaneous nerves**. During injection at this location, distension of the fascial sheath should be observed.

Complexity level:

- Intermediate

Clinical pearl:

- The needle can be advanced in-plane (IP) from either a cranial- or caudal direction toward the target nerve(s). In many cases, a caudal-to-cranial trajectory is easier to perform since the needle only needs to pass through muscle, as opposed to navigating around the humerus. For a caudal approach, the puncture site is located on the caudal aspect of the brachial region, over the long belly of the lateral head of the *m. triceps brachii*.

- This block **will** produce motor paralysis of the carpus +/− the elbow.

WHAT DO WE ALREADY KNOW?

The ultrasound-guided "RUMM" block (sometimes referred to as a "distal RUMM" block) targets the four primary nerves of the distal thoracic limb at two sites – the **radial nerve** at one location, and the **ulnar**, **median**, and **musculocutaneous nerves** together at a second location (Portela et al. 2013). The **radial nerve** is visualized and blocked midway between

Small Animal Regional Anesthesia and Analgesia, Second Edition. Edited by Matt Read, Luis Campoy, and Berit Fischer.
© 2024 John Wiley & Sons, Inc. Published 2024 by John Wiley & Sons, Inc.

the mid-humerus and the lateral epicondyle after it separates from the other three nerves and crosses from the medial aspect of the limb towards the lateral aspect of the limb. The **ulnar**, **median**, and **musculocutaneous nerves** are blocked on the medial aspect of the limb where they are contained within a fascial sheath together with the brachial artery and vein.

Different approaches to performing RUMM (radial, ulnar, median, and musculocutaneous) blocks in dogs either blindly or with the use of nerve stimulation have been described with varying levels of success (Lamont and Lemke 2008; Trumpatori et al. 2010; Bortolami et al. 2012). Portela et al. (2013) first described the use of a two-step (i.e. two needle punctures) ultrasound-guided approach to the RUMM block as part of the successful anesthetic management for surgical correction of a carpal luxation in a dog. Those authors approached the **radial nerve** with the ultrasound transducer placed on the lateral aspect of the limb. Using an in-plane (IP) approach, cranial to caudal needle trajectory, ropivacaine 0.1 ml kg^{-1} was administered around the **radial nerve** at this location. To block the remaining target nerves, the needle was withdrawn, the operative limb was abducted, and the transducer was placed on the medial aspect of the limb. A second skin puncture was performed, with the needle again approaching the nerves from a cranial direction. Ropivacaine 0.1 ml kg^{-1} was first administered around the **ulnar** and **median nerves** and then 0.05 ml kg^{-1} was deposited around the **musculocutaneous nerve**.

In 2015, Castiñeiras et al. described the use of a single-step (i.e. one needle puncture) out-of-plane (OP) approach to performing an ultrasound-guided RUMM block in a dog that presented for radius and ulna fractures. Placing the transducer on the medial aspect of the affected limb, they initially blocked the **ulnar** and **median nerves** with a single injection of ropivacaine at their location between the brachial artery and vein, followed by redirection of the needle to access the **musculocutaneous nerve** cranial to the artery and the **radial nerve** at its more lateral location. Successful blockade was obtained with this technique using a total volume of 0.18 ml kg^{-1} ropivacaine. The authors suggested that the main advantage of their technique over that used by Portela et al. (2013) was the ability to perform blockade of all four nerves without altering the patient's recumbency or manipulating the limb, both of which could potentially be detrimental in patients with complex fractures.

The first report on using ultrasound to perform RUMM blocks in cats was by Leung et al. (2019) who compared two different needle approaches. Using feline cadavers, they compared single-step (i.e. one needle puncture) IP or OP needle approaches with the ultrasound transducer positioned laterally on the limb. They found that the IP needle technique resulted in more successful staining of all the target nerves, with the **radial nerve** being successfully stained in 18/18 (IP) versus 14/18 injections (OP) and the **ulnar**, **median**, and **musculocutaneous nerves** being successfully stained in 17/18 (IP) versus 12/18 (OP). "Failed" attempts resulted in the

dye being located within the medial head of the **m. triceps brachii**. They concluded that the OP approach, while successful in a single dog (Castiñeiras et al. 2015), was challenging to perform in cat cadavers and resulted in higher failure rates when assessed by staining of target nerves. However, as this technique has not been examined in live cats, its success in a clinical scenario using a local anesthetic solution is not currently known.

It remains much to be learned about the use, efficacy, and safety of "distal" RUMM blocks in small animal patients. Since most of the current literature surrounding RUMM blocks is based on case reports, letters to the editor, and cadaver studies, larger case series and prospective and blinded studies are needed to learn more about this potentially useful approach to providing anesthesia and analgesia for painful procedures involving the distal thoracic limb in dogs and cats.

This chapter describes a variation of previously published techniques, with the approach to all nerves involving a single needle puncture from the lateral aspect of the limb.

PATIENT SELECTION

INDICATIONS FOR THE BLOCK

Surgical procedures that may benefit from the use of an ultrasound-guided RUMM block, include repair of radius and ulna fractures, radial ostectomies for angular limb deformity correction, stabilization of carpal fractures, and carpal arthrodesis.

CONTRAINDICATIONS

- Skin infection or other lesions at the intended puncture site.

- Peripheral nerve disease affecting the thoracic limb.

- Small patient sizes (i.e. small breed dogs and cats, approx. <5 kg) can present technical challenges. Use of a small-footprint linear ultrasound transducer (25 mm or "hockey stick") and/or standoff may be necessary.

- Allergic reactions to local anesthetics.

POTENTIAL SIDE EFFECTS AND COMPLICATIONS

- Due to the presence of the brachial vessels within the brachial sheath, there is potential for the needle to puncture the artery and/or vein as is advanced towards the **ulnar**, **median**, and **musculocutaneous nerves**, resulting in hemorrhage and/or hematoma formation.

- If a vessel is punctured without the anesthetist recognizing the issue and a local anesthetic is administered at an excessive dose, there is potential for local anesthetic systemic toxicity (LAST).

- Visualization of the needle as it is being advanced toward the target nerves located in the medial aspect of the limb (**ulnar**, **median**, and **musculocutaneous nerves**) can be challenging due to the steep angle that this approach sometimes requires relative to the transducer. It is important that the needle tip is able to be identified as it is being advanced.

- Depending on the level along the brachium where the block is executed, motor function of the elbow may be lost. However, since shoulder function will be maintained, patients will still be able to stabilize themselves in sternal recumbency.

TIP

If the needle tip cannot be clearly identified, injection of small volumes of saline may help reveal its location. As the needle tip contacts the neurovascular sheath, a deflection of this sheath as well as slight resistance will be noticed. As the needle tip penetrates the sheath, a "click or pop" will usually be felt.

GENERAL CONSIDERATIONS
CLINICAL ANATOMY

The **radial nerve** crosses from the medial aspect of the limb (in the axillary area) to the lateral aspect of the limb between the *medialis* and *lateralis capitis* of the *m. triceps brachii* and the *m. brachialis* at the level of the mid-humerus. The **ulnar**, **median**, and **musculocutaneous nerves** and the brachial vessels are contained within the brachial sheath and run together along the medial aspect of the limb (Figure 10.1).

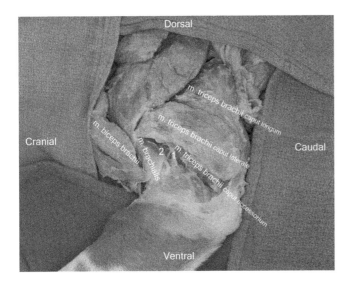

FIGURE 10.1   Dissection of the left tricipital region of a dog in right lateral recumbency. The *m. triceps brachii caput laterale* has been retracted caudally to expose the **radial nerve** (1) **deep branch**; (2) **superficial branches, lateral, and medial**) visible between *m. brachialis*, *mm. triceps brachii-caput accessorium* and *caput laterale*.

EXPECTED DISTRIBUTION OF ANESTHESIA

A successful RUMM block will provide anesthesia for procedures involving structures distal to the elbow.

LOCAL ANESTHETIC: DOSE, VOLUME, AND CONCENTRATION

Any local anesthetic (e.g. bupivacaine, ropivacaine, and levobupivacaine) can be used to perform a RUMM block, with or without the coadministration of an adjuvant (e.g. dexmedetomidine, dexamethasone, and buprenorphine).

Portela et al. (2013) recommended using volumes of $0.1\,ml\,kg^{-1}$ for the **radial nerve** and $0.05\,ml\,kg^{-1}$ for the **ulnar**, **median**, and **musculocutaneous nerves**. Castiñeiras et al. (2015) used $0.18\,ml\,kg^{-1}$. The authors most commonly use bupivacaine 0.5% or ropivacaine 0.5% at a total volume of 0.2–$0.4\,ml\,kg^{-1}$, with or without the addition of dexmedetomidine ($1\,\mu g\,ml^{-1}$), depending on the size of the patient (i.e. lower relative volumes for larger patients).

PATIENT PREPARATION AND POSITIONING

The patient should be positioned in lateral recumbency with the leg to be blocked uppermost and extended in a natural position. The leg should be clipped free of hair and standard surgical preparation of the skin over the injection site should be performed.

STEP-BY-STEP PERFORMANCE
SURFACE ANATOMY AND LANDMARKS TO BE USED

The ultrasound transducer should initially be positioned on the lateral aspect of the thoracic limb at the level of mid-humerus, centered over the *m. triceps brachii* (Figure 10.2). The transducer should be positioned perpendicular to the humerus to provide a short-axis view of the bone and radial nerve with the marker oriented cranially. This allows the needle to have the same orientation on the ultrasound screen as it is advanced in a caudal-to-cranial trajectory (i.e. for right-handed anesthetists).

ULTRASOUND ANATOMY

The **radial nerve** should be observed at its location between the *mm. brachialis, triceps brachii caput laterale, mediale,* and **accessorium** (Figure 10.3). Deep to the **radial nerve** (i.e. on the medial aspect of the limb), the neurovascular sheath that is formed by the *fascia brachialis* should be identified containing the brachial vessels and the **ulnar**, **median**, and **musculocutaneous nerves**. Depending on

(a)

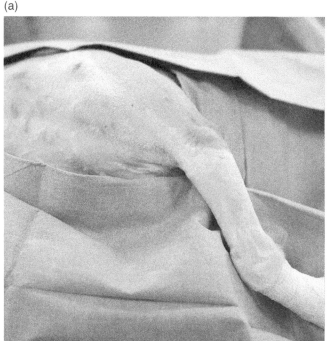

(b)

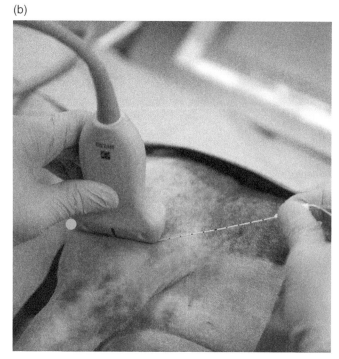

FIGURE 10.2   (a) Dog positioned in lateral recumbency for a left RUMM block. The leg is extended in a natural position. (b) Transducer and in-plane needle position for a left RUMM block. The ultrasound transducer is positioned over the tricipital region (*m. triceps brachii*) with the marker (green circle) oriented cranially.

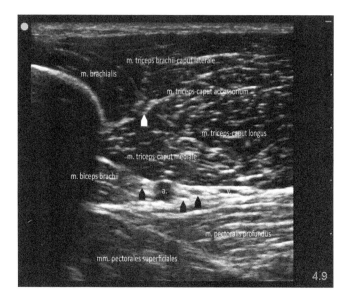

FIGURE 10.3   Ultrasound image showing the relevant anatomy for a RUMM block in a dog. The marker (green circle) is oriented cranially. Observe the position of the radial nerve (white arrowhead) between the *m. brachialis, mm. triceps brachii – caput laterale, caput accesorium*, caput longus, and *caput mediale*. Deep to the radial nerve, the neurovascular sheath can be seen containing the brachial artery (a.) and brachial vein (v.) as well as the **musculocutaneous** (cranial to the artery), **median**, and **ulnar nerves** (located between the artery and vein) (black arrowheads).

the amount of pressure being applied to the transducer on the limb, the vein may be compressed and may not always be seen. At this level, the **musculocutaneous nerve** can usually be identified cranial to the artery, whereas the **ulnar** and **median nerves** will be found caudal to it. The *m. biceps brachii* can be observed cranial to the neurovascular sheath whereas the *m. triceps brachii caput longum* can be observed caudal to it (or maybe outside the field of view, depending on the size of the patient). Color Doppler can be used to highlight the location of the brachial vessels.

NEEDLE INSERTION TECHNIQUE

The needle puncture will be on the lateral aspect of the mid-humerus (Figure 10.2b). The needle should initially be advanced on a caudal-to-cranial trajectory toward the **radial nerve** (Figure 10.4). A caudal approach avoids the humerus, making needle advancement easier.

After injection around the **radial nerve** is completed, the needle should be slightly withdrawn and redirected medially toward the neurovascular sheath that was previously identified on the medial aspect of the limb. At this point, increasing the depth on the ultrasound machine may be necessary to visualize the medial aspect and the neurovascular sheath. The tip of the needle should be carefully introduced into neurovascular sheath, avoiding the brachial (a)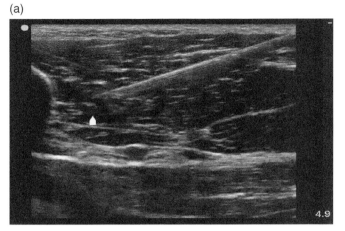

(b)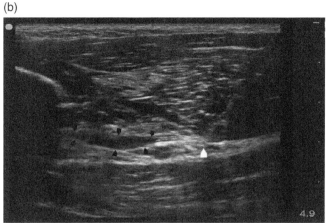

FIGURE 10.4   (a) Ultrasound image of a **radial nerve** block in a dog. The marker (green circle) is oriented cranially. Observe the tip of the needle in proximity to the radial nerve (white arrowhead). The local anesthetic injected (seen as a hypoechoic pocket) is surrounding the nerve. (b) Ultrasound image of an **ulnar**, **median**, and **musculocutaneous** nerve block in the same dog. Observe the tip of the needle (white arrowhead) penetrating the neurovascular sheath. Note that some of the local anesthetic is located outside the sheath (black arrowheads).

vessels. A palpable "click" or "pop" sensation may be appreciated by the anesthetist as the needle tip penetrates the sheath, which may also be simultaneously visualized occurring on the ultrasound screen.

EXPECTED MOTOR RESPONSES FROM NERVE STIMULATION

If nerve stimulation is being used, when the needle tip comes in close proximity to the **radial nerve**, extension of the carpus and/or digits may be observed. Depending on the position of the needle tip within the neurovascular sheath and whether the **ulnar**, **median**, and **musculocutaneous nerves** are being stimulated, either elbow flexion (i.e. **musculocutaneous nerve**) or internal rotation of the antebrachium, and/or carpal or digital flexion (i.e. **median** and/or **ulnar nerves**) may be observed.

ADMINISTRATION OF LOCAL ANESTHETIC – WHAT TO LOOK FOR, WHAT TO FEEL FOR, AND DECISION POINTS

Once the tip of the needle is positioned adjacent to the **radial nerve** and a negative aspiration test has been performed, 0.1–0.15 ml kg^{-1} of local anesthetic solution can be administered. No resistance to injection should be appreciated and the needle can be carefully manipulated to make sure that the local anesthetic disperses around the nerve. After the needle has been repositioned within the brachial sheath to block the **musculocutaneous**, **median**, and **ulnar nerves**, distention of the sheath should be appreciated as 0.05 ml kg^{-1} of local anesthetic solution is injected around each of the nerves (Figure 10.4b).

BLOCK EFFECTS AND PATIENT MANAGEMENT

This block will cause paralysis of the carpus and perhaps the elbow. Until the block has worn off, larger patients may require assistance (e.g. use of a sling) when being walked.

COMPLICATIONS AND HOW TO AVOID THEM

Close monitoring of needle position using ultrasound is crucial to patient safety and success of this block. As described, since the use of a steep trajectory can make a needle hard to visualize (Figure 10.4b), it is possible to inadvertently puncture the brachial vessels (especially the vein) as the needle is being advanced into the neurovascular bundle during performance of the **UMM** (**ulnar**, **median**, and **musculocutaneous**) **nerve** block. Use of color Doppler may be helpful for verifying the location of the brachial vessels before advancing the needle into this location.

Negative blood aspiration should be verified prior to drug administration to minimize the chances of inadvertently performing an intravascular injection.

COMMON MISTAKES AND HOW TO AVOID THEM

A common mistake is to inject the local anesthetic solution outside the neurovascular sheath into the ***m. triceps*** during the second part of this block (i.e. blockade of the **UMM nerves**). Injection of a small amount of injectate can be used to distend the sheath, verifying correct needle position prior to administration of the full volume of local anesthetic at this location.

HOW TO TALK TO CLIENTS/PROFESSIONAL COLLEAGUES

- For an experienced anesthetist, a RUMM block should take less than five minutes to perform.

- Depending on the local anesthetic solution that is used, a RUMM block will provide analgesia to the affected area for up to 18–24 hours.

- Additional pain management in the postoperative period should include icing of the incision site (e.g. 15 minutes, 3–4 times a day) and administration of oral analgesics (e.g. NSAIDs and pregabalin) for the following 5–7 days.

- Patients are usually able to walk immediately following recovery from anesthesia and can eat four to six hours post recovery and should be able to void.

- Motor deficits will be observed at the level of the carpus, and perhaps the elbow. Since the block is performed at the mid-brachium, shoulder function will be preserved.

REFERENCES

Bortolami E, Love EJ, Harcourt-Brown TR et al. (2012) Use of a midhumeral block of the radial, ulnar, musculocutaneous and median (RUMM block) nerves for extensor carpi radialis muscle biopsy in a conscious dog with generalized neuro-muscular disease. Vet Anaesth Analg 39, 446–447.

Castiñeiras D, Viscasillas J, Seymour C (2015) A modified approach for performing ultrasound-guided radial, ulnar, median and musculocutaneous nerve block in a dog. Vet Anaesth Analg 42, 659–661.

Lamont, L, Lemke K (2008) The effects of medetomidine on radial nerve blockade with mepivacaine in dogs. Vet Anaesth Analg 35, 62–68.

Leung JBY, Rodrigo-Mocholi D, Martinez-Taboada F (2019) In-plane and out-of-plane needle insertion comparison for a novel lateral block of the radial, ulnar, median and musculocutaneous nerves in cats. Vet Anaesth Analg 46, 523–528.

Portela DA, Raschi A, Otero PE (2013) Ultrasound guided mid-humeral block of the radial, ulnar, median and musculocutaneous (RUMM block) nerves in a dog with traumatic exposed metacarpal luxation. Vet Anaesth Analg 40, 552–554.

Trumpatori BJ, Carter JE, Hash J et al. (2010) Evaluation of a midhumeral block of the radial, ulnar, musculocutaneous and median (RUMM block) nerves for analgesia of the distal aspect of the thoracic limb in dogs. Vet Surg 39, 785–796.

The Thoracic Spinal Nerves: Overview and Functional Anatomy

Diego A. Portela and Marta Romano

OVERVIEW

Thoracic spinal nerves are responsible for the somatic, visceral and motor innervation of the thorax and the cranial abdomen. The cutaneous sensory innervation of each spinal nerve supplies a variable area which overlaps with the area of innervation of the immediate cranial and caudal spinal nerves (Bailey et al. 1984). Similar to spinal nerves that serve other anatomical regions, the thoracic spinal nerves can be divided into four anatomical segments – roots, main trunk, primary branches, and peripheral branches (Evans and de Lahunta 2013) (Figure 11.1). Thoracic **spinal nerves** give off four main branches – a **meningeal branch**, a **dorsal primary branch**, the **ramus communicans**, and a **ventral primary branch** (Figure 11.2). Each pair of thoracic spinal nerves is named based on the vertebral body that lies cranial to the intervertebral foramen through which they leave the vertebral canal (i.e. the T12 spinal nerve leaves the spinal canal through the intervertebral foramen located between T12 and T13).

The thoracic spinal nerves send muscular and sensory branches to the thoracic wall, including the skin, muscles, ribs, and the underlying parietal pleura. The last six or seven thoracic spinal nerves also provide innervation to the abdomen, including the skin of the cranial and ventrolateral abdominal wall, the abdominal muscles, and the underlying parietal peritoneum. The thoracic spinal nerves also supply the innervation of the visceral contents of the thorax and abdomen via the sympathetic trunk.

SPINAL NERVE ANATOMY

In dogs and cats, there are 13 pairs of thoracic spinal nerves. In addition to their other functions, the first two pairs of nerves (i.e. T1 and T2) participate in the formation of the brachial plexus, while the 9th, 10th, 11th, 12th, and 13th (the costoabdominal nerve) spinal nerves contribute to the innervation of the cranial abdominal wall.

The spinal nerves originate from the dorsal and ventral nerve roots, which transmit afferent and efferent information, respectively. The dorsal root (with its corresponding spinal ganglion) and ventral root connect to the spinal cord via the spinal rootlets lying within the spinal canal. Before leaving the intervertebral foramen, the dorsal and ventral roots converge to form the main trunk of the spinal nerve, which therefore contains both sensory and motor fibers (Figure 11.1).

The main trunk of the spinal nerve gives off a meningeal branch before leaving the vertebral canal. The meningeal branch, also known as the **sinu-vertebral nerve,** provides sensory and sympathetic innervation of the dura mater, the dorsal longitudinal ligament, the annulus fibrosus of the intervertebral disk, and blood vessels located within the vertebral canal (Evans and de Lahunta 2013). The meningeal branch connects to the sympathetic trunk through the *ramus communicans* and this circuitry seems to participate in nociceptive transmission in humans with chronic back pain (Raoul et al. 2003).

After the main trunk of the spinal nerve emerges from the intervertebral foramen, it runs through the thoracic paravertebral space, giving off the **dorsal primary branch** and the *ramus communicans* before continuing laterodistally as the **ventral primary branch** (Figure 11.2). When the main trunk leaves the intervertebral foramen, it is covered by evaginations of the periosteum that lines the vertebral canal (the epidural membrane), which forms a circumferential sleeve around the spinal nerve. In dogs, the length of these evaginations ranges from 0.5 to 2 cm in the lumbar spinal nerves (Breit et al. 2013). The deep layer of the thoracolumbar fascia forms the superficial layer of the circumferential sleeve and continues as the epineurium of the spinal nerve.

The **dorsal primary branch** leaves the main trunk of the spinal nerve and runs dorsocaudally between *mm. multifidus thoracis* and *levator costalis* where it gives off **medial** and **lateral branches** (Figure 11.3). In some dogs, an intermediate **muscular branch** can be found innervating the *m. longissimus thoracis* (Forsythe and Ghoshal 1984).

The **medial branch** travels dorsally between *mm. multifidus thoracis* and *longissimus thoracis* (Chua and Bogduk 1995), providing sensory innervation to the vertebral lamina, ligaments, and facet joints. The medial branch also provides motor supply to *mm. multifidus thoracis*, *longissimus thoracis*, *spinalis,* and *semispinalis* but does not provide any cutaneous innervation (Forsythe and Ghoshal 1984; Binder and Nampiaparampil 2009).

Small Animal Regional Anesthesia and Analgesia, Second Edition. Edited by Matt Read, Luis Campoy, and Berit Fischer.
© 2024 John Wiley & Sons, Inc. Published 2024 by John Wiley & Sons, Inc.

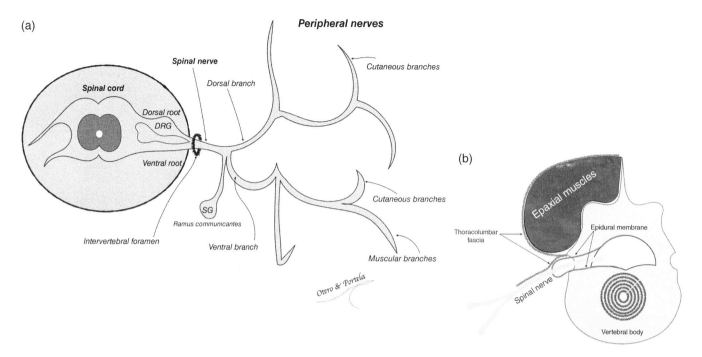

FIGURE 11.1   (a) Schematic representation of the components of a thoracic spinal nerve, indicating the rootlets, roots, main trunk, and the four primary branches. DRG, dorsal root ganglion; SG, sympathetic ganglion. (b) Schematic representation of the perineural sleeve that covers the spinal nerve formed by the epidural membrane (continuation of the internal periosteum from the vertebral canal) and the thoracolumbar fascia. Source: (b) based on Breit et al. (2013).

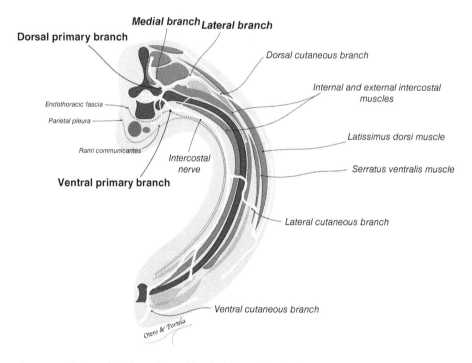

FIGURE 11.2   Schematic representation of the branching of the fifth thoracic spinal nerve.

The **lateral branch** is the direct continuation of the primary dorsal branch of each spinal nerve and runs caudolaterally with a slight dorsal orientation between the *mm. longissimus thoracis*, *levator costalis*, and *iliocostalis thoracis* (Figure 11.3). The lateral branch pierces the thoracolumbar fascia and the *mm. serratus dorsalis*, *latissimus dorsi*, and *cutaneous trunci*, providing motor innervation to these muscles before finally reaching the skin where it divides into **dorsal**

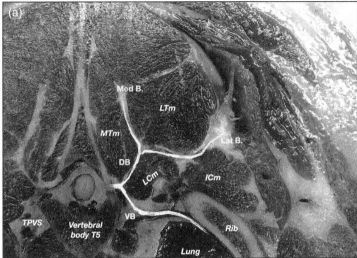
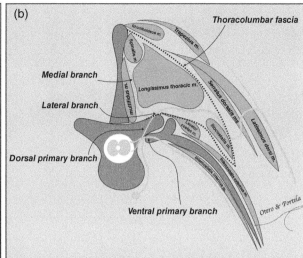

FIGURE 11.3   (a) Cross section of the trunk at the level of the fifth thoracic vertebra and (b) schematic representation of the branching of the fifth thoracic spinal nerve. DB, **dorsal branch**; ICm, *m. iliocostalis thoracis*; Lat B, **lateral branch**; LCm, *m. levator costalis*; LTm, *m. longissimus thoracis*; Med B, **medial branch**; MTm, *m. multifidus thoracis*; TPVS, thoracic paravertebral space; VB, **ventral branch**. Source: Image by Pablo Otero and Diego Portela (author).

and **ventral cutaneous branches** (Bailey et al. 1984) (Figure 11.3). These two sensory cutaneous branches supply the skin of the dorsal and dorsolateral aspects of the thoracic body wall.

After the main trunk of the spinal nerve gives off the **dorsal primary branch**, it continues laterally into the thoracic paravertebral space where it gives off the preganglionic fibers (*ramus communicans*) to the sympathetic trunk. The *rami communicantes* and the sympathetic trunk are part of the sympathetic nervous system and carry general visceral afferent and efferent axons to and from thoracic and abdominal visceral structures (Evans and de Lahunta 2013). They also participate in the autonomic innervation of the blood vessels and in the transmission of visceral pain. Autonomic innervation is primarily responsible for maintaining visceral functions and controlling vascular tone.

It is well-recognized in humans that the sympathetic nervous system also plays a role in the generation and persistence of pain in clinical conditions such as complex regional pain syndrome (Rho et al. 2002; Jänig and Baron 2007). In fact, neuroablation of the sympathetic chain has been successfully used to treat visceral (Day 2008) and non-visceral chronic pain such as lower back pain (Rigaud et al. 2012).

The role of the sympathetic nervous system in the modulation of chronic pain seems to depend on the preexistence of primary afferents sensitized by trauma or inflammation, with no effect on acute pain (Bantel and Trapp 2011). Acute nociceptive pain was believed to be transmitted only through the somatic nervous system; however, this concept has been challenged by McDonnell et al. (2011) who showed that preoperative blockade of the sympathetic stellate ganglion in humans undergoing major upper limb surgery resulted in a significant reduction in postoperative pain scores and opioid

consumption. At present, the contributions of the sympathetic nervous system to the modulation of acute pain are not fully understood and more studies are needed to understand if sympathetic blockade has a clinical effect on the management of acute pain in companion animals.

The **ventral primary branch** is the continuation of the main trunk of each spinal nerve and travels laterally across the thoracic paravertebral space, dorsal to the endothoracic fascia, and ventral to the internal intercostal membrane to reach the caudal aspect of the corresponding rib where it becomes the **intercostal nerve** (Figure 11.4). The **intercostal nerves** are initially embedded in the deep fibers of *mm. intercostalis internus* before they emerge at their deep surface, superficial to the endothoracic fascia which lies interposed between the nerves and the parietal pleura. Distal to this, the **intercostal nerves** are located along the caudomedial aspect of their corresponding ribs within neurovascular bundles, where their associated intercostal arteries and veins can also be found (Figure 11.4).

The **intercostal nerves** provide motor innervation to *mm. serratus dorsalis*, *intercostalis internus,* and *intercostalis externus*. The last eight **intercostal nerves** also supply motor innervation to the muscles of the abdominal wall.

At the level of the axillary line, the T2–T12 **intercostal nerves** give off lateral cutaneous branches, which run distally between the *mm. intercostalis internus* and *intercostalis externus*. These **lateral cutaneous branches** then pierce the *m. intercostalis externus* and the ventral insertion of the *m. serratus ventralis* before continuing distally, deep to the *m. latissimus dorsi*. At the level of the ventral margin of the *m. latissimus dorsi*, the **lateral cutaneous branch** divides into dorsal and ventral branches that innervate the lateroventral aspects of the thoracic wall, except for a narrow

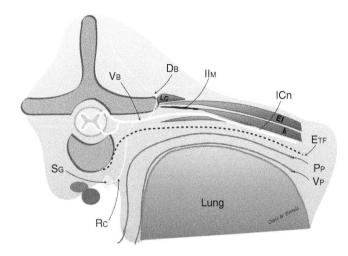

FIGURE 11.4 Schematic representation of the cross section of the thoracic paravertebral space at the level of the fifth thoracic vertebra. EI: *m. intercostalis externus*; ETF: endothoracic fascia; ICn: **intercostal nerve**; Ii: *m. intercostalis internus*; IIM: internal intercostal membrane; LC: *m. levator costalis*; PP: parietal pleura; RC: **ramus communicans**; SG: sympathetic ganglion; VP: visceral pleura. Source: Image by Pablo Otero and Diego Portela (author).

strip over the ventral midline (Bailey et al. 1984) (Figure 11.2). The dorsal branches of the lateral cutaneous branch do not extend dorsally beyond the axillary line. The caudal-most **intercostal nerves** (T8–T12 nerves) cross the costal arch and course towards the ventral abdominal midline between the *m. transversus abdominis* and the *mm. obliquus internus abdominis* or *rectus abdominis* in this region of the body.

The **intercostal nerves** that arise from the T2–T4 spinal nerves form the **cranial** and **caudal intercostobrachial**

nerves. These nerves innervate the caudolateral aspect of the scapula and brachium, the thoracic wall, and a small portion of the medial aspect of the brachium (Bailey et al. 1984).

The ventral cutaneous branches are the distal continuations of the T2–T10 **intercostal nerves** (Figure 11.2). Depending on the spinal level, the ventral cutaneous branches penetrate the belly or tendon of the *m. rectus abdominis* then pierce the superficial thoracic fascia and *mm. pectorales superficiales* and *pectoralis profundus,* before arborizing in the skin along the ventral thoracic midline (Bailey et al. 1984). The perforating branches of the internal thoracic artery run together with the ventral cutaneous branches of the **intercostal nerves**. It should be noted that there are no ventral cutaneous branches from the T11–L3 nerves and sensory innervation to the ventral midline at this location is supplied by the ventral extensions/branches of their respective lateral cutaneous branches.

There are a couple of exceptions to the aforementioned general descriptions of the anatomy of the thoracic spinal nerves. The first (T1) thoracic spinal nerve has a different anatomical configuration as it contributes to the formation of the brachial plexus and does not have a thoracic cutaneous branch like other thoracic nerves do (Evans and de Lahunta 2013). Additionally, the ventral branch of the last thoracic spinal nerve (T13) is referred to as the **costoabdominal nerve,** and it runs between the *mm. transversus abdominis* and *obliquus internus abdominis*, with anatomical features that more closely resemble those of the lumbar spinal nerves (Castañeda-Herrera et al. 2017). The **costoabdominal nerve** gives off a lateral cutaneous branch that divides into dorsal and ventral branches that supply the areas caudal and adjacent to the last rib, extending towards the ventral midline (Bailey et al. 1984).

REFERENCES

Bailey CS, Kitchell RL, Haghighi SS et al. (1984) Cutaneous innervation of the thorax and abdomen of the dog. Am J Vet Res 45, 1689–1698.

Bantel C, Trapp S (2011) The role of the autonomic nervous system in acute surgical pain processing - what do we know? Anaesthesia 66, 541–544.

Binder DS, Nampiaparampil DE (2009) The provocative lumbar facet joint. Curr Rev Musculoskelet Med 2, 15–24.

Breit S, Giebels F, Kneissl S (2013) Foraminal and paraspinal extraforaminal attachments of the sixth and seventh lumbar spinal nerves in large breed dogs. Vet J 197, 631–638.

Castañeda-Herrera FE, Buriticá-Gaviria EF, Echeverry-Bonilla DF (2017) Anatomical evaluation of the thoracolumbar nerves related to the transversus abdominis plane block technique in the dog. Anat Histol Embryol 46, 373–377.

Chua WH, Bogduk N (1995) The surgical anatomy of thoracic facet denervation. Acta Neurochir 136, 140–144.

Day M (2008) Sympathetic blocks: the evidence. Pain Pract 8, 98–109.

Evans HE, de Lahunta A (2013) Chapter 17 – The spinal nerves. In: Miller's Anatomy of the Dog, 4th edition. Evans HE, de Lahunta A (ed.) Elsevier Saunders, St Louis, MI, USA. pp. 611–657.

Forsythe WB, Ghoshal NG (1984) Innervation of the canine thoracolumbar vertebral column. Anat Rec 208, 57–63.

Jänig W, Baron R (2007) Sympathetic nervous system and pain. In: Encyclopedia of Pain. Schmidt R., Willis W. (eds.) Springer, Heidelberg, Berlin.

McDonnell JG, Finnerty O, Laffey JG (2011) Stellate ganglion blockade for analgesia following upper limb surgery. Anaesthesia 66, 611–614.

Raoul S, Faure A, Robert R et al. (2003) Role of the sinuvertebral nerve in low back pain and anatomical basis of therapeutic implications. Surg Radiol Anat 24, 366–371.

Rho RH, Brewer RP, Lamer TJ et al. Complex regional pain syndrome. Mayo Clin Proc 2002; 77, 174–80.

Rigaud J, Riant T, Labat JJ et al. (2012) Is section of the sympathetic rami communicantes by laparoscopy in patients with refractory low back pain efficient? Eur Spine J 22, 775–781.

Introduction to Fascial Plane Blocks

Berit L. Fischer

CHAPTER 12

INTRODUCTION

As ultrasound-guided locoregional anesthesia has increased in popularity, the ability to perform a special group of blocks, known as fascial plane blocks (FPBs), has followed. These blocks involve the deposition of local anesthetic solution into potential spaces between opposing sheets of connective tissue (i.e. fasciae), that serve as conduits or channels for nerves as they travel from the spinal cord to their sites of innervation (Elsharkawy et al. 2018; Chin et al. 2021b). The theory behind targeting fascial planes, as opposed to individual peripheral nerves themselves, is that the injectate will spread widely within the space with limited outward diffusion, bathing the nerves and inducing conduction blockade across a larger area than would otherwise be blocked (Chin et al. 2021b). While FPBs were historically attempted using blind techniques that relied solely on "feel," the use of ultrasound guidance has exponentially advanced our understanding of these techniques, allowing them to be performed with more precision and higher success rates. The following chapters describe several of the FPBs that are already in relatively widespread clinical use in small animal anesthesia, as well as some of those that are still in development. This chapter will introduce the reader to FPBs, their proposed mechanisms of action, and what their utility may be within the realm of locoregional anesthesia.

WHAT IS FASCIA?

Grossly, fasciae are sheets of connective tissue that surround and encompass all the structures of the body (Figure 12.1). Anatomical descriptions most often refer to three different layers of fasciae – superficial fasciae that lie just under the dermis, deep fasciae that encase muscles and neurovascular structures, eventually terminating as tendons, ligaments, and periosteum, and visceral fasciae that overly the organs of the body (Benjamin 2009; Chin et al. 2021b). Some variations of these descriptions exist; however, the nomenclature is less important than understanding that, when performing FPBs, it is the space between the two layers of deep fasciae that is the target.

Histologically, this connective tissue is formed from a varying number of organized collagen layers intermixed with adipose tissue, fibroblasts, and hyaluronic acid (Chin et al. 2021b). In dogs, similar to humans, these layers are loosely connected to one another by additional collagen fibers that are organized in transverse and/or oblique orientations, acting as scaffolds. This loose arrangement allows the layers to be easily separated through hydrodissection when performing regional blocks and plays a role in the dispersion of the local anesthetic solution (Ahmed et al. 2019; Chin et al. 2021b).

Species differences exist as demonstrated by Ahmed et al. (2019), who compared gross and histologic samples of fasciae from horses, dogs, and humans. They found that the arrangement of layers, presence or absence of adipose tissue, and number of contractile elements were very similar between dogs and humans, but that they differed from those found in horses. These differences were attributed to the different biomechanical needs of each species, with horses demonstrating a more compact collagen arrangement, less insulating adipose tissue, and more contractile elements that are made to withstand large amounts of force transmission throughout the body (Ahmed et al. 2019).

From a functional standpoint, fasciae have traditionally been viewed as shock absorbers, allowing muscles to glide along one another and transmit ground forces. They are thought to also play a role in proprioception and coordination of muscle function, as well as assisting blood and lymphatic flow via a "muscle pump" mechanism (Benjamin 2009; Willard et al. 2012). More recently, fasciae have started to become thought of almost as a separate organ that is richly innervated with both sensory and proprioceptive nerve fibers. While not fully elucidated in veterinary species, this innervation may allow fasciae to become a source of pain when they are inflamed or constricted (Benjamin 2009; Willard et al. 2012).

FASCIAL PLANE BLOCKS

FPBs were originally developed as alternatives to neuraxial techniques for providing regional analgesia to the trunk. The primary difference between these techniques is that several FPBs target spinal nerve branches at distal sites along their course after they exit the vertebral foraminae, and often after the *ramus communicans* has left the ventral branch to connect with the sympathetic chain in thoracolumbar spinal segments (Figure 12.2). This may be viewed as beneficial since neuraxial techniques can be associated with undesirable side effects

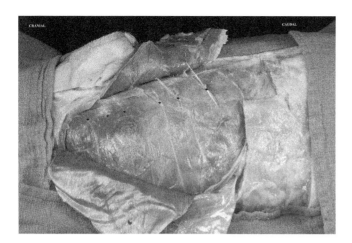

FIGURE 12.1   The thorax of a dog cadaver. The lateral cutaneous branches of thoracic spinal nerves (black stars) are visualized running from dorsal to ventral. The ***mm. cutaneous trunci*** and ***latissimus dorsi*** have been reflected dorsally.

such as hypotension and bradycardia, that result from widespread blockade of sympathetic efferent nerves (Holte et al. 2004).

Many of the body's fascial sheets become contiguous with one another, both cranial to caudal and dorsal to ventral (e.g. endothoracic, transversalis, and thoracolumbar fasciae). As a result, the same target fascial plane (and spinal nerves) can usually be accessed by using one of several different approaches, albeit with possible variations in the structures, level, and degree of sensory block achieved (Shao et al. 2022). As opposed to neuraxial anesthesia, this allows the anesthetist to exert a degree of titration with regards to block effects, by depositing local anesthetics closer to the area of interest.

The interest in and use of FPBs in veterinary medicine has increased dramatically over the past decade, as demonstrated by rapid growth in the number of research studies and related publications. Prior to 2013, only three articles, all relating to transversus abdominis plane (TAP) blocks, had been published on these types of locoregional blocks in veterinary literature (Schroeder et al. 2010, 2011; Bruggink et al. 2012). From 2013 to 2023, however, this number increased exponentially to more than eighty citations dedicated to the subject (Google Scholar). While small in comparison to the 900+ publications in human medicine during the same time period, it is worth noting that ultrasound-guided FPBs in humans were just beginning to be described in the mid-2000s (Hebbard et al. 2007; Machi and Joshi 2019). It would, therefore, be expected that veterinary publications will follow suit and continue to be of growing interest over the next decade.

RELEVANT ANATOMY FOR FASCIAL PLANE BLOCKS

As with any peripheral nerve block, the performance of ultrasound-guided FPBs requires a thorough understanding of anatomy and the innervation that is associated with the

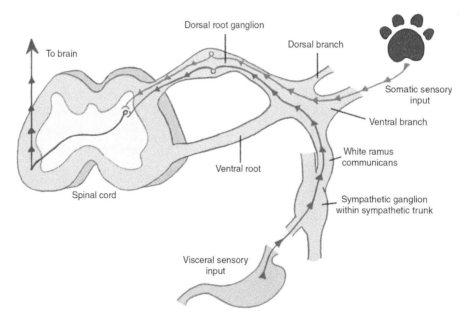

FIGURE 12.2   Diagram of a spinal nerve. Dorsal and ventral roots converge prior to exiting the vertebral foramen to form the spinal nerve. Somatic afferent fibers with their cell bodies in the dorsal root ganglion travel via dorsal and ventral branches to their sites of innervation including skin, muscle, and bone. Visceral afferents travel from their organ of origin through autonomic ganglia, entering the sympathetic chain and traveling through the *rami communicantes* to join somatic afferent sensory nerves before entering the dorsal horn of the spinal cord. Source: Image from Abigail L. Fischer. Used with permission.

area of interest. Fortunately, the anatomy of the trunk in dogs and cats is somewhat similar, with innervation of the thorax and abdomen being supplied by the branches of the T2–L3 spinal nerves (Hekmatpanah 1961; Hermanson et al. 2020; Garbin et al. 2022) (Figures 12.3). Although this arrangement is similar in most cases, minor anatomical differences, both within and between species, exist.

To date, the most studied differences in small animals relate to the anatomic variations of the spinal nerves that are located within the TAP. In a study that examined the spinal nerve contributions to the TAP in 10 dog cadavers, Castañeda-Herrera et al. (2017) found that T10–L3 were consistently present within the transversus abdominus plane, with varying contributions from T9 (95%), T8 (60%), and T7 (20%). Similar findings were demonstrated in cats, where anatomical dissections demonstrated that T9 was located within the TAP in 12/16 cats, and L3 was only observed reaching the abdomen in 1/16 cats (Garbin et al. 2022). While other factors can also impact overall block efficacy, these studies suggest that anatomic variations will also undoubtedly contribute to the success of a block. Variations in thoracic innervation are possible, however, literature documenting them in veterinary species is still lacking. For a full description of the anatomic features of thoracic spinal nerves, the reader is referred to Chapter 11.

MECHANISMS OF ACTION

Currently, much of what is known and assumed in the veterinary literature regarding sensory blockade following FPBs is the result of dye studies in cadavers. After injections have been completed, dissections are performed, and investigators use the number of stained nerves and the degree of stain uptake to predict which dermatomes would have likely been desensitized in a live animal (Figure 12.4). Randomized, controlled trials in humans following FPBs have found that, despite evidence of variable cutaneous blockade, patients

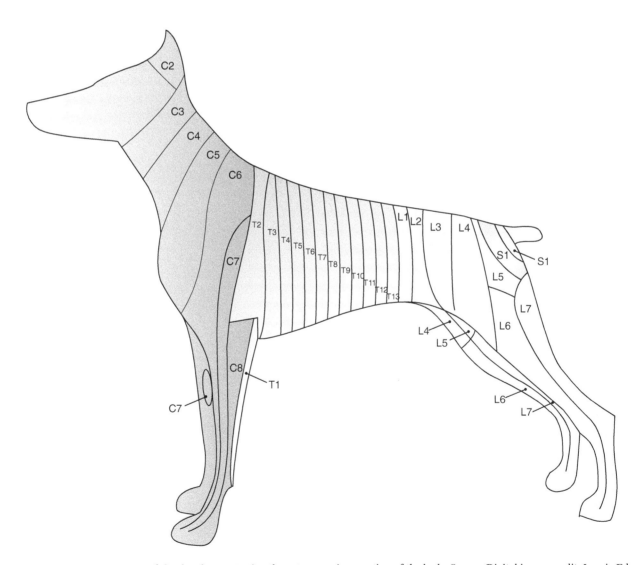

FIGURE 12.3   Dermatome map of the dog demonstrating the cutaneous innervation of the body. Source: Digital image credit: Laurie Edge Hughes and Peter Jenkins. Used with permission.

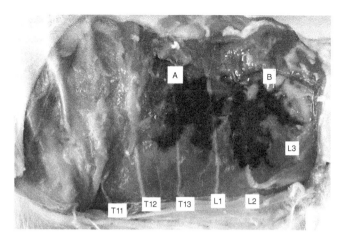

FIGURE 12.4 Dissection of the abdominal wall of a canine cadaver following injection of methylene blue within the transversus abdominis plane. Two separate injections (A and B) were performed, resulting in staining of T13–L3. Source: From Johnson et al. (2018). Used with permission.

often demonstrate good pain control and decreased opioid consumption during surgery and post-operatively (Baeriswyl et al. 2015; Støving et al. 2015; Visoiu and Scholz 2019). This suggests that FPBs may provide some of their analgesic effects through alternative mechanisms.

Several possible mechanisms for these analgesic effects have been proposed. Each proposed mechanism stems from the assumption that local anesthetic molecules behave in one of three ways following injection into the fascial plane – local spread within the confines of the fascial plane, diffusion across the fascia into surrounding tissues, or absorption by the vasculature to elicit effects at distant sites (Chin et al. 2021a).

LOCAL SPREAD

One aspect of FPBs that is undisputed is that the spread of a local anesthetic solution around the nerves lying within an interfascial plane leads to cutaneous sensory blockade. The spread and the subsequent block may be variable and are determined by several factors, including the bulk flow of the injectate, the specific composition and confines of the fascia itself, and the concentration and volume of the local anesthetic solution that was used (Bruggink et al. 2012; Elsharkawy et al. 2018; Chin et al. 2021a).

Bulk flow

The bulk flow of the injectate (i.e. movement of the injected volume of local anesthetic over time) is determined by fluid dynamics and the presence of pressure differences (Davis and Kenny 2005). Since fluid flows down the path of least resistance, the specific fascial plane, the degree of muscle tone, and the injection velocity may all act as external influences that determine the final spread of the injectate (Elsharkawy et al. 2018).

Volume

Logically, one would assume that if a larger volume of solution is injected, it should result in more widespread distribution within the targeted fascial plane. This finding was confirmed by Bruggink et al. (2012) who documented that increasing the volume of dye injectate (0.25 ml kg^{-1}, 0.5 ml kg^{-1}, 0.75 ml kg^{-1}, or 1.0 ml kg^{-1}), for single, lateral TAP blocks in dog cadavers, resulted in a greater number of nerves being stained. However, this finding is not consistent among studies and may speak to fascial constraints specific to each block. For example, a feline cadaver study examined local anesthetic spread following either a single lateral or a combination of subcostal and lateral injections for TAP blocks. Those authors determined that, despite splitting the total volume in half, the use of two injections stained a significantly greater number of nerves versus a single, larger volume injection (Garbin et al. 2022).

Concentration and dose of local anesthetic

How different volumes of injectate spread within interfascial spaces is important in determining potential block efficacy, but efficacy is also influenced by other factors. In fact, several studies have found that block efficacy may be affected more by the concentration of the local anesthetic and the total dose administered, as opposed to the volume that was injected.

During TAP blocks in humans, Forero et al. (2015) showed that the same dose of ropivacaine, diluted to three different concentrations (20 ml at 0.5%, 30 ml at 0.33%, and 40 ml at 0.25%) did not significantly affect cephalad spread, and the subsequent number of nerves that were blocked. Decreasing concentrations, however, resulted in shorter duration and faster regression of the desensitized area. These results were similar to those from a study that examined the use of the same volume, but different concentrations, of ropivacaine for transversalis FPBs, with higher concentrations (0.5% and 0.6%), resulting in faster onset, longer duration, and reduced opioid consumption when compared to the lower concentration that was evaluated (0.4%) (Tian et al. 2022).

Location of FPB block

The location within the fascial plane where the local anesthetic solution is injected also plays an important role in regard to which dermatomes will be desensitized, independent of drug volume and concentration. Studies in humans have demonstrated this effect by assessing the areas of sensory block following the performance of FPBs in awake subjects. In those studies, responses to pinprick and cold stimuli are used to help determine the extent of the blocks. Investigators have found that human volunteers who received lateral TAP blocks performed with 20 ml ropivacaine (0.75%) had sensory blockade that was limited primarily to the lateral abdomen, with some inferior extension but minimal blockade of the ventral midline (Støving et al. 2015). These findings were different from those of Chen et al. (2018) who assessed the use of single, subcostal TAP blocks with the same volume and concentration of ropivacaine and found consistent desensitization of the ventral midline in all cases.

Differences in the local spread of injectate may be related to the intrinsic characteristics of the fasciae. In healthy tissue, some fascial planes are noted to converge, forming "lines of fusion" that can produce anatomical barriers (Black et al. 2021). This is best illustrated by the linea alba which acts to prevent the spread of injectate across midline, thereby necessitating the performance of bilateral FPBs in order to desensitize the abdomen. Fasciae are multi-layered and most ultrasound machines do not provide the degree of resolution that would be necessary to see the individual layers. It is therefore unknown whether the location of local anesthetic deposition within these layers could impact resistance and prevent the spread of injectate as well (Brenner et al. 2018). In addition to these inherent "natural" obstacles, barriers can also be created as demonstrated by the formation of fascial adhesions following inflammation and/or trauma (Black et al. 2021). For that reason, the efficacy of FPBs in patients with known previous trauma may be unreliable.

DIFFUSION INTO SURROUNDING TISSUES

While bulk flow principles restrict the movement of the local anesthetic within the target fascial plane, the slower process of diffusion allows local anesthetic molecules to migrate across the fasciae along their concentration gradient into neighboring tissues (Chin et al. 2021a). It is postulated that the extent of this diffusion may not be fully appreciated in cadaver studies and could be time-dependent. This effect was demonstrated in a human study that evaluated the diffusion of bupivacaine mixed with contrast (i.e. gadolinium) using MRI following unilateral T10 erector spinae plane (ESP) blocks, and correlated those results with the degree of cutaneous sensory blockade that was present (Schwartzmann et al. 2020). MRI documented the presence of contrast within the *mm. longissimus* and *multifidus*, as well as in a variable number of paravertebral (PV) spaces. Abdominal and pelvic pain was abolished in all subjects, with sensory blockade consistent with local anesthetic diffusion to the ventral rami as noted by decreased sensation to the anterior (ventral) thorax and abdomen, in addition to the expected lateral and posterior (dorsal) aspects. To further demonstrate that the spread of injectate occurs by diffusion, not just bulk flow, Visoiu and Scholz (2019) used thoracoscopic imaging of PV spaces during the performance of ESP blocks to determine if local anesthetic could be visualized entering the spaces during injection. No bulging of the PV spaces was observed. However, the patient had sensory block consistent with diffusion of local anesthetic to the ventral rami within 30 minutes of injection.

Veterinary cadaver studies have thus far failed to demonstrate consistent migration of dye through the internal intercostal membrane into PV spaces following ESP blocks, despite a retrospective study suggesting that somatic and visceral nociception was decreased during sternotomy in 10 dogs

(Ferreira et al. 2019; Otero et al. 2020; Portela et al. 2020; Ferré et al. 2022). Interestingly, Otero et al. (2020) visualized dye uptake by the prevertebral lymph nodes in pigs following ESP block. From this observation, these authors hypothesized that this uptake could point towards the lymphatic system being intimately involved with the analgesia produced by this block through its known interactions with nociceptor neurons. The results of these studies suggest that the behavior of injectate following FPBs in live subjects may differ from that of injecting dye solutions in cadavers, demonstrating that further research into the use of these blocks in animals is required.

Differential block of sensory nerves

When nerves are exposed to low concentrations of local anesthetics, some fiber types may be more sensitive to conduction blockade than others, a phenomenon known as differential or selective block. Which nerve types are most sensitive is a source of debate and is likely to be dependent on the individual local anesthetic and the concentration used (Chin et al. 2021a).

The long-acting local anesthetics commonly used for FPBs, bupivacaine and ropivacaine, demonstrate differential sensory blockade with nociceptive C-fibers being blocked prior to Aσ- (fast, pricking pain), or Aβ-fibers (light touch, pressure) (Ford et al. 1984). An experimental study in cats demonstrated this by applying two concentrations of bupivacaine (0.025% and 0.05%) to isolated saphenous nerves with recording electrodes. It was determined that when 100% of the C-fibers were effectively blocked, only ~50% and 75% of Aσ-fibers at the respective bupivacaine concentrations were blocked (Ford et al. 1984).

Clinically, this difference in sensitivity has been observed following epidural administration of local anesthetics where the dermatomal level that patients experience loss of temperature discrimination and analgesia extends further than complete sensory block (cutaneous anesthesia) (White et al. 1998). With FPBs, it has been hypothesized that this difference in nerve fiber sensitivity could explain how analgesia may exist in locations beyond that of complete sensory blockade. This discrimination of different sensations has been able to be performed in humans, however, similar clinical studies in veterinary studies are likely to be challenging.

SYSTEMIC UPTAKE OF LOCAL ANESTHETICS

Antinociceptive effects from intravenous administration of lidocaine are reported in humans and animals (Smith et al. 2004; Robertson et al. 2005; Chin et al. 2021a). Studies propose that its analgesic effects may result from multiple mechanisms of action that likely extend beyond just sodium channel blockade, including activity on multiple receptors (e.g. NMDA, muscarinic, GABA), ion channels (e.g. potassium, calcium), and the inhibition of several inflammatory mediators (Lee and Schraag 2022).

Relatively large volumes of local anesthetic solutions are often used when performing FPBs, which can lead to variable amounts of systemic uptake depending on the vascularity of the target site. It has been proposed, therefore, that systemic uptake of the local anesthetic could contribute to a supraspinal analgesic effect (Chin et al. 2021a). It is currently unknown if the long-acting local anesthetics that are commonly used for FPBs have systemic analgesic effects similar to lidocaine because of their inherently higher risk of cardiotoxicity and the lack of studies investigating their systemic use. Recently, however, ropivacaine (1.5 mg kg^{-1}) was investigated in dogs for IV regional anesthesia and found to provide longer-lasting and more complete sensory blockade following tourniquet removal than lidocaine. However, those investigators reported clinical signs compatible with CNS toxicity in 4/6 dogs in the ropivacaine group, after tourniquet release with an associated maximum mean plasma concentration (Cmax) of 1.36 µg ml^{-1} (Rastabi et al. 2021). Surprisingly, this value was below the previously reported dose and plasma concentrations of ropivacaine associated with the onset of seizures (4.88 mg kg^{-1} and 11.4 µg ml^{-1}, respectively) (Feldman et al. 1989). Garbin et al. (2022) evaluated plasma concentrations of bupivacaine in cats following TAP blocks with either 2 or 2.5 mg kg^{-1}; doses that are higher than the commonly recommended range of 1–2 mg kg^{-1}. Those authors demonstrated systemic uptake of the bupivacaine, with a Cmax of 1.17 and 1.81 µg ml^{-1} respectively, which were one-third and one-half of plasma concentrations reported to cause seizures (Garbin et al. 2022).

The relevance of these findings with regard to a systemic analgesic effect have yet to be determined in a clinical setting. As of now, whether long-acting local anesthetics provide systemic analgesia and, if so, what plasma concentration imparts these effects, is unknown.

ADVANTAGES OF FASCIAL PLANE BLOCKS

FPBs offer several benefits when compared to specific peripheral nerve blocks and neuraxial blocks.

- *Less risk of direct neural damage* –Needle insertion sites and subsequent injections are often distant from the nerves themselves.

- *Less risk of systemic side effects* –Neuraxial techniques can lead to variable degrees of sympathetic blockade, resulting in hypotension and bradycardia. FPBs are generally more selective and often performed distal to where the *ramus communicans* exits to join the sympathetic chain, thereby leaving autonomic innervation intact. The use of opioids in neuraxial blocks has also been associated with urinary retention and nausea, both of which can prolong hospital stays.

- *Minimal number of injections to block a large number of dermatomes* –Unlike other types of peripheral nerve blocks, FPBs depend on relatively large volumes of dilute local anesthetic solutions, and the continuity between fascial sheets allows for the ability to efficiently block multiple nerves with fewer injections.

- *Potential contribution to "enhanced recovery after surgery" (ERAS) protocols* – ERAS protocols have been established in human medicine as a means to improve the perioperative experience of patients, resulting in patients returning to normal function more quickly and allowing hospital discharges to occur sooner (Campoy 2022). Like other nerve blocks, FPBs are now recognized as an important part of ERAS protocols. As this concept gains further traction in veterinary medicine, it would be expected that FPBs would show similar importance.

LIMITATIONS OF FASCIAL PLANE BLOCKS

While FPBs demonstrate numerous advantages, the anesthetist needs to remain cognizant of their limitations as well.

- *Variability of sensory blockade* –As described above, local anesthetic spread within the target FP is influenced by numerous factors, including fluid dynamics and location of the injection. These factors are not always able to be predicted and individual variation should be expected. Other factors that might affect block success may include the experience of the anesthetist performing the block, the positioning of the patient, the depth of anesthesia, and changes in intrathoracic pressure that can occur during mechanical ventilation.

- *Risk of local anesthetic systemic toxicity (LAST)* –Large volumes and high doses of local anesthetics may predispose a patient to a higher risk of LAST. Patient monitoring, including ECG and arterial blood pressure, is recommended during performance of these blocks. It is important that the anesthetist be aware of clinical signs associated with CNS and cardiovascular toxicity and be ready to intervene should they occur (see Chapter 28).

- *May not provide complete analgesia* –Based on studies and clinical experience, many of the FPBs that are currently being used in veterinary medicine, specifically TAP, rectus sheath, parasternal, and serratus plane blocks, may only provide analgesia for pain arising from somatic sources (i.e. from skin, muscle, bone, etc.). For this reason, the use of these blocks as part of a multimodal analgesic approach to patient management is still recommended at this time. Further clinical studies are needed to make further recommendations.

SUMMARY

FPBs offer an alternative to neuraxial techniques for providing anesthesia and analgesia to the trunk. While many techniques are still considered to be relatively early in their development, these techniques show promise in their ability to provide more selective analgesia while minimizing side effects. Anesthetists should familiarize themselves with each of the FPBs with respect to the associated anatomy and mechanism of analgesia (Table 12.1). Further research in the form of randomized, controlled clinical studies is still needed in veterinary medicine to reveal the full potential of FPBs.

Table 12.1   Fascial plane blocks used in veterinary medicine. The reader is referred to individual chapters for full-block descriptions.

Block	Location	Nerve(s) blocked	Areas desensitized/indications
Serratus plane block Superficial/deep approaches	Perpendicular to ribs 4–5 at the level of shoulder joint *Superficial*: Fascial plane between **mm. latissimus dorsi** and **serratus ventralis thoracis**. *Deep*: Fascial plane between **mm. serratus ventralis thoracis** and **mm. intercostales externi**.	Lateral cutaneous branches of intercostal nerves T1–T6.	Somatic analgesia of hemithorax extending 4–5 rib spaces (T1–6). Mastectomies, flail chest, rib fractures, thoracotomy, thoracoscopy.
Transversus abdominis plane block	Ventral abdomen *Subcostal* approach: Fascial plane between the **mm. rectus abdominus** and **transversus abdominus** just caudal and parallel to the costal arch. *Lateral* approach: Fascial plane between **mm. internus abdominus obliquus** and **tranversus abdominus**.	Ventral branches of T9–L3 spinal nerves as they course caudoventrally.	Somatic analgesia of the ventral abdomen from T9–L3. Any procedure requiring an abdominal incision (e.g. exploratory laparotomy, ovariohysterectomy).
Rectus sheath block	Abdominal midline just cranial to the umbilicus. Fascial plane between **m. rectus abdominus** and the internal rectus sheath.	Ventral branches of spinal nerves (T11–T13) as they emerge from **m. transversus abdominus** and enter the dorsal border of **m. rectus abdominus**.	Somatic analgesia to the periumbilical region. Procedures involving periumbilical abdominal midline incision (e.g. umbilical hernia repair, laparoscopy)
Quadratus lumborum block	Just caudal to the last rib, at the level of the hypaxial musculature. Several approaches described targeting the thoracolumbar fascia as it surrounds **m. quadratus lumborum**.	Ventral rami of (T12, T13) L1–L3 (L4). Blocks visceral afferents in the sympathetic chain to provide visceral analgesia.	Somatic and visceral analgesia of the cranial abdomen. Any procedure requiring an abdominal incision (e.g. ovariohysterectomy cholecystectomies, nephrectomy, cystotomy); abdominal pain caused by pancreatitis, cholelithiasis, etc . . .
Erector spinae plane block	Lateral to the spine at the level of the spinal nerve desired to be blocked. Fascial plane between **mm. erector spinae** and the transverse or the mamillary process of the vertebra.	Medial and lateral branches of the dorsal rami from thoracic and/or lumbar spinal nerves. Possible spread to PVS and ventral rami.	Somatic analgesia to the dorsal spine and associated muscles. (**mm. multifidus, iliocostalis, longissimus**). Somatic +/– visceral analgesia of lateral and ventral thorax/abdomen (human). Currently limited to hemilaminectomy and procedures of the dorsal spine in veterinary species.
Parasternal blocks (i.e. transversus thoracis plane (TTP) block; pecto-intercostal fascial plane (PIFP) block	Ventral aspect of the hemithorax, lateral to midline. *TTP* block: Fasical plane between **mm. transversus thoracis** and **intercostales interni**. *PIFP* block: Fascial plane between **mm. pectoralis profundus** and **intercostales externi**.	Ventral cutaneous branches of T2–T6 intercostal nerves.	Somatic analgesia to the sternum and associated soft tissues. Procedures involving the ventral thorax (e.g. median sternotomy).

REFERENCES

Ahmed W, Kulikowska M, Ahlmann T et al. (2019) A comparative multi-site and whole-body assessment of fascia in the horse and dog: a detailed histological investigation. J Anat 235, 1065–1077.

Baeriswyl M, Kirkham KR, Kern C et al. (2015) The analgesic efficacy of ultrasound-guided transversus abdominis plane block in adult patients: a meta-analysis. Anesth Analg 121, 1640–1654.

Benjamin M. (2009) The fascia of the limbs and back – a review. J Anat 214, 1–18.

Black ND, Stecco C, Chan VWS (2021) Fascial plane blocks: more questions than answers? Anesth Analg 132, 899–905.

Brenner D, Mahon P, Iohom G et al. (2018) Fascial layers influence the spread of injectate during ultrasound-guided infraclavicular brachial plexus block: a cadaver study. Brit J Anaesth 121, 876–882.

Bruggink SM, Schroeder KM, Baker-Herman TL et al. (2012) Weight-based volume of injection influences cranial to caudal spread of local anesthetic solution in ultrasound-guided transversus abdominis plane blocks in canine cadavers. Vet Surg 41, 455–457.

Campoy L (2022) Development of enhanced recovery after surgery (ERAS) protocols in veterinary medicine through a one-health approach: the role of anesthesia and locoregional techniques. J Am Vet Med Assoc 260, 1751–1759.

Castañeda-Herrera FE, Buritica-Gaviria EF, Echeverry-Bonilla DF (2017) Anatomical evaluation of the thoracolumbar nerves related to the transversus abdominus plane block technique in the dog. Anat Histol Embryol 46, 373–377.

Chen Y, Shi K, Xia Y et al. (2018) Sensory assessment and regression rate of bilateral oblique subcostal transversus abdominis plane block in volunteers. Reg Anesth Pain Med 43, 174–179.

Chin KJ, Lirk P, Hollmann MW et al. (2021a) Mechanisms of action of fascial plane blocks: a narrative review. Reg Anesth Pain Med 46, 618–628.

Chin KJ, Versyck B, Elsharkawy H et al. (2021b) Anatomical basis of fascial plane blocks. Reg Anesth Pain Med 46, 581–599.

Davis PD, Kenny GNC (2005) Fluid flow. In: Basic Physics and Measurement in Anaesthesia, 5th edition. Davis PD, Kenny GNC (eds.) Butterworth-Heinemann, United Kingdom. pp. 11–22.

Elsharkawy H, Pawa A, Mariano ER (2018) Interfascial plane blocks: back to basics. Reg Anesth Pain Med 43, 341–346.

Feldman HS, Arthur GR, Covino BG (1989) Comparative systemic toxicity of convulsant and supraconvulsant doses of intravenous ropivacaine, bupivacaine, and lidocaine in the conscious dog. Anesth Analg 69, 794–801.

Ferré BMI, Drozdzynska M, Vettorato E (2022) Ultrasound-guided bilateral erector spinae plane block in dogs undergoing sternotomies anaesthetised with propofol-dexmedetomidine continuous infusion. Vet Res Commun 46, 1331–1337.

Ferreira TH, St James M, Schroeder CA et al. (2019) Description of an ultrasound-guided erector spinae plane block and the spread of dye in dog cadavers. Vet Anaesth Analg 46, 516–522.

Ford DJ, Raj PP, Singh P et al. (1984) Differential peripheral nerve block by local anesthetics in the cat. Anesthesiology 60, 28–33.

Forero M, Heikkila A, Paul JE et al. (2015) Lumbar transversus abdominis plane block: the role of local anesthetic volume and concentration-a lot, prospective, randomized, controlled trial. Pilot Feasibility Stud 1:10. doi: 10.1186/s40814-015-0002-6. eCollection 2015

Garbin M, Marangoni S, Finck C et al. (2022) Anatomical, sonographic, and computed tomography study of the transversus abdominis plane block in cat cadavers. Animals 12, 2674.

Hebbard P, Fujiwara Y, Shibata Y et al. (2007) Ultrasound-guided transversus abdominis plane (TAP) block. Anesth Intensive Care 35, 616–617.

Hekmatpanah J (1961) Organization of tactile dermatomes C1 through L4 in cat. J Neurophysiol 24, 129–140.

Hermanson JW, de Lahunta A, Evans HE (2020) The spinal nerves. In: Miller and Evans' Anatomy of the Dog, 5th edition. Hermanson JW, de Lahunta A, Evans HE (eds.) Elsevier, USA. pp. 704–756.

Holte K, Foss NB, Svensen C et al. (2004) Epidural anesthesia, hypotension, and changes in intravascular volume. Anesthesiology 100, 281–286.

Johnson EK, Bauquier SH, Carter JE et al. (2018) Two-point ultrasound-guided transversus abdominis plane injection in canine cadavers – a pilot study. Vet Anaesth Analg 45, 871–875.

Lee IWS, Schraag S (2022) The use of intravenous lidocaine in perioperative medicine: anaesthetic, analgesic and immune-modulatory aspects. J Clin Med 11, 3543

Machi A, Joshi GP (2019) Interfascial plane blocks. Best Pract Res Clin Anaesthesiol 33, 303–315.

Otero PE, Fuensalida SE, Russo PC et al. (2020) Mechanism of action of the erector spinae plane block: distribution of dye in a porcine model. Reg Anesth Pain Med 45, 198–203.

Portela DA, Castro D, Romano M et al. (2020) Ultrasound-guided erector spinae plane block in canine cadavers: relevant anatomy and injectate distribution. Vet Anaesth Analg 47, 229–237.

Rastabi HI, Mirzaani R, Givi ME et al. (2021) Comparison of intravenous regional anaesthesia with lidocaine and ropivacaine in dogs. Vet Med Sci 7, 2135–2143.

Robertson SA, Sanchez LC, Merritt AM et al. (2005) Effect of systemic lidocaine on visceral and somatic nociception in conscious horses. Equine Vet J 37, 122–127.

Schroeder CA, Snyder LBC, Tearney CC et al. (2011) Ultrasound-guided transversus abdominis plane block in the dog: an anatomical evaluation. Vet Anaesth Analg 38, 267–271.

Schroeder CA, Schroeder KM, Johnson RA (2010) Transversus abdominis plane block for exploratory laparotomy in a Canadian lynx (*Lynx canadensis*). J Zoo Wildl Med 41, 338–341.

Schwartzmann A, Peng P, Maciel MA et al. (2020) A magnetic resonance imaging study of local anesthetic spread in patients receiving an erector spinae plane block. Can J Anesth 67, 942–948.

Shao P, Li H, Shi R et al. (2022) Understanding fascial anatomy and interfascial communication: implications in regional anesthesia. J Anesth 36, 554–563.

Smith LJ, Bentley E, Shih A et al. (2004) Systemic lidocaine infusion as an analgesic for intraocular surgery in dogs: a pilot study. Vet Anaesth Analg 31, 53–63.

Støving K, Rothe C, Rosenstock CV et al. (2015) Cutaneous sensory block area, muscle-relaxing effect, and block duration of the transversus abdominis plane block. A randomized, blinded, and placebo-controlled study in healthy volunteers. Reg Anesth Pain Med 40, 355–362.

Tian Y, Zhan Y, Liu K et al. (2022) Analgesic effect of different concentrations of ropivacaine in transversalis fascia plane block during laparotomy. BMC Anesthesiol 22, 54.

Visoiu M, Scholz S (2019) Thoracoscopic visualization of medication during erector spinae plane blockade. J Clin Anesth 57, 113–114.

White JL, Stevens RA, Kao TC (1998) Differential sensory block: spinal vs. epidural with lidocaine. Can J Anaesth 45, 1049–1053.

Willard FH, Vleeming A, Schuenke MD et al. (2012) The thoracolumbar fascia: anatomy, function and clinical considerations. J Anat 221, 507–536.

Ultrasound-Guided Thoracic Paravertebral Block

CHAPTER 13

Diego A. Portela

BLOCK AT A GLANCE

What is it used for?

- To supplement anesthesia for surgeries involving the thorax, including the thoracic body wall and visceral contents.

- To provide analgesia in animals with fractured ribs or other thoracic trauma.

- Caudal thoracic paravertebral blocks (i.e. caudal to T10) can be used to provide cranial abdominal analgesia.

Landmarks/transducer position:

- The ultrasound transducer is placed parasagittal to the dorsal midline, at the level of the thoracic spine, where the blockade is intended. Sonographic landmarks include the thoracic transverse processes, the internal intercostal membrane, and the parietal pleura.

- The needle should be introduced in-plane on a caudal-to-cranial trajectory.

What equipment and personnel are required?

- 20G 90 mm (3.5 in.) Tuohy (or similar) blunt atraumatic needle

- T-port

- Syringe of drug(s)

- Ultrasound machine

- High frequency (15–6 MHz) linear array transducer +/− protective sleeve

- Gloves

- Coupling agent (e.g. alcohol)

- Assistant to help perform the injection

When do I perform the block?

- Prior to surgery, after the patient has been clipped and skin preparation is complete. Final skin preparation before surgery is still required.

What volume of local anesthetic is used?

- $0.05–0.1\,\mathrm{ml\,kg^{-1}}$ per injection site (i.e. per spinal nerve)

Goal:

- During ultrasound-guided injection, the local anesthetic should spread within the thoracic paravertebral space.

- Ventral displacement of the parietal pleura during injection verifies the correct location of the injectate.

Complexity level:

- Advanced

Clinical pearl:

- The injectate may spread to the sympathetic trunk.

WHAT DO WE ALREADY KNOW?

The aim of thoracic paravertebral (TPV) blocks is to block the **thoracic spinal nerves** within the TPV space after they leave their respective intervertebral foramina (Karmakar 2001). Injections of local anesthetic into the TPV space result in blockade of the **ventral primary branch** of the corresponding spinal nerve, with potential spread towards the rami communicantes and the sympathetic trunk. This technique is commonly used to provide high-quality perioperative analgesia in people undergoing thoracotomies, sternotomies, breast surgery, abdominal surgery, herniorrhaphy, and renal surgery (Richardson and Lönnqvist 1998). Randomized clinical studies show that TPV blocks result in similar perioperative analgesia, but better hemodynamic stability and lower risk of complications, when compared with epidural analgesia in people (Pintaric et al. 2011; Yeung et al. 2016).

Ultrasound (US) guidance has become the gold standard for performing TPV blocks in humans by improving the safety and success of the technique (O Riain et al. 2010). In veterinary medicine, approaches for performing US-guided TPV blocks have been described in dogs (Portela et al. 2017; Ferreira et al. 2018) and foxes (Monticelli et al. 2017).

The incidence of intrapleural injectate migration, in canine cadaveric studies, has been reported as 0% and 50% following a US-guided parasagittal longitudinal approach (Portela et al. 2017; Ferreira et al. 2018) or transverse approach (Monticelli et al. 2017), respectively.

Local anesthetic injected into the TPV space produces reversible blockade of the **ventral primary branches** of the spinal nerves, the rami communicantes, and the sympathetic trunk. Studies in human volunteers have shown that single TPV injections using a large volume of local anesthetic can spread, cranial and caudal producing a multimetameric analgesic effect; however, the extension of sensory blockade after single injections may be unpredictable (Marhofer et al. 2013). A clinical study performed in women undergoing unilateral mastectomies showed that single TPV injections provided equivalent dermatomal spread and duration of analgesia compared with multiple injections using the same total volume of local anesthetic (Uppal et al. 2017).

Experimental studies performed in canine cadavers failed to find multisegmental spread (Portela et al. 2012, 2017; Monticelli et al. 2017). However, the injected solution was found in several contiguous spinal segments along the

sympathetic trunk following a US-guided technique (Portela et al. 2017; Ferreira et al. 2018). Using the loss of resistance technique to identify the TPV space, Santoro et al. (2021) found that 0.6 ml kg^{-1} of dye solution spread over five spinal segments into the ventral compartment of the TPV space.

The TPV space is divided into dorsal and ventral compartments by the endothoracic fascia (Stopar Pintaric et al. 2012). In people, injections performed dorsal to the endothoracic fascia resulted in a limited spread that was confined to the injection site only, whereas injections performed ventral to the endothoracic fascia resulted in longitudinal multisegmental distribution of the injectate (Naja et al. 2004). A similar spread pattern has been observed in dogs, where injections performed in the ventral compartment of the TPV space (between the endothoracic fascia and parietal pleura) resulted in multisegmental spread of the injectate over several segments of the sympathetic trunk, yet only affected the spinal nerve at the injection site (Portela et al. 2017; Ferreira et al. 2018; Santoro et al. 2021). This can be explained anatomically because the ventral compartment of the TPV space (which contains the sympathetic trunk) communicates with the contiguous TPV spaces, whereas the dorsal compartment does not (Figure 13.1). This same type of injectate spread was observed using volumes ranging from 0.05 to 0.3 ml kg^{-1} per injection (Monticelli et al. 2017; Portela et al. 2017; Ferreira et al. 2018).

A recent clinical study performed in dogs undergoing unilateral radical mastectomy showed that a single TPV injection at the level of T13 resulted in lower perioperative opioid requirements, better recovery quality, and lower postoperative

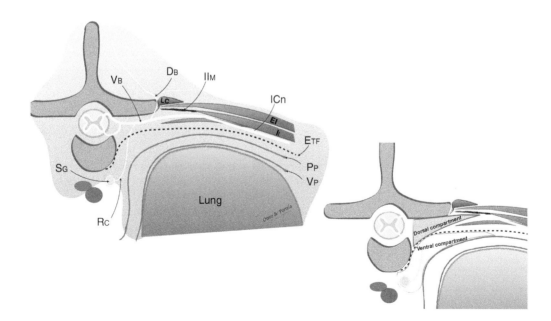

FIGURE 13.1 Schematic representation of a transverse view of a thoracic paravertebral space, showing the dorsal (red) and ventral (green) compartments divided by the endothoracic fascia (ETF). EI, *mm. intercostales externi*; ICn, **intercostal nerve**; II: *mm. intercostales interni*; IMM, internal intercostal membrane; LC, *mm. levatores costa*; PP, parietal pleura; RC, ramus communicans; SG, sympathetic ganglion; VB, ventral branch; VP, visceral pleura.

pain scores when compared with dogs not receiving the block (Santoro et al. 2022). Likewise, the use of a TPV catheter inserted at the T10 level was successfully used to control severe trauma-related pain of the caudal thoracic and cranial abdominal body wall in a dog (Thomson and Portela 2021).

PATIENT SELECTION
INDICATIONS FOR THE BLOCK

This block is typically used to provide intra- and postoperative analgesia in small animals undergoing intercostal thoracotomies (Garbin et al. 2021), surgical repair of the thoracic wall, or thoracic wall mass removals. Additionally, it can be implemented as part of a multimodal analgesic approach to relieve pain originating from rib fractures, or any traumatic injury to the thoracic wall (Thomson and Portela 2021). Caudal thoracic paravertebral blocks (i.e. caudal to T10) have been used in humans to provide perioperative abdominal pain relief (Sondekoppam et al. 2019). In dogs, caudal TPV blocks have been reported to provide analgesia to the caudal thoracic and cranial abdominal wall in trauma patients (Thomson and Portela 2021) and in dogs undergoing radical mastectomies (Santoro et al. 2022).

CONTRAINDICATIONS

- Skin infection or other lesions at the intended puncture site.

- Neoplastic processes invading the TPV space or the planned needle path.

- Caution should be used for patients with coagulation problems.

- Allergic reactions to local anesthetics.

POTENTIAL SIDE EFFECTS AND COMPLICATIONS

- Intercostal vessel puncture with subsequent paravertebral hematoma formation has been reported in humans (Song et al. 2018).

- Neuraxial spread of local anesthetic resulting in bilateral blockade and hypotension (sympathetic blockade).

- Local anesthetic spread towards the cranial sympathetic trunk can result in the blockade of the second-order neurons that participate in the innervation of the eye structures, producing Horner's syndrome (Viscasillas et al. 2013). This problem usually resolves when the local anesthetic effect wears off without further complications.

- Mediastinal spread of the injectate with unknown clinical consequences has been reported in cadaveric studies (Monticelli et al. 2017; Portela et al. 2017).

- Iatrogenic intrapleural punctures and injections can occur if the needle perforates the parietal pleura. The occurrence

of pneumothorax has not been reported in animals, but it can result from pleural puncture if the technique is not performed correctly.

- In obese dogs, the adipose tissue contained between the epaxial muscles and the thoracolumbar fascia produces a considerable amount of sound attenuation, reducing the quality of the image obtained from high-frequency transducers and interfering with needle visualization.

GENERAL CONSIDERATIONS
CLINICAL ANATOMY

The **thoracic spinal nerves** leave the intervertebral foramina and run into the TPV space where they divide into **dorsal** and **ventral primary branches**. The spinal nerves also give off the rami communicantes, which connect to the sympathetic trunk.

The TPV spaces are located alongside the vertebral column, immediately lateral to the intervertebral foramina and between two consecutive transverse processes, covered by the epaxial muscles, the *m. levatores costarum* and the *mm. intercostales externi* (Figure 13.2).

The internal intercostal membrane, the axial continuation of the *mm. intercostales interni*, is considered the roof (i.e. dorsal limit) of the TPV space. The vertebral bodies, the intervertebral foramina and the intervertebral disks constitute the medial boundary of the TPV space, while the ventral limit is formed by the parietal pleura (Figures 13.1 and 13.2). The TPV space tapers laterally and continues as the intercostal space, without a clear lateral limit (Portela et al. 2012, 2017; Monticelli et al. 2017).

Each TPV space is anatomically divided into a dorsal and a ventral compartment by the endothoracic fascia. The dorsal compartment contains the spinal nerve, with the **dorsal** and **ventral primary branches**, and the origin of the rami communicantes. The ventral compartment of the TPV space contains the rami communicantes and the sympathetic trunk and communicates with the dorsal mediastinum, and with the ventral compartment of the adjacent TPV spaces (Figure 13.1). The TPV space also contains the intercostal arteries and veins, lymphatics, and a variable amount of fat.

EXPECTED DISTRIBUTION OF ANESTHESIA

The distribution of the somatic locoregional anesthesia will depend on the number of spinal nerves blocked. For each nerve blocked, the desensitized area will extend from the dorsolateral aspect of the thoracic and cranial abdominal body wall to the ventral midline of the respective dermatome level, and it will include the skin, muscles, joints, bones, and the underlying parietal pleura/peritoneum.

Because there is some overlap in the innervation of the thoracic wall, it is recommended to block the nerves involved in the surgical field plus one to two adjacent spaces (i.e. cranially and caudally) (Bailey et al. 1984).

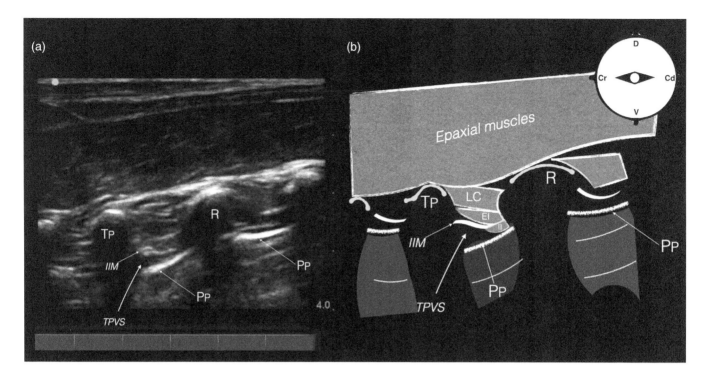

FIGURE 13.2   Sonoanatomy of the TPV space in a dog (a) and schematic representation (b). The transducer is positioned on a parasagittal plane, lateral to the dorsal midline at the level of the fifth thoracic vertebra, with a slight oblique orientation (cranial aspect of transducer slightly more medial, caudal aspect slightly more lateral). Cd, caudal; Cr, cranial; D, dorsal; EI, ***mm. intercostales externi***; II, ***mm. intercostales interni***; IIM, internal intercostal membrane; LC, ***mm. levatores costa***; PP, parietal pleura; R, rib; TP, transverse process; TPVS, thoracic paravertebral space; V, ventral.

The role of unilateral and multimetameric sympathetic trunk blockade in small animals is unclear, but it may be involved in reducing visceral thoracic and abdominal pain and preventing the development of chronic pain after thoracotomies (Kairaluoma et al. 2006; Richardson et al. 2011).

LOCAL ANESTHETIC: DOSE, VOLUME, AND CONCENTRATION

Any local anesthetic (e.g. bupivacaine, ropivacaine, and levobupivacaine) can be used, with or without the coadministration of an adjuvant (e.g. dexmedetomidine, dexamethasone, and buprenorphine).

Using US guidance, volumes of 0.05–0.1 ml kg^{-1} per nerve are recommended (Portela et al. 2012, 2017). Higher volumes, up to 0.3 ml kg^{-1}, have not shown any benefit in terms of multimetameric spread in small animals compared with lower volumes (Ferreira et al. 2018). However, in live animals, volumes up to 0.6 ml kg^{-1} using a single injection technique were reported to be safe, and potentially provide multisegmental analgesia in dogs (Thomson and Portela 2021; Santoro et al. 2022).

PATIENT PREPARATION AND POSITIONING

The patient should be positioned in sternal recumbency with the cervical and thoracic columns in alignment (Figure 13.3).

Creating a degree of kyphosis, by placing a small rolled-up towel under the sternum, can help identify the anatomical landmarks. Additionally, a small cushion should be positioned under the head to support the head and neck. In deep-chested dogs, a V-trough may help maintain the patient in sternal recumbency. The dorsal midline should be clipped free of hair, and standard surgical preparation of the skin over the injection site should be performed (Figure 13.3).

STEP-BY-STEP PERFORMANCE

SURFACE ANATOMY AND LANDMARKS TO BE USED

The target TPV space can be identified by simultaneously palpating and counting the dorsal spinous processes; however, this technique usually leads to inaccurate identification of the correct level (Ferreira et al. 2018). An easier way is to use the ultrasound to count the ribs, starting at the last (13th) rib, and counting forwards as the transducer is moved cranially until the desired intercostal space is identified. After identifying the target level, the transducer is moved towards the dorsal midline until the two transverse processes of the target space can be identified. Ultrasonographically, the transverse processes can be differentiated from the corresponding ribs based on their irregular (as opposed to round) contour (Figure 13.2).

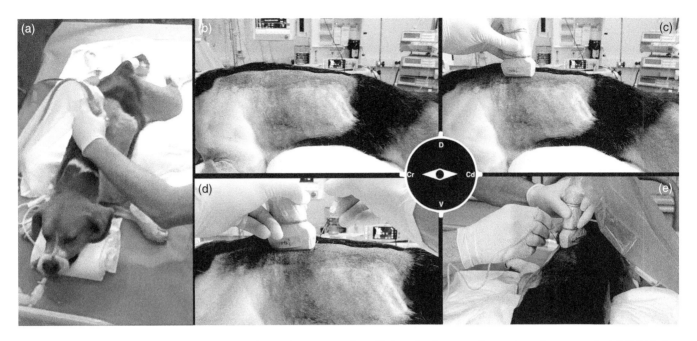

FIGURE 13.3   Sequence of dog positioning, transducer placement, and needle introduction to perform a thoracic paravertebral (TPV) block. (a) Dog positioned in sternal recumbency with a cushion under the head and under the sternum. The ultrasound transducer is positioned in a sagittal orientation, lateral to the dorsal midline. (b) Lateral view of a dog positioned to perform a TPV block. Note the slight kyphosis created by the cushion under the sternum, which helps move the scapula cranially. (c) Ultrasound transducer positioned lateral to the dorsal midline with a slight oblique orientation with the marker facing cranially. A mild oblique orientation of the transducer facilitates directing the needle toward the TPV space. (d) Lateral and (e) caudal views of the in-plane needle introduction to perform a TPV block at the level of the fifth thoracic TPV space. Note the needle puncture site located on the caudal margin of the transducer and the steep angle used for needle introduction.

To perform this block, the transducer should initially be positioned on a parasagittal plane relative to the dorsal midline. Next, the transducer can be rotated into a slightly oblique orientation by moving the caudal aspect of the transducer laterally. This position will facilitate the optimal needle orientation and allow easier access to the TPV space (Figures 13.3 and 13.4).

Alternatively, the transducer can be positioned perpendicular to the spine to obtain a transverse view of the TPV space, as described by Monticelli et al. (2017).

ULTRASOUND ANATOMY

Spinal nerves are usually not able to be visualized with standard ultrasound machines. However, the features defining the boundaries of the TPV space can be echographically identified.

In dogs, a "penetration" setting should be used when the spinous processes are taller than 4 cm. However, this setting may reduce the quality (resolution) of the image. When the TPV spaces are located deeper than 6 cm, the use of a low-frequency convex transducer may be necessary to obtain the penetration needed to visualize the relevant sonoanatomy.

The main sonographic landmarks for this block are the transverse processes, the parietal pleura, and the internal intercostal membrane (Figure 13.2). Two consecutive transverse processes should be identified as hyperechoic

structures with acoustic shadows projecting underneath (Figure 13.2). When the transducer is positioned with a slight oblique orientation, a transverse process will be observed cranially, and the proximal end of a rib tubercle will be observed caudally. Ventral to these hyperechoic structures, the parietal pleura is visible as a bright hyperechoic line. The sliding sign of the visceral pleura in close contact with the parietal pleura can also be observed during respiratory movements.

The intermuscular fascial plane between the **m. levatores costarum** and the **mm. intercostales externi** can be seen as a relatively echogenic line connecting two transverse processes or a transverse process with the caudal rib (i.e. when the oblique orientation of the transducer is used) (Figure 13.2). The internal intercostal membrane (roof of the TPV space) is seen as a thin echogenic line located between the parietal pleura and the **mm. intercostales externi**. It may be possible to visualize intercostal vessels in some animals using the color doppler settings.

NEEDLE INSERTION TECHNIQUE

Once the anatomical features of the target TPV space are identified, the transducer should be rotated slightly until the caudal border of the transducer lies over the rib immediately caudal to the target space (Figure 13.3). Although not necessary, in some patients this oblique orientation will

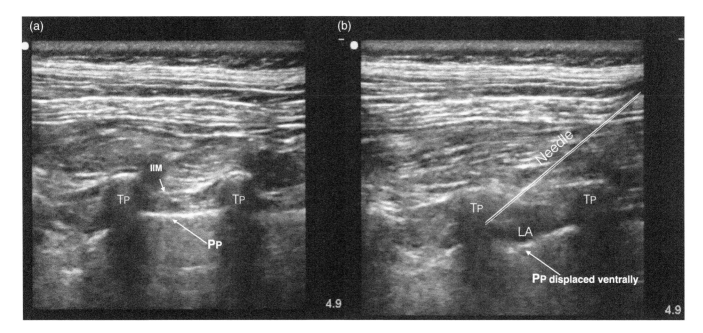

FIGURE 13.4 (a) Ultrasound image of the fifth thoracic paravertebral space in a dog obtained with a linear transducer positioned laterally to the dorsal midline with a slight oblique orientation and with the marker facing cranially. (b) Ventral displacement of the parietal pleura after injection of local anesthetic (LA). A line has been drawn over the needle to highlight its trajectory. The tip of the needle enters the thoracic paravertebral space between two consecutive transverse processes (TP), and its tip is located between the internal intercostal membrane (IIM) and the parietal pleura (PP).

"spread out" the available space between the two bony landmarks, facilitating the introduction of the needle.

Introduce the needle in-plane from the caudal border of the transducer with a caudodorsal to cranioventral direction (Figures 13.3 and 13.4). The needle should be advanced slowly through the epaxial muscles, the ***m. levatores costarum***, the ***mm. intercostales externi,*** and, finally, the internal intercostal membrane (Figure 13.4). Advancement of the needle should be stopped immediately after puncturing the internal intercostal membrane before it reaches the parietal pleura. A subtle "pop" sensation may be felt when the needle pierces the internal intercostal membrane.

EXPECTED MOTOR RESPONSES FROM NERVE STIMULATION

If an insulated needle connected to a nerve stimulator is being used to perform the US-guided TPV block, an intercostal or abdominal muscular response can be elicited upon needle entrance into the TPV space. However, since the spinal nerve is located in the dorsal compartment of the TPV space, injections performed when the muscular response is observed may not result in a multisegmental spread along the sympathetic chain (Portela at al. 2012). The contraction of intercostal muscles can be difficult to visualize in obese patients, therefore placing the nondominant hand on the thoracic wall facilitates perception of the muscular response.

ADMINISTRATION OF LOCAL ANESTHETIC – WHAT TO LOOK FOR, WHAT TO FEEL FOR, DECISION POINTS

Following the verification of a negative aspiration test, the local anesthetic should be injected slowly into the space between the parietal pleura and the internal intercostal membrane. When the injection is performed correctly, ventral displacement of the parietal pleura is generally noted (Figure 13.4). The technique is repeated at each TPV space to be blocked.

BLOCK EFFECTS (SENSORY, MOTOR, ETC.) AND PATIENT MANAGEMENT

This block produces motor blockade of the affected **intercostal nerves**. However, there is no evidence that this effect will have a clinical impact on the ability to maintain normal ventilation. In people with multiple rib fractures, the use of TPV blocks results in less respiratory function impairment when compared with patients receiving only systemic analgesics. It is suspected that this is due to better pain control (Yeying et al. 2017).

The extension of the analgesic effect will depend on the number of spinal nerves blocked. Cardiovascular and respiratory function should be monitored following the injections to promptly detect any potential side effects or complications resulting from the block.

COMPLICATIONS AND HOW TO AVOID THEM

Bilateral blockade resulting from epidural spread has been observed in people (Cowie et al. 2010; Pace et al. 2016). However, the clinical impact of the epidural spread is not clear, and it may actually contribute to the analgesic effect of this block. When using electrostimulation to perform this block in dogs, a 15% incidence of epidural spread was reported (Portela et al. 2012). In contrast, a 0% incidence of epidural spread was reported following an in-plane, ultrasound-guided technique (Portela et al. 2017; Ferreira et al. 2018). In a study in foxes, using a transverse approach to the TPV space resulted in an 8% incidence of epidural spread (Monticelli et al. 2017). Injecting a low volume at each TPV space, rather than a high-volume single injection, may reduce the chances of epidural spread.

Total spinal anesthesia may result if the needle is unintentionally positioned into an intervertebral foramen, or if the intervertebral nerve cuff is pierced during TPV injection (Albi-Feldzer et al. 2016).

If needle advancement is not stopped in the TPV space, it could potentially reach the dorsal mediastinum and puncture a large mediastinal vessel. As with other ultrasound-guided blocks, the needle should never be advanced if the precise location of its tip cannot be readily identified.

When using nerve stimulation alone, pleural puncture was reported with an incidence of 45% in dogs (Portela et al. 2012). The use of ultrasound allows visualization of the parietal pleura and the needle in real time, reducing the incidence of pleural puncture. Using an in-plane and longitudinal approach (see above), the incidence of pleural puncture was 0% in canine cadaveric studies (Portela et al. 2017; Ferreira et al. 2018). Using a transverse approach to the TPV space in foxes, however, a 50% incidence of intrapleural contamination was observed as well as the presence of contrast solution in the vena cava and into the right atrium (Monticelli et al. 2017).

The incidence of intrapleural injection can be higher when visualization of the landmarks and the needle tip is poor (i.e. large breed or obese dogs, transverse needle approach). This complication can result in block failure and/or pneumothorax. Therefore, it is not recommended to perform the block when the landmarks and the needle position cannot be determined. To reduce the chances of producing a pneumothorax, it is recommended to keep the T-port and syringe connected to the injection needle so as to avoid the introduction of air into the pleural cavity should a pleural puncture occur.

An incomplete or failed block can also be considered a potential complication, therefore, the clinician should be ready to provide rescue analgesia, if needed.

COMMON MISTAKES AND HOW TO AVOID THEM

In some animals, the US-guided approach can be technically challenging. This may be the case in animals with tall spinous processes and deep TPV spaces where the needle trajectory travels at a steeper angle and impairs visualization of the tip.

Using echogenic needles and making small needle movements back and forth to produce tissue disturbances may help improve needle tip recognition and the success of the block.

Another challenge that is associated with the described technique is difficulty advancing the needle because of angle limitations imposed by the transducer and the transverse process located just caudal to the target TPV space, producing a double-fulcrum effect. This can be remedied by sliding the transducer cranially until the target TPV space is located under the caudal edge of the transducer (i.e. instead of centering the target TPV space on the ultrasound screen, it will be located "off side"), and is closer to the entrance point of the needle (Figure 13.5) (Abdallah and Brull 2014).

In some dogs, TPV injections cranial to T4 can be challenging because the scapula interferes with transducer placement and needle path. In these cases, a cushion under the sternum can help to facilitate visualization of the T3 and T4 TPV space. Alternatively, the most cranial TPV space that can be visualized can be injected with a larger volume of local anesthetic to try and take advantage of the potential multisegmental analgesic effect. However, the effect on the cranial dermatomes is unpredictable.

HOW TO TALK TO CLIENTS/PROFESSIONAL COLLEAGUES

- When planning to include the block as part of perioperative pain management, it is important to recognize and communicate with surgeons the time needed to perform this block. At the beginning of the learning curve, the TPV block may take longer than other routinely performed blocks, so it is recommended to have 10–15 minutes available to complete this technique properly.

- Another important aspect to discuss with surgeons is postoperative analgesic expectations. This block provides excellent postoperative analgesia that may last up to eight hours when long-acting local anesthetics are used. However, rescue analgesia should always be available and given promptly based on the results of an analgesic scoring system (e.g. Glasgow Pain Scale-Short Form).

- Respiratory depression from **intercostal nerve** block is not a concern after TPV block; therefore, surgeons may be reassured that patients will not have respiratory compromise as a consequence of the block.

- Horner's syndrome is a potential complication that can be seen following this block. Therefore, clinicians should alert surgeons about this side effect before performing the block. Horner's syndrome resolves spontaneously within a few hours.

- In patients with traumatic lesions of the thoracic or abdominal wall, a TPV block and a catheter placement could be offered to improve pain management.

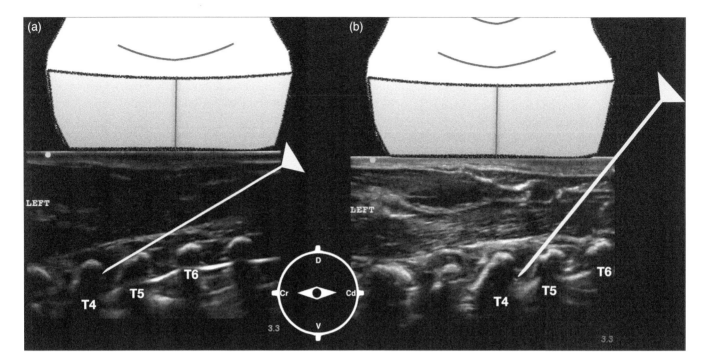

FIGURE 13.5 "Off-side" transducer position to facilitate needle introduction towards the thoracic paravertebral (TPV) space. (a) Illustration of the "double-fulcrum" effect whereby the caudal end of the transducer and the transverse process immediately caudal to the target TPV space limit the needle's range of motion. (b) To remedy this, the transducer is moved cranially so that the target TPV space is moved from the center of the screen to the right side of the screen. This "off-side" transducer position improves the range of motion for the needle, facilitating needle introduction towards the target TPV space. Cd, caudal; Cr, cranial; D, dorsal; T4, T5, and T6, fourth to sixth thoracic transverse processes; V, ventral.

REFERENCES

Abdallah FW, Brull R (2014) Off side! A simple modification to the parasagittal in-plane approach for paravertebral block. Reg Anesth Pain Med 39, 240–242.

Albi-Feldzer A, Duceau B, Nguessom W et al. (2016) A severe complication after ultrasound-guided thoracic paravertebral block for breast cancer surgery: total spinal anaesthesia: a case report. Eur J Anaesthesiol 33, 949–951.

Bailey CS, Kitchell RL, Haghighi SS, Johnson RD (1984) Cutaneous innervation of the thorax and abdomen of the dog. Am J Vet Res 45, 1689–1698.

Cowie B, McGlade D, Ivanusic J et al. (2010) Ultrasound-guided thoracic paravertebral blockade: a cadaveric study. Anesth Analg 110, 1735–1739.

Ferreira TH, Teixeira LBC, Schroeder CA et al. (2018) Description of an ultrasound-guided thoracic paravertebral block technique and the spread of dye in dog cadavers. Vet Anaesth Analg 45, 811–819.

Garbin M, Bertolizio G, Portela DA (2021) The thoracic paravertebral block for an opioid-free thoracotomy in a dog. Vet Anaesth Analg 48, 622–623.

Kairaluoma PM, Bachmann MS, Rosenberg PH et al. (2006) Preincisional paravertebral block reduces the prevalence of chronic pain after breast surgery. Anesth Analg 103, 703–708.

Karmakar MK (2001) Thoracic paravertebral block. Anesthesiology 95, 771–780.

Marhofer D, Marhofer P, Kettner SC et al. (2013) Magnetic resonance imaging analysis of the spread of local anesthetic solution after ultrasound-guided lateral thoracic paravertebral blockade: a volunteer study. Anesthesiology 118, 1106–1112.

Monticelli P, Jones I, Viscasillas J (2017) Ultrasound-guided thoracic paravertebral block: cadaveric study in foxes (Vulpes vulpes). Vet Anaesth Analg 44, 968–972.

Naja MZ, Ziade MF, Rajab ME et al. (2004) Varying anatomical injection points within the thoracic paravertebral space: effect on spread of solution and nerve blockade. Anesthesia 59, 459–463.

O Riain SC, Donnell BO, Cuffe T et al. (2010) Thoracic paravertebral block using real-time ultrasound guidance. Anesth Analg 110, 248–251.

Pace MM, Sharma B, Anderson-Dam J et al (2016) Ultrasound-guided thoracic paravertebral blockade. Anesth Analg 122, 1186–1191.

Pintaric TS, Potocnik I, Hadzic A et al. (2011) Comparison of continuous thoracic epidural with paravertebral block on perioperative analgesia and hemodynamic stability in patients having open lung surgery. Reg Anesth Pain Med 36, 256–260.

Portela DA, Campoy L, Otero PE et al. (2017) Ultrasound-guided thoracic paravertebral injection in dogs: a cadaveric study. Vet Anaesth Analg 44, 636–645.

Portela DA, Otero PE, Sclocco M et al. (2012) Anatomical and radiological study of the thoracic paravertebral space in dogs: iohexol distribution pattern and use of the nerve stimulator. Vet Anaesth Analg 39, 398–408.

Richardson J, Lönnqvist P (1998) Thoracic paravertebral block. Brit J Anesth 81, 230–238.

Richardson J, Lönnqvist PA, Naja Z (2011) Bilateral thoracic paravertebral block: potential and practice. Br J Anaesth 106, 164–171.

Santoro F, Franci P, Grandis A et al. (2021) Distribution of injectates in the thoracic paravertebral space of the dog and cat: a cadaveric study. Open Vet J 11, 27–35.

Santoro F, Debidda P, Franci P (2022) Single-injection caudal thoracic paravertebral block improves pain control and recovery quality in female dogs undergoing unilateral radical mastectomy: a randomized controlled trial. J Am Vet Med Assoc 260, S53–S58.

Sondekoppam RV, Uppal V, Brookes J et al. (2019) Bilateral thoracic paravertebral blocks compared to thoracic epidural analgesia after midline laparotomy: a pragmatic noninferiority clinical trial. Anesth Analg 129, 855–863.

Song L, Zhou Y, Huang D (2018) Inadvertent posterior intercostal artery puncture and haemorrhage after ultrasound-guided thoracic paravertebral block: a case report. BMC Anesthesiol 18, 196.

Stopar Pintaric T, Veranic P, Hadzic A et al. (2012) Electron-microscopic imaging of endothoracic fascia in the thoracic paravertebral space in rats. Reg Anesth Pain Med 37, 215–218.

Thomson ACS, Portela DA (2021) Use of a thoracic paravertebral catheter to control severe trauma-related pain in a dog. Vet Anaesth Analg 48, 809–811.

Uppal V, Sondekoppam RV, Sodhi P et al. (2017) Single-injection versus multiple-injection technique of ultrasound-guided paravertebral blocks: a randomized controlled study comparing dermatomal spread. Reg Anesth Pain Med 42, 575–581.

Viscasillas J, Sanchis-Mora S, Hoy C et al. (2013) Transient Horner's syndrome after paravertebral brachial plexus blockade in a dog. Vet Anaesth Analg 40, 104–106.

Yeung JHY, Gates S, Naidu BV et al. (2016) Paravertebral block versus thoracic epidural for patients undergoing thoracotomy. Cochrane Database Syst Rev 2, CD009121.

Yeying G, Liyong Y, Yuebo C et al. (2017) Thoracic paravertebral block versus intravenous patient-controlled analgesia for pain treatment in patients with multiple rib fractures. J Int Med Res 45, 2085–2091.

Ultrasound-Guided Intercostal Nerve Block

Alexander C. S. Thomson

CHAPTER 14

BLOCK AT A GLANCE

What is it used for?

- The **intercostal nerve** block (INB) is used to desensitize the thoracic body wall for surgeries such as lateral thoracotomy or median sternotomy and to provide analgesia for painful conditions such as trauma.

Landmarks/transducer position:

- Position the dog in lateral recumbency.

- The ultrasound transducer should be positioned on the lateral thoracic body wall, perpendicular to the ribs, and dorsal to the midaxillary line.

- The transducer is moved cranially and caudally to visualize each rib and its associated structures.

What equipment and personnel are required?

- 21G 100 mm (or similar) blunt atraumatic needle with an extension line or T-connector

- Syringe of drug(s)

- Ultrasound machine

- High frequency (15–6 MHz) linear array transducer +/− protective sleeve

- Gloves

- Coupling agent (e.g. alcohol)

- Assistant to help perform the injection

When do I perform the block?

- After the lateral thorax is clipped and skin preparation is complete. The final skin preparation should be performed after the block and prior to the surgery.

What volume of local anesthetic is used?

- 0.03–0.05 ml kg^{-1} per injection site

Goal

- During injection, the parietal pleura should be displaced medially away from the transducer, and the injectate should not be seen dissecting/spreading within the *mm. intercostales*.

Complexity level

- Easy

Clinical pearl

- When performing multiple adjacent INBs, the needle can be redirected subcutaneously to avoid multiple punctures through the skin.

WHAT DO WE ALREADY KNOW?

Intercostal nerve blocks (INBs) provide segmental anesthesia of the ventral two-thirds of the thoracic body wall. The neurovascular bundle containing each **intercostal nerve** is bounded by robust fascial planes medially and laterally which, together with the ribs, serve as sonographic landmarks when using ultrasound guidance to perform this technique.

INBs have been performed in companion animals for many years, typically using a blind technique in which a needle is inserted through the skin caudal to a rib and is slowly advanced cranially until the rib is contacted. Alternatively, the needle can be "walked off" the caudal margin of the rib into an area that is assumed to be in close proximity to the **intercostal nerve** (Thompson and Johnson 1991; Pascoe and Dyson 1993; Duke 2000). While simple and fast to perform, the blind technique is relatively inaccurate, with a reported success rate of less than 60% per nerve (Thomson et al. 2021).

While INBs are commonly performed in practice, literature pertaining to companion animals remains scarce, particularly regarding outcomes, efficacy measures, and complications. A study comparing morphine and oxymorphone to

INBs in dogs undergoing thoracotomy found that postoperative hypoventilation was observed in the opioid groups but not in the INB group (Berg and Orton 1986). However, it is unclear whether this result can be attributed to superior analgesia imparted by INBs, opioid-mediated respiratory depression, or a combination of these factors.

Using a blind approach with bupivacaine, Flecknell et al. (1991) found INBs may provide analgesia for more than eight hours in dogs, based on assessments of respiratory function that have previously been correlated to the degree of analgesia in humans. Dogs administered nalbuphine at four hours and eight hours after thoracotomy demonstrated an improvement in arterial oxygenation, believed to be due to its analgesic effect and provision of more comfortable respiratory movements. Dogs that received INBs, however, did not have an improvement in arterial oxygenation after nalbuphine administration at 4 and 8 hours, only showing a change at 16 hours, presumably once the INBs were no longer providing effective analgesia.

Pascoe and Dyson (1993) compared bupivacaine INBs to morphine epidural in dogs undergoing lateral thoracotomy and found that fewer dogs in the INB group required additional postoperative analgesics.

Ultrasound guidance improves the accuracy of INBs in both humans and dogs (Bhatia et al. 2013; Thomson et al. 2021). In dogs, the ultrasound-guided technique has been reported to yield a 91.4% success rate per nerve, with the most significant source of error being miscounting of the ribs, rather than off-target intramuscular injection (Thomson et al. 2021). With greater accuracy, smaller volumes of local anesthetic can be used for each nerve, reducing the risk of local anesthetic systemic toxicity (LAST), and improving the efficacy and duration of blockade. More recently, the use of INBs in combination with transversus abdominis plane (TAP) block was reported to reduce postoperative opioid requirements in dogs undergoing laparoscopic ovariectomy (Paolini et al. 2022).

Several fascial plane techniques that target the distal extensions of the **intercostal nerves** (the *ventral cutaneous branches*) have been investigated in canine cadavers as possible analgesic strategies for median sternotomy (Zublena et al. 2021; Escalante et al. 2022). These parasternal approaches only desensitize the ventral thoracic body wall distal to the site of injection and do not anesthetize areas innervated by the **lateral cutaneous branches** of the **intercostal nerves**. Therefore, they would be inadequate for lateral thoracotomies or for providing analgesia to more proximal rib fractures. While these techniques reliably stained the **ventral cutaneous branches** of the **intercostal nerves** in the canine cadavers, the spread of injectate was variable. Until fascial plane techniques are further refined, the performance of multiple INBs bilaterally remains a reasonable option for providing analgesia of the mid- to ventral thorax.

PATIENT SELECTION
INDICATIONS FOR THE BLOCK

INBs can be used for any painful condition of the ventrolateral thoracic body wall, such as lateral thoracotomy, median sternotomy, or thoracic body wall trauma.

CONTRAINDICATIONS

- Skin infection or other lesions at the intended needle puncture site.

- Inability to identify the relevant anatomy during ultrasound scanning.

- Uncontrolled coagulopathy or anticoagulation therapy are relative contraindications.

- INBs should be performed with caution in dyspneic patients, or in those with known diaphragmatic dysfunction, since the respiratory function of the intercostal muscles may be impaired. Similarly, these blocks should be performed with caution in patients with abdominal distention (e.g. patients with uncontrolled hyperadrenocorticism) since the diaphragm may be unable to compensate for a reduced ventilatory contribution from the *mm. intercostales*.

POTENTIAL SIDE EFFECTS AND COMPLICATIONS

- Laceration or puncture of the intercostal artery or vein can result in clinically significant hemorrhage and/or the potential for hemothorax if the parietal pleura is also penetrated.

- If the needle enters the thorax, laceration of the lung and/or pneumothorax is also possible. The incidence of pneumothorax after **INB** has been estimated at 5.6% in a retrospective study of human patients with rib fractures (Shanti et al. 2001). Reports of pneumothorax in companion animals are scarce; one study reported pneumothorax in 1 out of 24 dogs undergoing INB and lateral thoracotomy but did not specify the cause of the pneumothorax (Thompson and Johnson 1991). To avoid these complications, the tip of the needle should always be visualized using ultrasound, as the needle is being advanced in-plane. Color Doppler flowmetry can assist with identifying and avoiding vascular structures. Inadvertent puncture of the parietal pleura is more likely if the needle is misaligned with the transducer, or if the tip of the needle is positioned within the acoustic shadow of the rib.

- Severe ventilatory depression has been reported in humans receiving bilateral INBs (Cory and Mulroy 1981; Casey 1984). Careful patient selection is important to avoid respiratory complications. While the contribution of the *mm. intercostales* to ventilation is minor in a normal animal, patients with diaphragmatic dysfunction may be more dependent on the accessory muscles of respiration.

GENERAL CONSIDERATIONS
CLINICAL ANATOMY

The **intercostal nerves** arise from the ventral branch of each spinal nerve and course ventrally along the caudomedial border of the first 12 pairs of ribs. They are mixed-function nerves containing sensory, motor, and sympathetic fibers. Each **intercostal nerve** is contained within a loose neurovascular bundle, roughly triangular in cross-section. This bundle is bordered cranially by the caudal surface of the rib, laterally by the thin aponeurosis of the *m. intercostales interni* at its insertion on the caudal margin of the rib (referred to as the *internal intercostal membrane*), and medially by the fused endothoracic fascia and parietal pleura. Unlike humans, dogs lack *m. intercostalis intimus* between the neurovascular bundle and the endothoracic fascia. However, more distally between the costochondral junction and the sternum, the *m. transversus thoracis* lies between the *m. intercostales interni* and the parietal pleura. Within the neurovascular bundle, the intercostal vein is located most cranially, the intercostal artery is located in the center, and the **intercostal nerve** is located caudally. The neurovascular structures are surrounded by a small amount of loose connective and adipose tissue.

At the midaxillary line, each **intercostal nerve** gives off a **lateral cutaneous branch**, which emerges through the *mm. intercostales* to ramify within the subcutaneous tissues (Bailey et al. 1984). The **lateral cutaneous branch** of the second **intercostal nerve** gives rise to the **intercostobrachial nerve**, which contributes sensory innervation to the soft tissues overlying the axilla and medial surface of the thoracic limb. Blocks performed ventral to the **lateral cutaneous branches** may fail to desensitize the superficial structures of the thoracic body wall, so performing INBs as dorsal as possible results in the most consistent effects.

The layers of muscle overlying the ribs and intercostal musculature vary based on the injection site. The *m. cutaneous trunci* is most superficial, followed by *m. latissimus dorsi*, which spans from the teres tubercle on the humerus to the dorsal midline over the lumbar spine, covering the dorsal half of the thoracic body wall. The *m. serratus ventralis* overlies intercostal spaces 5–7, in between the *mm. latissimus dorsi* and *intercostales externi*.

The ventral branch of the 13th spinal nerve forms the **costoabdominal nerve**, which does not run along the border of the 13th rib, and instead crosses *m. quadratus lumborum*, continuing caudally between *m. transversus abdominis* and the transversalis fascia.

EXPECTED DISTRIBUTION OF ANESTHESIA

INBs provide segmental anesthesia of the ventral two-thirds of the thoracic body wall, including the skin, musculature, ribs, and parietal pleura. The **intercostal nerves** associated with the asternal ribs, along with the **costoabdominal nerve**, also provide sensory innervation to the cranioventral abdominal body wall and peritoneum within the costal arch. The cranial and caudal extent of anesthesia is dependent on the number of **intercostal nerves** blocked. For lateral thoracotomy, it is commonly recommended to block at least two **intercostal nerves** cranial and two **intercostal nerves** caudal to the site of the planned surgical incision. For median sternotomy, bilateral INBs of the sternal ribs (through the ninth rib) are recommended. A parasternal approach may be preferred, since the first two ribs are inaccessible from a lateral approach.

INBs are not expected to provide analgesia to the dorsal third of the thoracic body wall, which is innervated by the **dorsal branches** of the spinal nerves.

LOCAL ANESTHETIC: DOSE, VOLUME, AND CONCENTRATION

Bupivacaine, ropivacaine, and levobupivacaine are preferred for performing INBs. Because of the proximity of the intercostal artery and vein to the associated **intercostal nerve**, additives such as dexmedetomidine or epinephrine may be considered to prolong the duration of the blockade, and reduce the systemic uptake and redistribution of the local anesthetic.

An injectate volume of $0.03–0.05\,\mathrm{ml\,kg^{-1}}$ per nerve is recommended. The total volume of local anesthetic administered will vary based on the number of intercostal nerves to be blocked, but the total bupivacaine dose should not exceed $2.5\,\mathrm{mg\,kg^{-1}}$. If ropivacaine is used, the total dose should not exceed $3\,\mathrm{mg\,kg^{-1}}$.

PATIENT PREPARATION AND POSITIONING

For the lateral (proximal) approach, the patient should be positioned in lateral recumbency with the side to be blocked facing upwards (Figure 14.1). The hair should be clipped over the required spaces, and the skin prepared using a standard aseptic technique. Final skin preparation should be performed after the block if the patient requires surgery.

STEP-BY-STEP PERFORMANCE
SURFACE ANATOMY AND LANDMARKS TO BE USED

The anesthetist should be positioned so that the dominant hand holding the needle is caudal and the nondominant hand holding the transducer is cranial, allowing a caudal-to-cranial in-plane needle approach to the neurovascular bundle. The

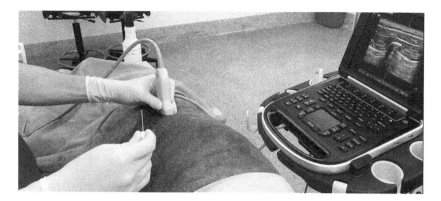

FIGURE 14.1 A canine patient is positioned for performance of **intercostal nerve** blocks. The patient is positioned in right lateral recumbency and the transducer is oriented perpendicular to the ribs with the marker facing cranially, dorsal to the mid-axillary line. The ultrasound machine is positioned directly in front of the anesthetist.

(a)

(b)

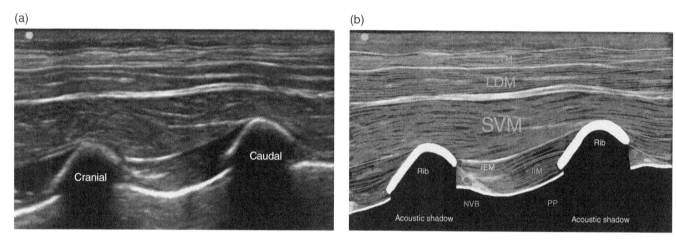

FIGURE 14.2 (a) Pre-block ultrasonographic image of the target area for intercostal nerve blocks in a dog. (b) Same image with labels. CTM, *m. cutaneous trunci*; IEM, *mm. intercostales externi*; IIM, *mm. intercostales interni*; LDM, *m. latissimus dorsi*; NVB, neurovascular bundle; PP, parietal pleura; R, rib; SVM, *m. serratus ventralis*.

ultrasound transducer should be positioned in the coronal plane on the lateral thoracic body wall, perpendicular to the ribs, and dorsal to the midaxillary line. From this position, the transducer can be glided cranially and caudally across each rib.

ULTRASOUND ANATOMY

The depth control on the ultrasound machine should be adjusted so that the rib lies within the focal zone of the transducer, which is usually in the center of the image for many point-of-care ultrasound machines (Figure 14.2). Gain is adjusted to achieve optimal contrast resolution between the *mm. intercostales* and the adipose tissue found within the neurovascular bundle. The distance from the skin surface to the rib will vary based on the rib number, the body condition, and the conformation of the patient. The cranial ribs are deeper,

and the thoracic limb often needs to be pulled cranially to expose the target anatomy.

Each rib will appear as a hyperechoic chevron shape with distal acoustic shadowing. Spanning adjacent ribs, from lateral to medial, are the *mm. intercostales externi* and the *mm. intercostales interni*. These thin muscles, elongated and roughly triangular in cross section, are separated by a thin oblique intermuscular fascial layer which appears as a hyperechoic line. This intermuscular fascia between the *mm. intercostales externi* and *intercostales interni* should not be mistaken for the internal intercostal membrane, which is formed by the insertion of *m. intercostales interni* on the caudal margin of the rib. Medial to these muscles, the parietal pleura is seen as a broader, brighter hyperechoic line spanning the space between the acoustic shadow under each rib and moving with each breath.

NEEDLE INSERTION TECHNIQUE

The needle is inserted caudal to the transducer and advanced in-plane in a cranial direction (Figure 14.3). The angle of insertion, approximately 30°–50°, depends on the depth of the target neurovascular bundle relative to the length of the ultrasound transducer. Deeper targets and shorter transducers typically require steeper insertion angles. Importantly, contact between the shaft of the needle and the adjacent rib may preclude an excessively shallow insertion angle. With the full length of the needle clearly visualized, the needle is advanced in-plane until the tip crosses the internal intercostal membrane.

EXPECTED MOTOR RESPONSES FROM NERVE STIMULATION

If nerve stimulation is used, motor responses will be detected either visually or palpably as the intercostal muscles contract.

ADMINISTRATION OF LOCAL ANESTHETIC – WHAT TO LOOK FOR, WHAT TO FEEL FOR, DECISION POINTS

Once the tip of the needle penetrates the internal intercostal membrane, and a negative aspiration test has been performed, a small volume (0.1–0.2 ml) of local anesthetic can be delivered

(a)

(b)

(c)

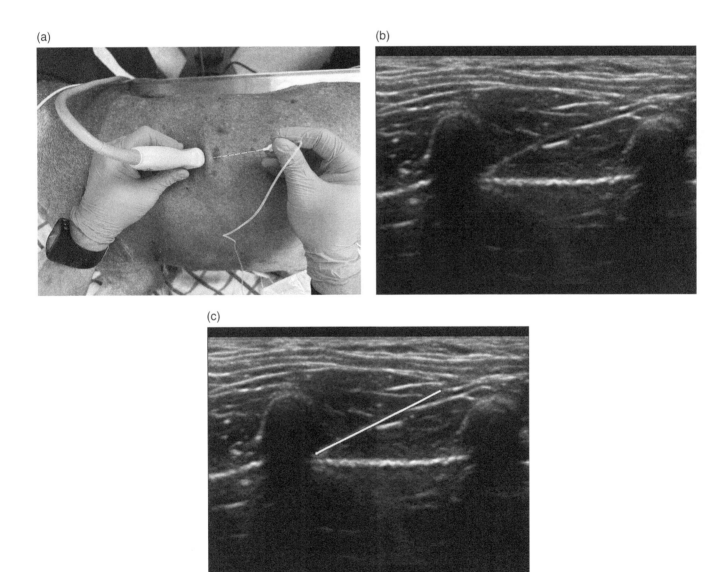

FIGURE 14.3 (a) An **intercostal nerve** block is being performed in a dog. The needle is being advanced in-plane on a caudal-to-cranial trajectory towards the neurovascular bundle. (b) Pre-block ultrasonographic image of the needle in the correct location prior to injection of the local anesthetic. (c) Same image, with yellow arrow showing position of the needle.

(a)

(b)

(c)

(d)

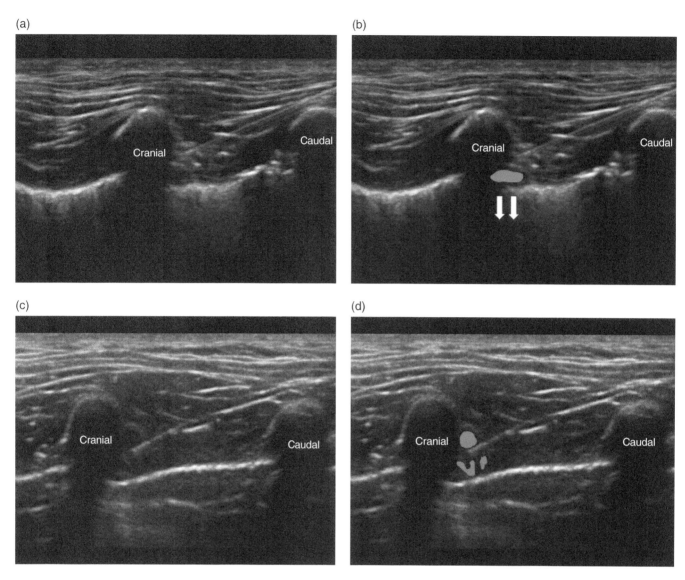

FIGURE 14.4   Ultrasonographic images of local anesthetic distributions following injections for **intercostal nerve** blocks. (a) Correct location of injectate. The needle penetrated the internal intercostal membrane and the local anesthetic solution has displaced the parietal pleura medially and is located within the neurovascular bundle caudal to the rib. (b) Same image, with annotations. Arrows show displacement of pleura; local anesthetic is represented in blue. (c) Incorrect location of injectate. The needle was not in the correct location so local anesthetic is seen intramuscular in multiple small areas outside of the neurovascular bundle. (d) Same image, with annotations. Local anesthetic is represented in blue.

as a "test" dose. The parietal pleura should be displaced medially (i.e. away from the transducer) by the injectate, and no local anesthetic should be seen dissecting within or between the *mm. intercostales* (Figure 14.4). If intramuscular injectate is observed, the tip of the needle should be carefully advanced or repositioned until the internal intercostal membrane is penetrated. If a blunt needle is used, this may be accompanied by a very subtle "click."

If no hypoechoic local anesthetic or deflection of the pleura is observed during the injection, the tip of the needle may have crossed the endothoracic fascia and entered the pleural cavity. In this situation, the needle should be withdrawn, and the patient monitored closely for signs of pneumothorax that might result from laceration of the lung.

BLOCK EFFECTS (SENSORY, MOTOR, ETC.) AND PATIENT MANAGEMENT

This block affects the sensory innervation of the ventral two-thirds of the thoracic body wall and the motor function of the intercostal muscles distal to the site of injection. The effect of INBs on respiratory function varies with the number of nerves blocked, and whether or not both sides were blocked (i.e. unilateral blockade for lateral thoracotomy versus bilateral blockade for median sternotomy). Animals with normal ventilatory function can compensate for the loss of intercostal muscle function by increasing the contraction of the abdominal muscles and diaphragm. However, this compensatory response may be blunted under anesthesia, requiring support with mechanical ventilation.

COMPLICATIONS AND HOW TO AVOID THEM

The most common complication of performing INBs is block failure, usually due to off-target, intramuscular injection. Ultrasound guidance improves the accuracy of INBs from approximately 60% to over 90% (Thomson et al. 2021).

Laceration of the intercostal artery is a rare but potentially life-threatening complication of INBs. Hemorrhage from the intercostal artery is usually self-limiting, but persistent hemorrhage could potentially result in hemothorax, requiring chest tube placement and transfusion of blood products. Ultrasonography and color Doppler flowmetry can sometimes identify the damaged intercostal artery, but thoracotomy or thoracoscopy may be required to identify the precise location of the hemorrhage. The treatment is proximal ligation of the intercostal artery with hemostatic clips or sutures. Laceration of intercostal vasculature is less likely when blunt needles designed for peripheral nerve blocks are used.

COMMON MISTAKES AND HOW TO AVOID THEM

- The first 3–4 **intercostal nerves** can be difficult to block due to their depth and overlying anatomical structures, such as the scapula. An assistant may be required to pull the thoracic limb cranially and expose the scanning site for the third **intercostal nerve**. The first and second **intercostal nerves** are only accessible by a distal or parasternal approach. Steep angles of needle insertion may impair needle visualization. In these cases, the needle tracking feature on the ultrasound unit (if equipped) may prove useful. If needle tracking is not available, laser-etched needles can be used to improve needle visibility.

- If the needle is inserted too far from the injection site, adjacent ribs may block the path of the needle to the target. The skin and needle can be pulled cranially to correct the insertion angle, without completely withdrawing the needle.

- When blocking multiple **intercostal nerves**, it is easy to lose track of the rib number. The ribs to be blocked can be marked with a surgical marker, or an assistant can be assigned to keep track of the rib number with each injection.

- A blunt-beveled needle is less likely to lacerate intercostal vasculature and may provide tactile feedback to the operator when the internal intercostal membrane is punctured.

- In patients with pneumothorax, a mirror artifact may be seen below the hyperechoic parietal pleura, creating the appearance of additional tissue layers. If this is not recognized, the operator may inadvertently advance the needle into the pleural cavity.

- In under-conditioned patients, the transducer may lose contact with the body wall in between protruding ribs. A gel stand-off pad can be fitted to the transducer to maintain adequate contact.

- A hypoplastic or missing 13th rib may cause the operator to miscount intercostal spaces if counting ribs from caudal to cranial (Morgan 1968).

HOW TO TALK TO CLIENTS/PROFESSIONAL COLLEAGUES

INBs contribute to a multimodal analgesic strategy for thoracic body wall pain, allowing for lower doses of systemic anesthetics and analgesics. This is especially valuable in compromised patients, in which high inhalant concentrations and large doses of systemic drugs may have deleterious effects. Depending on the local anesthetic used, the analgesia provided by INBs may last for several hours after surgery, improving the patient's comfort level, respiratory function, and postoperative recovery.

INBs are easy to perform, and the risk of serious complications is low. While the ultrasound-guided technique takes marginally longer to perform than the blind technique, this potential drawback is outweighed by a significant increase in accuracy, success, and safety. Ultrasound guidance allows a smaller injectate volume and a lower risk of local anesthetic systemic toxicity, as well as a reduced risk of damage to off-target structures such as vasculature and thoracic viscera.

REFERENCES

Bailey CS, Kitchell R, Haghighi SS et al. (1984) Cutaneous innervation of the thorax and abdomen of the dog. Am J Vet Res 45, 1689–1698.

Berg RJ, Orton EC (1986) Pulmonary function in dogs after intercostal thoracotomy: comparison of morphine, oxymorphone, and selective intercostal nerve block. Am J Vet Res 47, 471–474.

Bhatia A, Gofeld M, Ganapathy S et al. (2013) Comparison of anatomic landmarks and ultrasound guidance for intercostal nerve injections in cadavers. Reg Anesth Pain Med 38, 503–507.

Casey WF (1984) Respiratory failure following intercostal nerve blockade. Anaesthesia 39, 351–354.

Cory PC, Mulroy MF (1981) Postoperative respiratory failure following intercostal block. Anesthesiology 54, 418–419.

Duke T (2000) Local and regional anesthetic and analgesic techniques in the dog and cat: part II, infiltration and nerve blocks. Can Vet J 41, 949–952.

Escalante GC, Ferreira TH, Hershberger-Braker KL et al. (2022) Evaluation of ultrasound-guided pectointercostal block in canine cadavers. Vet Anaesth Analg 49, 182–188.

Flecknell PA, Kirk AJB, Liles JH et al. (1991) Post-operative analgesia following thoracotomy in the dog: an evaluation of the effects of bupivacaine intercostal nerve block and nalbuphine on respiratory function. Lab Anim 25, 319–324.

Morgan JP (1968) Congenital anomalies of the vertebral column of the dog: a study of the incidence and significance based on a radiographic and morphologic study. Vet Radiol Ultrasound 9, 21–29.

Paolini A, Santoro F, Bianchi A et al. (2022) Use of transversus abdominis plane and intercostal blocks in bitches undergoing laparoscopic ovariectomy: a randomized controlled trial. Vet Sci 9, 604.

Pascoe PJ, Dyson DH (1993) Analgesia after lateral thoracotomy in dogs: epidural morphine vs. intercostal bupivacaine. Vet Surg 22, 141–147.

Shanti CM, Carlin AM, Tyburski JG (2001) Incidence of pneumothorax from intercostal nerve block for analgesia in rib fractures. J Trauma 51, 536–539.

Thomson ACS, Portela DA, Romano M et al. (2021) Evaluation of the effect of ultrasound guidance on the accuracy of intercostal nerve injection: a canine cadaveric study. Vet Anaesth Analg 48, 256–263.

Thompson SE, Johnson JM (1991) Analgesia in dogs after intercostal thoracotomy: a comparison of morphine, selective intercostal nerve block, and interpleural regional analgesia with bupivacaine. Vet Surg 20, 73–77.

Zublena F, Briganti A, De Gennaro C et al. (2021) Ultrasound-guided parasternal injection in dogs: a cadaver study. Vet Anaesth Analg 48, 563–569.

Ultrasound-Guided Serratus Plane Block

Matt Read

CHAPTER 15

BLOCK AT A GLANCE

What is it used for?

- The Serratus Plane Block (SPB) is used to provide analgesia for a variety of thoracic wall injuries and surgical procedures, including multiple rib fractures, mastectomy, lateral thoracotomy, and thoracoscopy.

Landmarks/transducer position:

- The transducer is placed perpendicular to the fourth to fifth ribs at the level of the shoulder joint.

What equipment and personnel are required?

- 21G 100 mm (4 in.) (or similar) blunt atraumatic needle
- Syringe of drug(s)
- Ultrasound machine
- High frequency (15–6 MHz) linear array transducer +/− protective sleeve
- Gloves
- Coupling agent (e.g. alcohol)
- +/− Assistant to help perform the injection

When do I perform the block?

- Prior to the surgery, after the lateral thorax is clipped and the surgical skin preparation is complete. Final skin preparation will still be needed prior to surgery.

What volume of local anesthetic is used?

- 0.5–1 mL kg^{-1} (may dilute the local anesthetic in cases where the maximum recommended dose of the local anesthetic will not allow for this volume to be used).

Goal

- During the injection, the local anesthetic should be observed spreading and expanding the fascial plane between the *m. latissimus dorsi* and *m. serratus ventralis thoracis* ("*superficial*" approach), or between the *m. serratus ventralis thoracis* and *mm. intercostales externi* ("*deep*" approach).

Complexity level

- Easy to intermediate.

Clinical pearl

- If key structures are not able to be identified or the performance of the block is found to be difficult, instead of losing the benefits of regional anesthesia entirely, the anesthetist can quickly and easily perform multiple intercostal blocks using the same equipment and drugs.

WHAT DO WE ALREADY KNOW?

The Serratus Plane Block (SPB) is an ultrasound-guided fascial plane (compartmental) block that can be used to provide analgesia to the ventrolateral hemithorax. Like the more widely known Transversus Abdominus Plane (TAP) block that is used to provide analgesia to the abdominal wall, the SPB involves injecting a local anesthetic solution between two muscles into an interfascial space.

The SPB was first described for use in humans by Blanco et al. (2013) for breast surgery. Since its initial description, this block has been investigated as an alternative to thoracic epidural anesthesia, intercostal nerve blocks, thoracic paravertebral blocks, and erector spinae plane blocks as a means of providing analgesia for a range of procedures in humans and animals, including rib fractures, mastectomy, lateral thoracotomy, and thoracoscopy (Teixeira et al. 2018; Semyonov et al. 2019; Liu et al. 2020; Asorey et al. 2021; Hu et al. 2021; Bosak et al. 2022; Nair and Diwan 2022). Postoperative pain following any of these procedures can result in hypoventilation and hypoxemia and local anesthetic techniques can be used to complement or replace the use of systemic analgesics in these patients. SPBs have been found to carry a lower risk of adverse effects and complications than alternative regional anesthetic techniques for these procedures.

Small Animal Regional Anesthesia and Analgesia, Second Edition. Edited by Matt Read, Luis Campoy, and Berit Fischer.
© 2024 John Wiley & Sons, Inc. Published 2024 by John Wiley & Sons, Inc.

Two approaches to the SPB have been described in humans and dogs – *superficial* and *deep*. The *superficial* approach (i.e. "*anterior*" approach in humans) involves injecting a local anesthetic solution between the **m. latissimus dorsi** and **m. serratus ventralis thoracis**. The *deep* approach ("*posterior*" approach in humans) involves injecting a local anesthetic solution between the **m. serratus ventralis thoracis**. and **mm. intercostales externi**. In both cases, the goal of performing a SPB is to block the **lateral cutaneous branches** of the **intercostal nerves** that innervate the target area, rather than the **intercostal nerves** themselves (Mayes et al. 2016). In people, the **long thoracic nerve** and/or **thoracodorsal nerve** may also be blocked since they lie on the surface of the **m. serratus ventralis thoracis** (Mayes et al. 2016; Xie et al. 2021).

Both approaches to SPBs have been documented to provide varying degrees of analgesia intraoperatively, to reduce opioid requirements postoperatively, and to reduce postoperative nausea and vomiting (which is thought to be the result of lower opioid usage during the postoperative period) (Hu et al. 2021). Nair and Diwan (2022) reported the results of a literature review examining the efficacy of anterior SPBs for managing pain in people with multiple rib fractures. They found that ultrasound-guided SPBs could significantly decrease postoperative pain scores and opioid requirements without inducing notable adverse effects, and that continuous infusion of a local anesthetic using an indwelling catheter for three to five days was better than a single-shot injection. Hu et al. (2021) conducted a systematic review and meta-analysis of the efficacy of SPBs for postoperative pain in patients undergoing breast surgery and found that SPBs decreased opioid consumption and relieved pain postoperatively with no risk of complications. Liu et al. (2020) conducted a meta--analysis of randomized controlled trials to explore the efficacy of anterior SPBs for analgesia following thoracic surgery. Like other studies, those investigators found that SPBs significantly reduced postoperative pain scores and opioid consumption for up to 24 hours, as well as decreased the incidence of postoperative nausea and vomiting.

There are very few reports of using SPBs in animals to date. The use of SPBs was first described in dogs in a small case series by Teixeira et al. (2018). Those authors used *deep* SPBs in combination with TAP blocks in four dogs undergoing unilateral radical mastectomies, with the blocks being performed at the level of the fourth rib using bupivacaine 0.25% (0.3 ml kg⁻¹) with the ultrasound transducer oriented perpendicular to the long axis of the dog and the needle directed dorso-ventrally using an in-plane technique. None of their dogs required rescue analgesia during surgery, and all dogs had low scores on their postoperative pain scale at two and four hours. No complications were observed during the performance of the blocks, during anesthesia, or at follow-up.

Asorey et al. (2021) also reported their experiences using a *deep* approach for performing ultrasound-guided SPBs. A prior canine cadaver study by Drozdzynska et al. (2017) found that injection of 1 ml kg⁻¹ of a dye-contrast solution at two sites between the **m. serratus ventralis thoracis** and **mm. intercostales externi** (0.5 ml kg⁻¹ at a site ventral to the scapula at the fourth intercostal space and 0.5 ml kg⁻¹ at a site located more dorsally at the fifth intercostal space) resulted in the spread of the injected solution between the first and sixth intercostal spaces. Using this same 2-injection site approach to perform the block in clinical cases, Asorey et al. (2021) used SPBs to provide adjunctive analgesia to four dogs undergoing lateral thoracotomies. Total injection volumes ranged between 1 ml kg⁻¹ (0.25% levobupivacaine) and 1.9 ml kg⁻¹ (0.15% levobupivacaine), and each injection was confirmed to be in the correct location by observing hydro-dissection of the fascial plane deep to the **m. serratus ventralis thoracis** as the injection was being made. In that report, none of the dogs experienced intraoperative nociception (defined by the authors as 20% increases in heart rate or blood pressure above baseline), there was a low intraoperative requirement for opioids, and no complications were identified as a result of performing the blocks.

The use of *superficial* SPB injections has also been reported in dogs. Freitag et al. (2020) investigated the relevant anatomy and dispersion of three different volumes of a local anesthetic-dye solution in canine cadavers between the **m. latissimus dorsi** and **m. serratus ventralis thoracis**. In a formaldehyde-preserved cadaver, the **lateral cutaneous branches** of the **intercostal nerves** were identified in the serratus plane, which the authors concluded may result in partial thoracic wall analgesia if they could be blocked by a local anesthetic. In that study, to correctly inject their dye solutions in the serratus plane, the authors placed the ultrasound transducer perpendicular to the fourth and fifth ribs at the level of the shoulder joint and were able to identify the ribs, **m. cutaneous trunci**, **m. latissimus dorsi**, **m. serratus ventralis thoracis**, and **mm. intercostales externi**. Using an in-plane, cranio-caudal needle approach, three different volumes of injectate (0.3, 0.6, and 1.0 ml kg⁻¹) were administered into the plane between the **m. latissimus dorsi** and **m. serratus ventralis thoracis**. The cadavers were dissected 30 minutes later to assess the accuracy of their injections and to document the spread of the injectate around the target nerves. Although the **lateral cutaneous branches** of the **intercostal nerves** were only able to be located by dissection in three of the 26 cadaver thoracic walls studied, 26 out of 29 (90%) injections were successfully administered into the superficial serratus plane, suggesting that, if the same technique was performed *in situ*, blockade of these nerves would likely result. The spread of injectate resulting from the three volumes was not significantly different, with all three volumes resulting in a similar dermatomal distribution (consistently, four to five rib spaces). The authors concluded that the lower volume (0.3 ml kg⁻¹) could result in appropriate analgesia with a lower risk of toxicity than the higher volumes, but that clinical studies would need to be performed to understand the real analgesic potential of this technique.

Bosak et al. (2022) also reported on the use of a *superficial* approach to perform SPBs in a case series of three small breed dogs undergoing video-assisted thoracotomies for PDA ligation. They used an ultrasound-guided approach and injected 0.3 ml kg^{-1} of bupivacaine 0.5% ($n = 1$) or ropivacaine 0.75% ($n = 2$) into the superficial serratus plane. In their case series, all dogs received an opioid infusion during surgery and a non-steroidal anti-inflammatory postoperatively, which confounded their pain scoring. No complications related to the blocks were observed and the authors concluded that further studies are required.

Although these limited cadaver studies and case reports suggest that there is promise for more widespread use of this block, prospective, blinded, randomized, controlled studies are warranted to more definitively show whether there is value in incorporating SPBs into small animal anesthesia and pain management.

PATIENT SELECTION

INDICATIONS FOR THE BLOCK

A SPB can be used to provide partial analgesia to the hemithorax for a variety of potentially painful conditions or procedures. Most commonly, this technique is administered to trauma patients with multiple rib fractures and/or a flail chest, or those that will be undergoing surgical procedures of the trunk such as intercostal thoracotomy, thoracoscopy, mastectomy, mass removals, etc.

CONTRAINDICATIONS

- Skin infection or other lesions at the intended needle puncture site.
- Inability to identify the relevant anatomy during ultrasound scanning.

POTENTIAL SIDE EFFECTS AND COMPLICATIONS

When performed correctly, there are very few risks or side effects associated with this block. However, if the needle tip is not able to be visualized or is not adequately controlled while it is being advanced into the serratus plane, there may be a risk of the needle entering the chest and causing injury to either the lungs or the neurovascular bundle that contains the intercostal artery, vein, and nerve that lies immediately caudal to each rib. Regardless of the technique being employed (i.e. *superficial* or *deep*), if the needle stays superficial to the intercostal muscles, there is little risk of inadvertent patient injury, since the needle will not enter the pleural space.

GENERAL CONSIDERATIONS

CLINICAL ANATOMY

The *m. serratus ventralis thoracis* is an anti-gravity muscle that plays a role in supporting the trunk, stabilizing the body during movement, helping to maintain an upright posture, and supporting inspiration. The *m. serratus ventralis* is comprised of several thin, flat strips that originate on the medial aspect of the dorsal scapula (at the "facies serrata") before fanning out and inserting on either the transverse processes of the caudal five cervical vertebrae (*m. serratus ventralis cervicis*) or on the first to seventh or eighth ribs (*m. serratus ventralis thoracis*). It is the latter muscle that is of particular interest for this block.

The chest wall is composed of several layers of muscle, which must be able to be identified when using ultrasound to perform the SPB. The *m. cutaneous trunci* is the most superficial muscle of the lateral chest wall, and it lies in the superficial fascia of the trunk immediately under the skin. The *m. latissimus dorsi* lies deep to the cutaneous trunci on the dorsal aspect of the thorax, while the *m. obliquus externus abdominis* covers the ventral aspect of the thorax and the lateral and ventral aspects of the abdomen. The *m. serratus ventralis thoracis* covers the cranial half of the thoracic body wall, lying between the *m. latissimus dorsi* and the *mm. intercostales externi*.

At the ventral edge of the *m. serratus ventralis thoracis*, the **lateral cutaneous branches** of the **intercostal nerves** course laterally away from the ribs to provide sensory innervation to the ventrolateral aspect of the hemithorax (Figure 15.1). Following SPBs in humans, there is good evidence that only the lateral cutaneous branches are affected by the local anesthetic, not the **intercostal nerves** themselves (Mayes et al. 2016).

When performed at the level of the fourth rib, dye consistently spreads over the **lateral cutaneous branches** of the T2–T5 **intercostal nerves** and may affect the **long thoracic nerve** and the **thoracodorsal nerve**. The **lateral cutaneous branches** are the only sensory nerves of importance since the **long thoracic nerve** and the **thoracodorsal nerve** are strictly motor in function (to the *m. serratus ventralis* and *m. latissimus dorsi*, respectively).

EXPECTED DISTRIBUTION OF ANESTHESIA

Based on cadaver studies in dogs, the injection of 0.3–1 ml kg^{-1} of a dye solution into the serratus plane will result in the distribution of the injectate across four to five rib spaces in one hemithorax, suggesting that if a local anesthetic solution was injected, it would potentially block all the associated **lateral cutaneous branches** of the respective **intercostal nerves**. If a broader area of blockade is required, an additional site of injection can be made to increase the potential area of distribution.

LOCAL ANESTHETIC: DOSE, VOLUME, AND CONCENTRATION

Any local anesthetic (e.g. bupivacaine, ropivacaine, and levobupivacaine) can be used to perform a SPB. Depending on the size of the patient and the formulation of the local

(a)

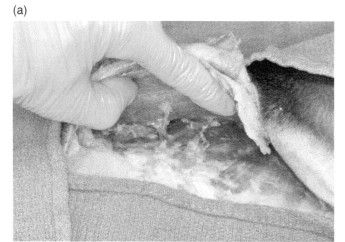

(b)

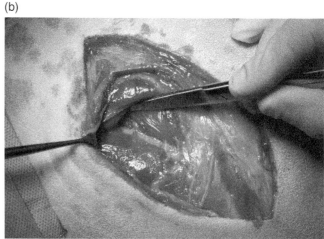

FIGURE 15.1 (a) Dissection of the right lateral chest wall of a canine cadaver. The *m. latissimus dorsi* has been transected and is being reflected caudally to show the location of the neurovascular bundles as they emerge from the fan-shaped *m. serratus ventralis* and occupy the "serratus plane" between the two muscles. Source: Luis Campoy. (b) Lateral thoracotomy being performed on the left side of a dog. The *m. latissimus dorsi* is being retracted dorsally, showing the location of the neurovascular bundle superficial to the *m. serratus ventralis*.

anesthetic that is available (i.e. 0.5% versus 0.75%), the local anesthetic may be diluted with saline to increase the effective volume that will be injected. The author most commonly uses a volume of 0.5–1 ml kg^{-1} with 0.5% ropivacaine.

PATIENT PREPARATION AND POSITIONING

The patient should be sedated or under general anesthesia and positioned in lateral recumbency, with the side of the thorax to be blocked positioned uppermost. The chest should be clipped free of hair to allow for transducer and needle placement as necessary for the planned procedure (i.e. patients undergoing lateral thoracotomy should be clipped from dorsal midline to ventral midline, and from the caudal aspect of scapula to behind costal arch), and standard surgical preparation of the skin should be performed over the planned injection site.

STEP-BY-STEP PERFORMANCE

SURFACE ANATOMY AND LANDMARKS TO BE USED

For a right-hand dominant individual who normally holds their needle in their right hand and the ultrasound transducer in their left hand, they should position themself beside the patient with the patient's head to their left, regardless of whether the patient's left side (i.e. its feet toward the anesthetist) or right side (i.e. its feet away from the anesthetist) is being blocked. For a left-hand dominant person, the opposite orientation should be used.

The ultrasound transducer should be positioned on the lateral aspect of the thorax at the level of the shoulder joint with the ultrasound marker positioned cranially (Figure 15.2).

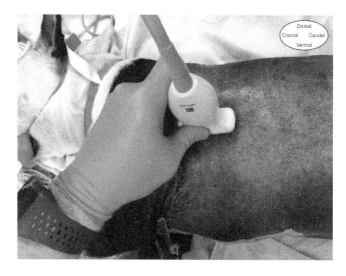

FIGURE 15.2 A dog has been positioned for Serratus Plane Block prior to lateral thoracotomy. The transducer has been placed perpendicular to the fourth and fifth ribs at the level of the shoulder joint. Blue circle indicates orientation of marker as seen in Figures 15.4, 15.5 and 15.6.

This way, as the needle is being advanced from right to left *in situ*, its movement will correspond to the needle trajectory that is being observed on the ultrasound monitor (Figure 15.3).

ULTRASOUND ANATOMY

The transducer should be oriented parallel to the long axis of the patient so a short-axis view of the ribs can be obtained (Figure 15.4). Using the depth and gain controls, the image should be optimized so that the ribs are positioned in the

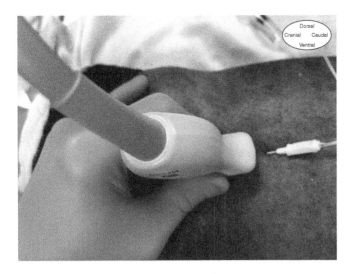

FIGURE 15.3   A regional nerve block needle has been inserted in-plane, in a caudo-cranial direction, towards the target location between the *m. latissimus dorsi* and *m. serratus ventralis thoracis*.

center (i.e. from top to bottom), or the bottom third of the ultrasound screen, and the ribs appear as round shadows with a superficial, hyperechoic rim. Since they are superficial to the ribs, this should result in the muscles of interest being located in the part of the screen with the highest resolution so small details will be easier to see. Next, glide the transducer on the skin cranially under the scapula (the upper limb may need to be pulled cranially to allow for this maneuver) until the first rib can be identified. Once the first rib is observed, glide the transducer caudally while identifying and counting each rib until the transducer is centered over the fourth and fifth ribs.

Tilt and rotate the transducer and adjust the gain and depth controls to further optimize the image over the area of interest.

Depending on the size of the patient and its body condition, the *m. cutaneous trunci* and *m. latissimus dorsi* should be able to be identified in the near field. The *m. serratus ventralis thoracis* should lie deep to the *m. latissimus dorsi* and usually appears x2–3 wider than the *m. latissimus dorsi* at this location. Glide the transducer dorsally and ventrally to assess the limits of the *m. serratus ventralis thoracis* relative to the planned surgical site. To successfully block the **lateral cutaneous branches** of the **intercostal nerves**, the local anesthetic solution will need to be injected at the level of, or just slightly dorsal to, the shoulder joint.

Next, glide the transducer caudally to confirm the identity of the *m. serratus ventralis thoracis*. It should appear as a thin triangular muscle that tapers off and disappears once the transducer reaches the seventh and eighth ribs (i.e. where it inserts on the ribs). Deep to the *m. serratus ventralis thoracis*, the *mm. external intercostalis* should be identified lying over/between the ribs.

Once all the relevant structures and the desired target location for injection are identified, and the ultrasound image has been optimized, this first image should be saved and stored to document the appearance of the anatomical structures of interest prior to needle placement and drug administration.

NEEDLE INSERTION TECHNIQUE

Although the needle can approach the serratus plane from any direction, it can be useful to perform the block so that the needle approaches the target area on a caudal-to-cranial trajectory (Figures 15.3 and 15.5). Since the **intercostal nerves**

(a)   (b)

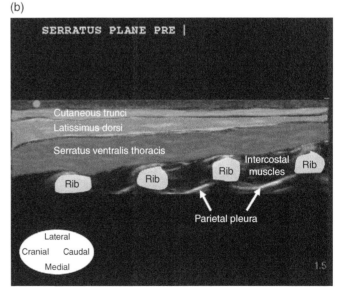

FIGURE 15.4   (a) Pre-block ultrasonographic image of the target area for a Serratus Plane Block in a dog. (b) Same image with labels. Note the positions and appearances of the *mm. cutaneous trunci*, *latissimus dorsi*, *serratus ventralis thoracis* and *intercostales externi* relative to the ribs and pleura.

(a)

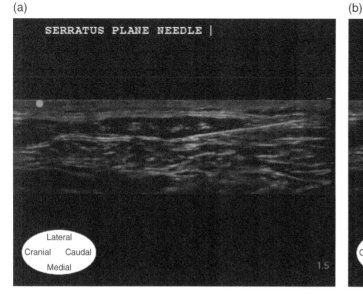

(b)

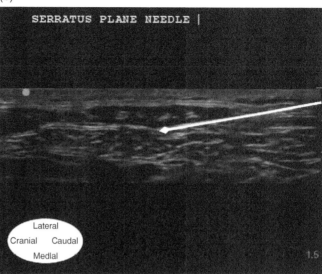

FIGURE 15.5   (a) Ultrasonographic image of "*superficial*" SPB. (b) Same image with white arrow representing position of needle. The needle tip has been advanced into its final position between the ***m. latissimus dorsi*** and ***m. serratus ventralis thoracis***.

lie caudal to their associated ribs, if the appropriate landmarks for an SPB are not able to be identified, and the block would otherwise be aborted, a caudal-to-cranial needle trajectory allows for easy conversion to performing multiple intercostal nerve blocks instead. If a cranial-to-caudal trajectory is used (i.e. the needle approaching the target area from the opposite direction), it will be more difficult to switch over and perform multiple intercostal blocks since the needle will be approaching the ribs and **intercostal nerves** from the wrong direction, adding time and risking patient injury and block failure.

EXPECTED MOTOR RESPONSES FROM NERVE STIMULATION

This block does not involve the use of nerve stimulation.

ADMINISTRATION OF LOCAL ANESTHETIC – WHAT TO LOOK FOR, WHAT TO FEEL FOR, DECISION POINTS

Like fascial plane blocks that are performed in other parts of the body, once the needle tip is thought to be in the correct location, it is useful to administer a small volume of the drug solution to distend the potential space between the two layers of fascia and confirm that the needle tip is in the correct location before the entire drug volume is administered. By using this method of hydrodissection to confirm that the tip of the needle is in the correct location, there is a higher likelihood of block success, rather than the local anesthetic inadvertently being injected into one of the adjacent muscles. During injection of the local anesthetic solution, it may be necessary to slightly reduce the pressure that the transducer applies to the skin since it is easy to inadvertently compress the space and

not recognize that the serratus plane is appropriately filling with the drug solution, especially in small patients.

In the ideal situation, the fascial plane that initially appears between the two target muscles as a single hyperechoic line will separate into two, with the hypoechoic local anesthetic solution dissecting them apart as it is being injected (Figure 15.6). Once the plane starts to distend, advance the needle into the space, and, depending on the volume to be administered, inject the local anesthetic slowly over 30–60 seconds. If desired, the needle can be advanced cranially within the space as it distends, allowing for the local anesthetic to be dispersed over a wider area cranially, caudally, dorsally, and ventrally.

BLOCK EFFECTS (SENSORY, MOTOR, ETC.) AND PATIENT MANAGEMENT

This block will primarily affect the sensory innervation to the ventrolateral chest wall. Since the goal is to block the **lateral cutaneous branches** of the **intercostal nerves**, motor supply to the ***mm. intercostales*** should remain intact and the patient should be able to ventilate normally. As described previously, blockade of the **thoracodorsal nerve** and/or **long thoracic nerve** is possible, but these provide motor innervation to the ***m. latissimus dorsi*** and ***m. serratus ventralis***, respectively, and motor paralysis in these muscles is unlikely to result in clinically recognized side effects for the duration of the block.

COMPLICATIONS AND HOW TO AVOID THEM

An in-plane needle technique is used to assist with visualizing the needle as it is advanced toward the target site. As long as the needle tip is observed while the needle is being advanced,

(a)

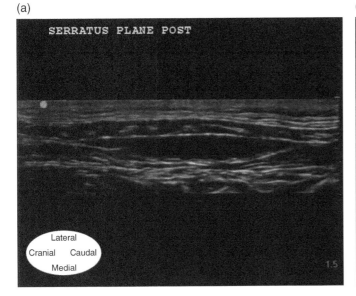

(b)

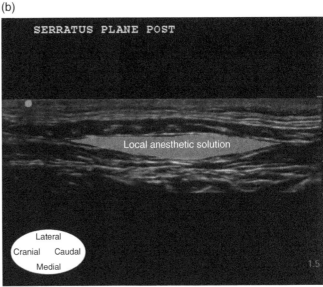

FIGURE 15.6   (a) Post-injection ultrasonographic image following a "*superficial*" Serratus Plane Block. (b) Same image with labels. Local anesthetic solution (hypoechoic) can be observed spreading between the ***m. latissimus dorsi*** and ***m. serratus ventralis thoracis***.

there is little risk of patient injury since the needle will only encounter muscle and not risk puncturing blood vessels, the pleural space, the lungs, etc. This is a relatively superficial regional anesthetic block and other than muscles, if it is performed correctly there are very few structures that will be encountered as the needle is advanced into the serratus plane.

If the needle tip cannot be visualized, stop moving the needle and manipulate the ultrasound transducer until the entire length of the needle can be observed in-plane. Make sure to identify the needle tip (e.g. by using markings), as opposed to simply observing the needle in an oblique cross-section and not confirming where the tip is located. Once the needle tip is identified, continue to move the needle toward the target location and complete the block.

Prior to injection, take a time-out to make sure the volume and concentration of the local anesthetic are appropriate for the patient. Although it would be rare to encounter a blood vessel in the target area, negative blood aspiration should be verified prior to drug administration to prevent an intravascular injection. Do not administer more than the recommended dose of local anesthetic or systemic toxicity may result.

COMMON MISTAKES AND HOW TO AVOID THEM

- It can be challenging to position the tip of the needle in the serratus plane between the fascia, especially in small patients. Use hydrodissection to verify the correct needle position prior to the administration of the full volume of local anesthetic solution. Alternatively, injecting saline as the "test-volume" during hydrodissection can minimize the total dose of local anesthetic that is administered. As is the case for other fascial plane blocks, asking an assistant to perform the injection can be helpful, allowing the anesthetist to manipulate the ultrasound transducer with

one hand and the needle with the other hand in real time, while the injection is being made under US observation.

- Make sure the injectate is being administered into the interfascial space and not into a muscle. If performed correctly, you should only be able to see local anesthetic solution between the thin white lines representing fascia, not inside the muscles themselves.

- It is easy to inadvertently apply too much pressure to the transducer as it is being positioned on the patient. This can result in compression of the interfascial space and the inability to see it being distended as the local anesthetic is being injected, especially in small patients. If the local anesthetic cannot be observed within the serratus plane, apply slightly less pressure to the transducer and confirm that the injection is being made in the correct location before additional local anesthetic is administered.

- In small patients (e.g. small breed dogs, cats), it can be difficult to optimize the ultrasound image due to them having such a thin body wall. In these cases, the use of a "stand-off" on the ultrasound probe can be helpful to place the area of interest in the center of the ultrasound screen. This will maximize the resolution of the image, improving the ability to position the needle tip in the ideal location prior to injection of the local anesthetic.

HOW TO TALK TO CLIENTS/PROFESSIONAL COLLEAGUES

A SPB will contribute to balanced anesthesia during a surgical procedure and to analgesia postoperatively for several hours, depending on the local anesthetic that is administered. Since many patients that have rib fractures or are scheduled to undergo thoracic surgery are often already compromised or expected to become physiologically unstable during surgery, being able to use less general anesthesia and/or systemic analgesics can be very beneficial and may contribute to better patient outcomes.

Although there is a learning curve to performing the SPB technique, once it is mastered, it is relatively easy to perform and can be performed quickly (i.e. less than five minutes). It does not involve clipping hair or preparing the patient anywhere beyond that of the planned surgical field and carries a low risk of complications or side effects.

One possible consideration to make the surgeon performing the procedure aware of is that, as they make their surgical approach to the chest (i.e. through a lateral intercostal incision), they may encounter slight tissue edema where the local anesthetic was deposited between muscles (i.e. between the ***m. serratus ventralis thoracis*** and ***m. latissimus dorsi*** when a "*superficial*" SPB is performed, or between the ***m. serratus ventralis thoracis*** and ***mm. intercostales externi*** when a "*deep*" SPB is performed). This does not affect their ability to identify relevant anatomy and is usually transient, having usually resolved prior to closure of the incision at the end of surgery.

REFERENCES

Asorey I, Sambugaro B, Bhalla RJ et al. (2021) Ultrasound-guided serratus plane block as an adjunct to systemic analgesia in four dogs undergoing thoracotomy. Open Vet J 10, 407–411.

Blanco R, Parras T, McDonnell JG et al. (2013) Serratus plane block: a novel ultrasound-guided thoracic wall nerve block. Anaesthesia 68, 1107–1113.

Bosak VL, Piontkovsky RJ, Mazur dos Santos A et al. (2022) Ultrasound-guided superficial serratus plane block in multimodal analgesia for three dogs undergoing surgical correction of persistent ductus arteriosus. Vet Anaesth Analg 49, 330–332.

Drozdzynska M, Fitzgerald E, Neilson D et al. (2017) Description of ultrasound-guided serratus plane block in dogs: cadaveric study. Abstracts presented at the Association of Veterinary Anaesthetists Meeting 14–17th September 2016, Prague, Czech Republic. Vet Anaesth Analg 44, 389–395.

Freitag FAV, Gaio TS, dos Santos AAM et al. (2020) Ultrasound-guided superficial serratus plane block in dog cadavers: an anatomical evaluation and volume dispersion study. Vet Anaesth Analg 47, 88–94.

Hu NQ, He QQ, Qian L et al. (2021) Efficacy of ultrasound-guided serratus anterior plane block for postoperative analgesia in patients undergoing breast surgery: a systematic review and meta-analysis of randomized controlled trials. Pain Res Manag 2021, 7849623.

Liu XC, Song TT, Xu HY ct al. (2020) The scrratus anterior plane block for analgesia after thoracic surgery: a meta-analysis of randomized controlled trials. Medicine 99, e20286.

Mayes J, Davison E, Panahi P et al. (2016) An anatomical evaluation of the serratus anterior plane block. Anesthesia 71, 1064–1069.

Nair A, Diwan S (2022) Efficacy of ultrasound-guided serratus anterior plane block for managing pain due to multiple rib fractures: a scoping review. Cureus 2022 Jan 17; 14(1), e21322.

Semyonov M, Fedorina E, Grinshpun J et al. (2019) Ultrasound-guided serratus anterior plane block for analgesia after thoracic surgery. J Pain Res 12, 953–960.

Teixeira LG, Pujol DM, Pazzim AF et al. (2018) Combination of transversus abdominis plane block and serratus plane block anesthesia in dogs submitted to mastectomy. Pesqui Vet Bras 38, 315–319.

Xie C, Ran G, Chen D et al. (2021) A narrative review of ultrasound-guided serratus anterior plane block. Ann Palliat Med 10, 700–706.

Ultrasound-Guided Parasternal Blocks

Matt Read

CHAPTER 16

BLOCK AT A GLANCE

What might they be used for?

- "Transversus thoracis plane" ("TTP") and "Pecto-intercostal fascial plane" ("PIFP") blocks aim to anesthetize the ventral cutaneous branches of the second through sixth intercostal nerves. Although slightly different in terms of how they are performed, each technique attempts to provide analgesia to the ventral thorax for procedures such as median sternotomy.

Landmarks/transducer position:

- The transducer is placed on the ventral aspect of each hemi-thorax, lateral to the midline.

What equipment and personnel might be required?

- 21G 100 mm (4 in.) (or similar) blunt atraumatic needle
- Syringe of drug(s)
- Ultrasound machine
- High frequency (15–6 MHz) linear array transducer +/− protective sleeve
- Gloves
- Coupling agent (e.g. alcohol)
- +/− Assistant to help perform the injection

When would you perform the block?

- Prior to the surgery, after the ventral thorax is clipped and surgical skin preparation is complete. Final skin preparation will still be needed prior to surgery.

What volume of local anesthetic might be used?

- 0.25–1.0 ml kg^{-1} per side, depending on the specific technique being used. The local anesthetic may need to be diluted in cases where the maximum recommended dose will not allow for this undiluted volume to be used.

Goal

- During injection, the local anesthetic should be observed spreading within and expanding the fascial plane between the ***m. transversus thoracis*** and ***mm. intercostales interni*** ("TTP" approach), or between the ***m. pectoralis profundus*** and ***mm. intercostales externi*** ("PIFP" approach).

Complexity level:

- Advanced

WHAT DO WE ALREADY KNOW?

Surgery involving the chest wall is relatively common and is frequently associated with patients manifesting intraoperative responses to surgical stimulation and experiencing postoperative pain. Although balanced anesthetic techniques that incorporate regional anesthesia would be expected to be advantageous for procedures involving this area of the body, blocks for use in people and small animals have not been described or investigated until relatively recently.

Several different techniques for performing ultrasound-guided interfascial plane blocks of the anterior/ventral thorax have been described in people (de la Torre et al. 2014; Liu et al. 2018; Bloc et al. 2021; Zhang et al. 2021) and these approaches have recently been extrapolated for use in dogs (Alaman et al. 2021; Alaman et al. 2022; Zublena et al. 2021; Escalante et al. 2022; Fernández Barrientos and Merlin 2022). Like other interfascial plane blocks, these newly described "parasternal" techniques involve injecting a local anesthetic solution into an interfascial space where the **ventral cutaneous branches** of the **intercostal nerves** are located between two muscles.

In a clinical setting, parasternal injection of local anesthetic solutions in people causes desensitization of the distal branches of the **intercostal nerves** near the sternum, contributing to intraoperative analgesia (for procedures such as median sternotomy), postoperative pain relief (as measured by reductions in pain scores and postoperative opioid use), improved ventilation and oxygenation (as measured by arterial blood gas analysis and electrical impedance tomography of the lungs), duration of ICU stay and hospitalization, and lower inflammatory responses in response to surgery (McDonald et al. 2005; Barr et al. 2007; de la Torre et al. 2014; Ozturk et al. 2016; Thomas et al. 2016; Liu et al. 2018; Zhang et al. 2021).

Two techniques have been extrapolated from their use in people, and have recently been investigated using canine cadavers (Alaman et al. 2021; Zublena et al. 2021; Escalante et al. 2022). To date, a single case report has also been published (Fernández Barrientos and Merlin 2022) but there have been no randomized, blinded clinical studies to assess the efficacy and safety of using parasternal regional anesthesia in animals. For this reason, this chapter will focus mainly on the relevant anatomy and expected effects based on what is known from studies in people and canine cadavers. Since the approaches to these blocks will undoubtedly be revised as further research is conducted and they are adopted for clinical use, step-by-step descriptions of these techniques, recommendations for drug doses, etc. will not be included here since that would be premature based on our limited current understanding.

Two approaches to providing parasternal analgesia through regional anesthesia have been investigated to date. The *transversus thoracis plane* ("TTP") approach involves injecting a local anesthetic solution lateral to the sternum between the *m. transversus thoracis* and the *mm. intercostales interni*. "Sagittal" and "transverse" techniques for performing TTP blocks (based on the orientation of the ultrasound transducer on a patient) have been reported in people and dogs (Alaman et al. 2021; Zublena et al. 2021) (Figures 16.1 and 16.2). The *pecto-intercostal fascial plane* ("PIFP") approach involves injecting a local anesthetic solution lateral to the sternum between the *m. pectoralis profundus* and the *mm. intercostales externi* (Escalante et al. 2022) (Figure 16.3).

Although the target site for local anesthetic deposition differs between the techniques, these approaches aim to provide analgesia to the ventral aspect of the thorax (i.e. anterior in humans) by blocking the **ventral cutaneous branches** of the **intercostal nerves** that serve the area. In the case of dogs, the **ventral cutaneous branches** of the second to sixth intercostal nerves are the primary target of these regional anesthetic techniques since these are the nerves that are responsible for providing sensory innervation to the sternum, midline skin, costal pleura, and related structures (Alaman et al. 2021) (Figure 16.4).

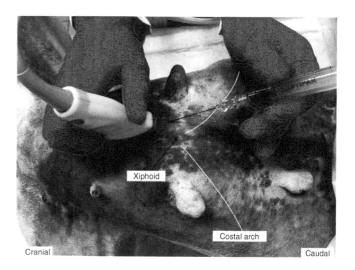

FIGURE 16.2 *Sagittal* ultrasound-guided approach to the transversus thoracis plane in a canine cadaver. The ultrasound transducer is placed in a parasternal position and the needle is advanced in-plane caudocranially. The yellow lines indicate the caudal border of the most caudal rib connected to the sternum. Source: From Zublena et al. 2021. Used with permission.

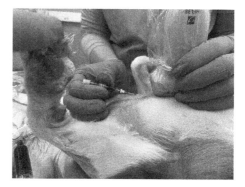

FIGURE 16.3 Ultrasound-guided approach to the pecto-intercostal fascial plane of a dog cadaver in dorsal recumbency. The ultrasound transducer is placed in a parasternal position and the needle is advanced in-plane craniocaudally. Source: From Escalante et al. (2022). Used with permission.

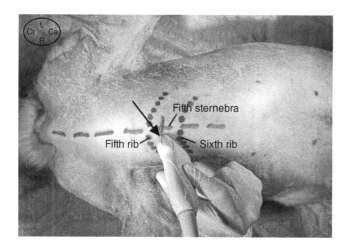

FIGURE 16.1 *Transverse* ultrasound-guided approach to the transversus thoracis plane at the level of the fifth interchondral space in a canine cadaver. The ultrasound transducer is positioned parallel to the fifth and sixth costal cartilages and oriented in a caudolateral to craniomedial direction. The black arrow indicates the direction of needle approach using an in-plane technique. Ca, caudal; Cr, cranial; L, left; R, right. Source: From Alaman et al. 2021. Used with permission.

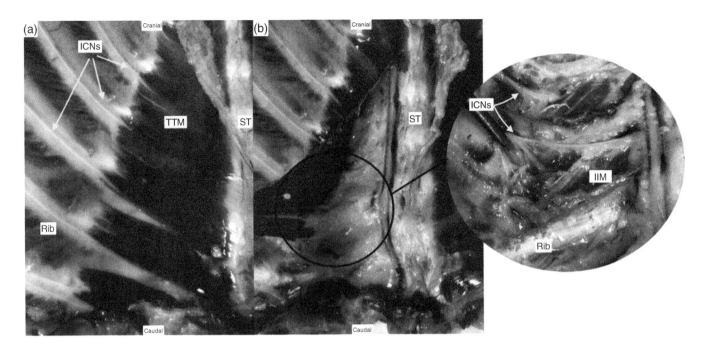

FIGURE 16.4   Inner visualization of the thorax before (a) and after (b) dissection of the *m. transversus thoracis* (TTM). In (b), the TTM has been removed and two branches of **intercostal nerves** (ICNs) are visible. IIM, *mm. intercostales interni*; ST, sternum. Source: From Zublena et al. 2021. Used with permission.

Anatomical studies in canine cadavers suggest that there may be a promise for more widespread use of these blocks, however, prospective, randomized, blinded, controlled studies are needed before widespread incorporation of them into small animal anesthesia and pain management.

PATIENT SELECTION
INDICATIONS FOR THE BLOCK

Based on their reported uses and benefits in people, parasternal block techniques would be expected to provide analgesia to the sternum and other structures of the ventral thorax for a variety of potentially painful conditions or procedures in animals. In people, these blocks provide analgesia to patients who are undergoing pericardiocentesis or cardiac procedures via median sternotomy, and to those who suffer from sternal fractures or chronic pain related to sternal lesions (McDonald et al. 2005; Barr et al. 2007; Ozturk et al. 2016; Thomas et al. 2016; Zhang et al. 2021). No clinical studies in small animals have been reported to date and, although the indications and benefits of these techniques might be expected to be similar to those that have been reported in people, further studies are required before definitive recommendations regarding indications for their use in dogs and cats can be made. A case report by Fernández Barrientos and Merlin (2022) documented the effects of performing a *transverse* TTP block as part of their multimodal analgesic plan for a dog undergoing median sternotomy for lung lobectomy. They concluded that

its use resulted in satisfactory operative conditions when only ketamine and lidocaine infusions were coadministered with propofol, and that the TTP block might be a useful adjuvant for surgeries such as median sternotomy in dogs, although further clinical studies are required.

CONTRAINDICATIONS

- Skin infection or other lesions at the intended needle puncture site.
- Inability to identify the relevant anatomy during ultrasound scanning.

POTENTIAL SIDE EFFECTS AND COMPLICATIONS

Parasternal block research in veterinary medicine is limited to only a few canine cadaveric studies that describe the relevant anatomy, investigate the use of various needle and transducer orientations, and document the distribution of different volumes of dye injectate (Alaman et al. 2021; Alaman et al. 2022; Zublena et al. 2021; Escalante et al. 2022). Although the results of these studies appear promising, only a single case report has been published, therefore, information about potential side effects and the incidence of clinically relevant complications is not yet known. Based on the few studies that have been published, some initial assumptions can be made about potential complications and aspects of the blocks to be mindful of.

In addition to the potential for complications that are related to the performance of any regional anesthetic technique (e.g. needle trauma, intravascular injections, etc.), parasternal techniques carry additional risks associated with the potential for inadvertent intrathoracic needle placement. Based solely on the relevant anatomy, the PIFP approach would be expected to carry less risk of this complication than the TTP approach since it is performed more superficially, and the needle stays outside the thoracic wall through its entire course.

Unlike the PIFP approach, the TTP approach involves penetrating the intercostal musculature and advancing the tip of the needle into its final location between the *m. transversus thoracis* and *mm. intercostales interni*, making it potentially a more precarious block, especially in patients whose chests are moving due to spontaneous or mechanical ventilation. If the needle tip is not able to be visualized while it is being advanced (or even if it can be), the needle could inadvertently penetrate the thoracic cavity and puncture the lungs, the apex of the heart, and/or the internal thoracic artery and vein (Escalante et al. 2022). To perform the TTP block safely, the anesthetist must be highly skilled with the use of ultrasound, have excellent hand–eye coordination, and have a good understanding of the sonoanatomy of the thoracic wall (Zublena et al. 2021).

GENERAL CONSIDERATIONS
CLINICAL ANATOMY

Innervation of the ventral thoracic wall is supplied by the terminal branches of the **intercostal nerves** that arise from the T2 to T6 spinal nerves. These nerves provide innervation to the sternum and adjacent tissues and are the primary target of the different regional anesthetic techniques described here. The *m. transversus thoracis* is a flat, fan-shaped muscle that is located ventral to the costochondral junctions on the innermost aspect of the thoracic wall (Alaman et al. 2021). The *m. transversus thoracis* arises from the sternum between the second sternebra and the xiphoid process and inserts on the medial aspect of the second to seventh costal cartilages. The medial aspect of the *m. transversus thoracis* is covered by the endothoracic fascia and parietal/costal pleura which then extend dorsally to cover the medial aspect of the *mm. intercostales interni*. The *mm. intercostales interni* insert on their cranial ribs via *internal intercostal membranes*, whose fibers course from one costal cartilage to another, extending between the interchondral spaces from the costochondral junctions to the lateral aspect of the sternum (Alaman et al. 2021). The *mm. intercostales interni* are covered laterally by the *mm. intercostales externi*; however, the *mm. intercostales externi* do not extend all the way ventrally and do not contact the sternum at the level of the first nine or ten intercostal spaces. The transversus thoracis plane is located between the *m. transversus thoracis* and the *mm. intercos-*

tales interni at the level of the second to seventh intercostal spaces. Along with variable amounts of fat, the internal thoracic artery and vein run parallel to the lateral aspect of the sternum within the transversus thoracis plane (Figures 16.4 and 16.5).

After emerging from the thoracic paravertebral space dorsally, the **intercostal nerves** run together with intercostal arteries and veins within neurovascular bundles on the caudomedial aspect of their associated ribs. In dogs, the T2–T6 **intercostal nerves** course through the transversus thoracis plane and are ultimately responsible for innervation of the ventral thoracic wall. After giving off muscular branches to the *m. transversus thoracis* and *m. rectus abdominis*, the **ventral cutaneous branches** of the **intercostal nerves** pass through the internal intercostal membrane just lateral to the midline, where they provide sensory innervation to the skin, sternum, mammary glands, and other structures on the ventral thorax (Alaman et al. 2021; Escalante et al. 2022).

EXPECTED DISTRIBUTION OF ANESTHESIA

The goal of using a parasternal regional anesthetic technique is to provide analgesia to the sternum and related structures. Like other interfascial plane blocks that are used to provide analgesia for procedures along the midline (i.e. TAP blocks for the abdomen), parasternal block techniques must be performed bilaterally to be effective.

Studies by Zublena et al. (2021) and Alaman et al. (2021, 2022) assessed different approaches to the TTP and the distribution of dye following the administration of multiple, small volume injections or single, large volume injections of dye (Figures 16.6, 16.7, 16.8). Zublena et al. (2021) showed that injections of $0.05\,\text{ml}\,\text{kg}^{-1}$ of dye at each intercostal space can result in high levels of success and that this technique may be an appropriate technique for blocking the sternum, despite the need for multiple needle sticks and the time to perform the block bilaterally. Alaman et al. (2021) showed that, although multiple nerves were successfully stained following a single injection into the transversus thoracis plane, the observed distribution of dye did not appear to be adequate to block the entire sternum if a local anesthetic had been used. Alaman et al. (2022) showed that lower volumes at two injections sites were effective for staining the majority of the target nerves.

Using a PIFP approach in canine cadavers, Escalante et al. (2022) showed that the injection of 0.25–$0.5\,\text{ml}\,\text{kg}^{-1}$ of a dye solution will result in the distribution of the injectate across several intercostal spaces over one hemithorax, with a greater number of ventral branches of intercostal nerves being stained by the higher volume of injectate (Figure 16.9). Despite this, not all the target nerves were stained by the dye and the investigators concluded that, if a local anesthetic solution was injected, the observed spread would likely be inadequate to provide effective analgesia to the entire sternum. Further investigation into the use of this technique is also needed.

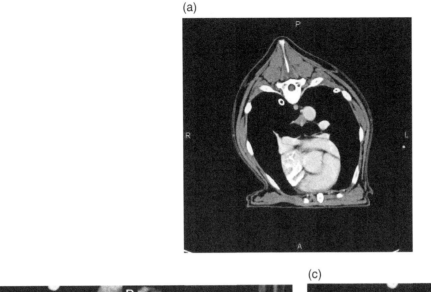

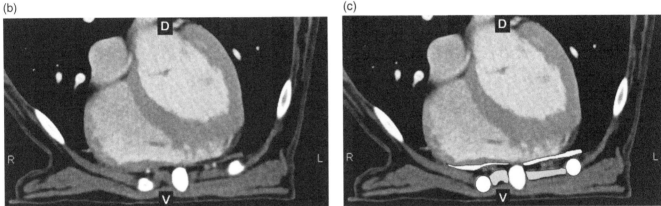

FIGURE 16.5   (a) Computed tomographic (CT) image of the thorax of a dog at the level of the fifth sternebra. (b) Enlarged view, with annotations (c). Note the *m. transversus thoracis* (yellow), *mm. intercostales* (orange), ribs (white circles) and internal thoracic arteries (red circles) and veins (blue circles). D, dorsal; L, left; R, right; V, ventral.

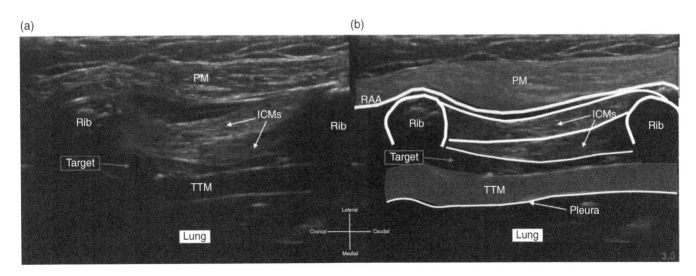

FIGURE 16.6   Sagittal ultrasound image of the intercostal space in the parasternal area of a canine cadaver (a), with relevant anatomical structures indicated (b). ICMs, intercostal muscles; PM, *mm. pectoralis*; RAA, *m. rectus abdominis* aponeurosis; TTM, *m. transversus thoracis*. Source: From Zublena et al. 2021. Used with permission.

(a)

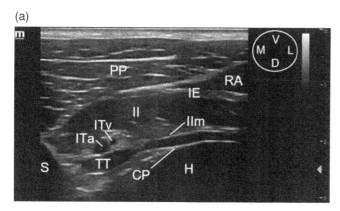

(b)

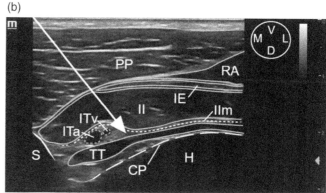

FIGURE 16.7 (a) Ultrasound image of the fifth interchondral space in a canine cadaver, showing the anatomical structures observed during the *transverse* approach to the transversus thoracis plane (TTP) (as shown in Figure 16.1). (b) The same ultrasound image with the edges of the muscular structures (solid grey lines), the internal intercostal membrane (short dashed white lines), fifth sternebra (solid white line), vascular structures (short dashed grey lines) and costal pleura (long dashed lines) superimposed to facilitate their identification. The white arrow shows the needle pathway and the needle tip located in the transversus thoracis plane. CP, costal pleura; D, dorsal; H, heart; IE, *mm. intercostales externi*; II, *mm. intercostales interni*; Im, internal intercostal membrane; ITa, internal thoracic artery; ITv, internal thoracic vein; L, lateral; M, medial; PP, *m. pectoralis profundus*; RA, *m. rectus abdominis*; S, sternum; TT, *m. transversus thoracis*; V, ventral. Source: From Alaman et al. 2021. Used with permission.

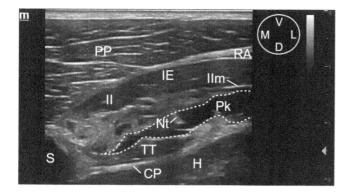

FIGURE 16.8 Ultrasound image showing the distribution of injectate following administration of a methylene blue-lidocaine solution using the *transverse* transversus thoracis plane (TTP) approach at the level of the fifth interchondral space. The pocket of fluid is delimited by the dotted line. CP, costal pleura; D, dorsal; IE, *mm. intercostales externi*; II, *mm. intercostales interni*; IIm, internal intercostal membrane; L, lateral; M, medial; Nt, needle tip; Pk, pocket of fluid; PP, *m. pectoralis profundus*; RA, *m. rectus abdominis*; S, sternum; TT, *m. transversus thoracis*; V, ventral. Source: From Alaman et al. 2021. Used with permission.

LOCAL ANESTHETIC: DOSE, VOLUME, AND CONCENTRATION

Any local anesthetic (e.g., bupivacaine, ropivacaine, levobupivacaine) could be used to perform a parasternal block. Depending on the size of the patient and the formulation of the local anesthetic that is available (i.e. 0.5% versus 0.75%), the local anesthetic could be diluted with saline to increase the volume that is injected.

The ideal volume of injectate for the TTP approach in dogs has not yet been established, but it has been investigated in

canine cadavers (Alaman et al. 2021; Alaman et al. 2022; Zublena et al. 2021). Using a transverse transducer orientation and an in-plane needle technique, Alaman et al. (2021) compared two volumes of injectate (0.5 ml kg^{-1} or 1.0 ml kg^{-1}) and found that the use of the higher volume resulted in more dye staining of the target intercostal nerves than the use of lower volume, suggesting that increasing the volume may result in more effective desensitization of the ventral chest wall. However, they also found that, although dye staining in the interchondral spaces could be extensive, staining of the corresponding intercostal nerves was variable. Following the use of their experimental TTP technique, they also documented the spread of dye under the costal pleura and into the mediastinum, which they attributed to the injectate spreading along the endothoracic fascia that exists between the *m. transversus thoracis* and the costal pleura. Using the transverse TTP approach described by Alaman et al. (2021), Fernández Barrientos and Merlin (2022) administered bupivacaine 0.25% 0.2 ml kg^{-1} bilaterally in a dog undergoing median sternotomy for lung lobectomy.

Using a parasagittal transducer orientation and an in-plane needle technique, Zublena et al. (2021) also investigated different volumes of injectate for TTP blocks using canine cadavers. Those investigators injected either 0.05 ml kg^{-1} of injectate at each of six sites (second through seventh intercostal spaces) in their "low-volume" group or 0.1 ml kg^{-1} at each of three sites (third, fifth, and seventh intercostal spaces) in their "high-volume" group. Although they found that injecting six spaces on each side of the sternum resulted in a more reliable and accurate spread of the dye solution (36/36 injections), the use of the larger volume at fewer spaces also resulted in reasonable spread to adjacent intercostal spaces through the TTP. The overall distribution of the dye solution was limited laterally by the

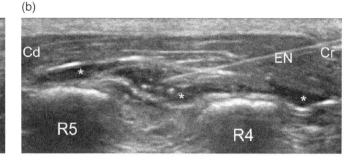

FIGURE 16.9 (a) Ultrasound image of the pecto-intercostal fascial plane (PIFP) in a canine cadaver. The targeted fascial plane (indicated by + + +) lies between the fourth (R4) and fifth (R5) ribs, superficial to the ***mm. intercostales externi*** (EIM) and deep to the ***m. pectoralis profundus*** (DP). (b) Ultrasound image following injection of methylene blue dye solution (indicated by * * *) into the PIFP of a canine cadaver, indicating a craniocaudal spread. Cd, caudal; Cr, cranial; EN, echogenic needle. Source: From Escalante et al. 2022. Used with permission.

insertion of the ***m. transversus thoracis*** onto the ribs and, as far as complications, there was a single case where dye was observed on the pleural surface of one lung.

The ideal volume of injectate for the PIFP approach has also been investigated. In a pilot study that used canine cadavers, Escalante et al. (2022) found that >0.5 ml kg⁻¹ of injectate may spread cranially toward the brachial plexus. Based on this observation, they more thoroughly investigated the spread of smaller volumes of injectate (0.25 and 0.5 ml kg⁻¹) following administration at a single site into the PIFP using a parasagittal transducer orientation and in-plane needle technique. Although they found no significant differences in the overall spread of dye between the two volumes, fewer **ventral cutaneous branches** of the **intercostal nerves** were stained with the lower volume, suggesting the higher volume may be more effective for providing analgesia *in vivo*. However, they found that the higher volume of injectate occasionally stained non-targeted structures such as the **subscapular** and **axillary nerves**. The investigators concluded that using a lower volume but administering it across several different sites might provide more complete analgesia with less concern for the potential complications that appear to be associated with the use of the higher volume of injectate at a single site of injection. However, this theory has not yet been tested.

CONCLUSIONS

How the results of these canine cadaver studies might translate into clinical practice when local anesthetics are used in live patients requires continued investigation. Further studies of the TTP and PIFP approaches are necessary to establish the optimum combination of injection technique, number of injection sites, and volume of injectate that will result in predictable, safe, and effective spread of injectate in the parasternal region of veterinary patients. In the author's experience (anecdotal, not peer-reviewed), use of a transvese TTP approach at two sites per side (2nd and 5th sternebra) contributes to balanced anesthesia that eliminates or reduces the need for additional systemic analgesics (e.g. constant rate infusions of ketamine and/or opioids) for canine patients that are anesthetized for median sternotomies. Parasternal techniques carry tremendous potential to contribute to perioperative care and further research and documentation of their risks and benefits are required.

REFERENCES

Alaman M, González-Marrón A, Lorente C et al. (2021) Description of an ultrasound-guided transverse approach to the transversus thoracis plane block and evaluation of injectate spread in canine cadavers. Animals (Basel) 11, 2657.

Alaman M, Bonastre C, González-Marrón A et al. (2022) A two-point ultrasound-guided injection technique for the transversus thoracis plane block: A canine cadaveric study. Animals (Basel) 12, 2165.

Barr AM, Tutungi E, Almeida AA. (2007) Parasternal intercostal block with ropivacaine for pain management after cardiac surgery: a double-blind, randomized, controlled trial. J Cardiothorac Vasc Anesth 21, 547–53.

Fernández Barrientos MA, Merlin T. (2022) Ultrasound-guided transversus thoracis plane block as part of multimodal analgesia in a dog undergoing median sternotomy. Vet Anaesth Analg 49, 674–676.

Bloc S, Perot BP, Gibert H et al. (2021) Efficacy of parasternal block to decrease intraoperative opioid use in coronary artery bypass surgery via sternotomy: a randomized controlled trial. Reg Anesth Pain Med 46, 671–678.

de la Torre PA, García PD, Alvarez SL et al. (2014) A novel ultrasound-guided block: a promising alternative for breast analgesia. Anesthet Surg J 34, 198–200.

Escalante GC, Ferreira TH, Hershberger-Braker KL et al. (2022) Evaluation of ultrasound-guided pecto-intercostal block in canine cadavers. Vet Anaesth Analg, 49, 182–188.

Liu V, Mariano ER, Prabhaka C. (2018) Pecto-intercostal fascial block for acute poststernotomy pain. A A Prac 10, 319–322.

McDonald SB, Jacobsohn E, Kopacz DJ et al. (2005) Parasternal block and local anesthetic infiltration with levobupivacaine after cardiac surgery with desflurane: the effect on postoperative pain, pulmonary function, and tracheal extubation times. Anesth Analg 100, 25–32.

Ozturk NK, Baki ED, Kavakli AS et al. (2016) Comparison of transcutaneous electrical nerve stimulation and parasternal block for postoperative pain management after cardiac surgery. Pain Res Manag 2016, 4261949.

Thomas KP, Sainudeen S, Jose S et al. (2016) Ultrasound-guided parasternal block allows optimal pain relief and ventilation improvement after a sternal fracture. Pain Ther 5, 115–122.

Zhang Y. Gong H. Zhan B et al. (2021) Effects of bilateral pecto-intercostal fascial block for perioperative pain management in patients undergoing open cardiac surgery: a prospective randomized study. BMC AnesthesiologyAnesthesiol 21, 175.

Zublena F, Briganti A, De Gennaro C et al. (2021) Ultrasound-guided parasternal injection in dogs: a cadaver study. Vet Anaesth Analg 48, 563–569.

Ultrasound-Guided Erector Spinae Plane Block

Tatiana H. Ferreira

CHAPTER 17

BLOCK AT A GLANCE

What is it used for?

- In the veterinary literature, erector spinae plane blocks (ESPBs) are primarily used to contribute to anesthesia and analgesia for surgical procedures involving the spine.

Landmarks/transducer position

- The ultrasound (US) transducer should be positioned in a parasagittal orientation lateral to dorsal midline.

- Once the target vertebra is identified with US guidance, the transducer can be tilted medially and laterally until the optimal acoustic shadows made by the target transverse processes are identified.

- Deposition of local anesthetic occurs between the target transverse process and the muscles of the erector spinae group.

- For the lumbar area, a transverse approach with different landmarks has been described in dogs. Injection of the local anesthetic in this case is between the accessory process and the lateral aspect of the mammillary process of the following vertebra.

- This chapter will focus on the traditional parasagittal approach due to limited information in the human and veterinary literature on other approaches.

What equipment and personnel are required?

- Short-bevel, Tuohy, or blunt atraumatic needle (21–22G, 5–10 cm (1½–3½ in.), depending on the size of the patient

- Syringe of drug(s)

- Ultrasound machine

- High frequency (15–6 MHz) linear array transducer +/− protective sleeve

- Gloves

- Coupling agent (e.g. alcohol)

- T-connector extension (optional, but recommended by the author)

- Assistant to help perform test injections and final drug administration

When do I perform the block?

- Prior to the surgery, after the skin over the injection sites is clipped and preparation is complete. Final skin preparation should be performed after the block and prior to the surgery.

- Postoperative administration or nonsurgical use may be used for patients with painful conditions that are not undergoing surgery. In these situations, heavy sedation or general anesthesia would be required.

What volume of local anesthetic is used?

- 0.3–0.5 ml kg^{-1} per injection site. Note that dilution of the local anesthetic may be required to achieve this volume without exceeding recommended doses.

Goal

- To visualize a linear cranial–caudal spread of local anesthetic between the transverse process and erector spinae muscles (ESM).

- In case of the transverse approach, injectate should be visualized separating **m. longissimus lumborum** from the mammillary process at the injection level.

Complexity level

- Intermediate

Clinical pearl

- ESPBs should be used as a component of a multimodal analgesic approach until prospective clinical studies in veterinary species better document their clinical effects and mechanism(s) of action. They should not be relied on as the sole source of analgesia.

Small Animal Regional Anesthesia and Analgesia, Second Edition. Edited by Matt Read, Luis Campoy, and Berit Fischer.
© 2024 John Wiley & Sons, Inc. Published 2024 by John Wiley & Sons, Inc.

WHAT DO WE ALREADY KNOW?

The ESPB is a novel US-guided fascial plane block that has gained significant popularity (e.g. over 1000 publications in seven years) since it was first reported in the human literature (Forero et al. 2016). The first description of this block in veterinary medicine was in dogs (Ferreira et al. 2019) and, since then, more than 15 reports have been published, including cadaveric studies, retrospective clinical studies, and case reports in different species, including dogs, cats, cows, horses, and pigs (Otero et al. 2020; Portela et al. 2020, 2021; Zannin et al. 2020; Alza Salvatierra et al. 2021; Bartholomew and Ferreira 2021; Delgado et al. 2021; Medina-Serra et al. 2021a, b; Rodriguez Mulet et al. 2021; Cavalcanti et al. 2022; Chiavaccinia et al. 2022; D'Anselme et al. 2022; Ferré et al. 2022; Rodriguez et al. 2022; Sambugaro et al. 2022; Viilmann et al. 2022). The growing popularity of this block may be related in part to its relative simplicity and good safety profile.

ESPBs were initially described in people for management of painful conditions associated with the thoracic area (Forero et al. 2016; Yao et al. 2020). However, potential indications in the human literature have been extended to include procedures involving the spine, abdomen, upper limb, pelvis, and lower limb (De Cassai et al. 2019a; Goel et al. 2021; Saadawi et al. 2021; Campbell and Chin 2022) depending on which thoracic or lumbar level the injection(s) is performed. There are also descriptions of cervical ESPBs in the human literature for shoulder and cervical procedures (Saadawi et al. 2021; Campbell and Chin 2022; Kanna et al. 2023).

Most of the publications in veterinary medicine are cadaveric anatomical studies (thoracic and lumbar ESPBs) and case reports (Otero et al. 2020; Portela et al. 2020; Zannin et al. 2020; Alza Salvatierra et al. 2021; Bartholomew and Ferreira 2021; Delgado et al. 2021; Medina-Serra et al. 2021a, b; Rodriguez Mulet et al. 2021; Cavalcanti et al. 2022; Chiavaccinia et al. 2022; D'Anselme et al. 2022; Rodriguez et al. 2022; Sambugaro et al. 2022). Considering the clinical descriptions, the majority of the reports in the veterinary literature focus on procedures involving the spine (Zannin et al. 2020; Alza Salvatierra et al. 2021; Portela et al. 2021; Rodriguez Mulet et al. 2021; Chiavaccinia et al. 2022; Rodriguez et al. 2022; Viilmann et al. 2022), with two exceptions being a case report describing its use as part of a multimodal analgesic plan for pancreatitis in a dog and a retrospective study for thoracotomies in dogs (Bartholomew and Ferreira 2021; Ferré et al. 2022). The application of this block in veterinary medicine is not currently as extensive as it is in the human literature.

The approach that was first described for performing ESPBs in the thoracic region of dogs involves the administration of local anesthetic dorsal to the target transverse process and ventral to the ESM (Ferreira et al. 2019; Saadawi et al. 2021). After a single-point injection, the local anesthetic is expected to spread cranio–caudally, resulting in blockade of multiple vertebral levels (Chin and El-Boghdadly 2021). Recently, a transverse approach for the lumbar region has been described whereby local anesthetic is injected between the accessory process of the target vertebra and the lateral aspect of the mammillary process of the following vertebra (Medina-Serra et al. 2021b).

The mechanism of action of ESPBs is not completely understood and is considered to be controversial (Ivanusic et al. 2018; Otero et al. 2020; Chin and El-Boghdadly 2021; Saadawi et al. 2021). Clinical efficacy and anatomical studies (cadaveric or contrast-based) suggest conflicting mechanisms of action of ESPBs related to the spread of the injectate. Some studies demonstrate spread to the **ventral rami** of the spinal nerves with potential involvement of the paravertebral and epidural space, whereas other studies show that spread of the injectate is mostly confined to the branches of the dorsal rami of the spinal nerves (Adhikary et al. 2018; Ivanusic et al. 2018; Schwartzmann et al. 2018; Tulgar et al. 2018b; Vidal et al. 2018; Yang et al. 2018; Choi et al. 2019; Dautzenberg et al. 2019; Ferreira et al. 2019; Portela et al. 2020; Chin and El-Boghdadly 2021). If this block is limited to affecting the **dorsal rami** (as the veterinary literature suggests), clinical application of this block would seemingly be restricted to procedures involving the dorso–lateral aspects of the trunk. However, studies in humans, one case report in dogs, and a retrospective study in dogs have demonstrated efficacy of this block as part of a multimodal analgesic approach for procedures and painful conditions involving the ventral aspect of the body and viscera, suggesting involvement of the **ventral rami** as well (De Cassai et al. 2019a; Bartholomew and Ferreira 2021; Saadawi et al. 2021; Ferré et al. 2022). These differing findings may be the result of using cadavers, the particular technique that was used, the level of injection along the spine, the timing of the injection in relation to the assessments, and/or the volume of injectate (Choi et al. 2019; Dautzenberg et al. 2019; De Cassai et al. 2020; Chin and El-Boghdadly 2021).

Intra- and interspecies anatomical variations should also be considered. Owing to the high volume/dose of local anesthetic used for ESPBs and its rapid absorption following administration (De Cassai et al. 2021a), the potential for a systemic analgesic effect cannot be ruled out. The degree of contribution from this mechanism, however, is likely to be minimal as the local anesthetic plasma concentrations achieved following an ESPB decrease to levels below range of analgesic IV dosing regimens within two to three hours following administration (De Cassai et al. 2021a).

In addition to a controversial mechanism of action (Chin and El-Boghdadly 2021), the literature also shows some variation regarding the degree of clinical efficacy and the extent of the sensory block achieved with ESPBs (De Cassai et al. 2019a; Tulgar and Balaban 2019; Byrne and Smith 2020; Kendall et al. 2020; Ferré et al. 2022). Regardless, most studies in humans and dogs result in lower opioid consumption and improved postoperative pain control and recovery quality (De Cassai et al. 2019a; Kendall et al. 2020; Bartholomew and

Ferreira 2021; Portela et al. 2021; Rizkalla et al. 2021; Rodriguez Mulet et al. 2021; Saadawi et al. 2021; Ferré et al. 2022; Jiao et al. 2022; Koo et al. 2022; Viilmann et al. 2022). Some human studies suggest comparable analgesia to other regional techniques, such as thoracic paravertebral blocks (Gürkan et al. 2020; Zhao et al. 2020) or epidurals (Nagaraja et al. 2018), however, these are limited in scope and not corroborated in the literature (Saadawi et al. 2021). These discrepancies have led to some authors to question the routine use of this block for postoperative analgesia, instead opting to reserve it for rescue analgesia should other more reliable techniques fail (Zhang et al. 2020).

When utilizing an ESPB, the clinical effects will depend on the vertebral level at which the local anesthetic is deposited (Tulgar et al. 2018b; Tulgar and Balaban 2019). In humans and dogs, anatomical differences between the thoracic and lumbar vertebrae likely contribute to this variable effect, including differences in the specific muscles that form the ESM complex in each region, the anatomy of the spinal nerves, their branches and distribution, the sizes of the vertebrae and transverse processes, the structure of the fascia between these two regions, and potential anatomical barriers for the injectate spread (Hermanson 2020a, b, c; Tulgar et al. 2020b).

In humans, irrespective of these anatomical differences, the classic site for injection of lumbar ESPBs is similar to the site used for thoracic ESPBs, with some minor variations in technique (Harbell et al. 2020; Tulgar et al. 2020b; Campbell and Chin 2022). These may include the position of the patient (sternal versus lateral recumbency), the approach used (transverse versus parasagittal) (Aksu and Gürkan 2019; De Cassai et al. 2019b), and the reported inclusion of the psoas major muscle (deep to the transverse processes), both as a landmark (Campbell and Chin 2022) and as a target for additional injections between it and the transverse processes (Tulgar et al. 2019b). The goal of using the latter technique is to desensitize the lumbar plexus, which would make the block also useful for hip and lower limb procedures (Tulgar et al. 2018b, 2019b). As with thoracic ESPBs, there are reports of variable injectate spread affecting the paravertebral, intervertebral foramina, and epidural spaces (De Lara González et al. 2019; Harbell et al. 2020; Tulgar et al. 2020b; Chin and El-Boghdadly 2021; Campbell and Chin 2022). Overall, information in the literature regarding sensory effects and clinical assessments including complications of lumbar ESPBs is scarce, as most publications are limited to case reports (Tulgar et al. 2020b).

In veterinary medicine, both transverse and parasagittal in-plane techniques have been described for performing lumbar ESPB injections in dog cadavers. Using a transverse, in-plane technique, injection of contrast dye between the accessory process of L4 and the lateral aspect of the mammillary process of L5 resulted in complete staining of the **dorsal rami** of the **lumbar spinal nerves** in 94% of injections whereas deposition of injectate between the ***m. multifidus***

and the ***mm. longissimus/iliocostalis*** at the level of L4 using a modified parasagittal approach resulted in complete staining in only 23% of injections (Medina-Serra et al. 2021b). Despite better staining, however, the authors reported epidural and intravascular injectate migration in three and four of the 17 injections, respectively, following the use of a transverse approach. The lumbar ESPB approach described by (Medina-Serra et al. 2021b) is located more superficial and medial than the approach described in humans where injections typically occur between the transverse process and ***mm. erector spinae.*** How the differences in anatomy between the thoracic and lumbar regions and the differences in technique affect block performance, success, complications, and the use of consistent terminology remains to be established in veterinary medicine.

The primary focus of the most recent veterinary literature has been on blocking the **dorsal rami** for procedures involving the dorso–lateral regions of the trunk, including spinal surgery (i.e. hemilaminectomies), which may explain this modified superficial approach. A study by Cavalcanti et al. (2022) compared a transverse approach at the level of T12 to the more traditional parasagittal approach (between the transverse process and ***mm. erector spinae***) in dogs. Interestingly, those authors found that the transverse approach resulted in more consistent staining of the **medial branches** of the **dorsal rami** whereas the parasagittal approach resulted in more consistent staining of the **lateral branches** of the **dorsal rami**. Based on the different paths of the branches of the **dorsal rami** in the caudal thoracic vertebrae and lumbar area and the more consistent staining of the **medial branches** of the **dorsal rami** (which desensitize more anatomic structures involved with spinal surgeries), those authors suggested that, caudal to T11, the transverse approach could result in better outcomes and analgesia for procedures such as hemilaminectomies in dogs (Cavalcanti et al. 2022).

Besides the clear anatomical differences in the areas (thoracic *versus* lumbar), there are significant variations regarding the technique of this block within and between the human and veterinary literature. This issue and the improper use of some anatomic landmarks (including muscles) were recently brought up with a call to the research community for standardization of technique and nomenclature revision (Elkoundi and El Koraichi 2020; Hamilton 2020; Tulgar et al. 2020a). The benefits would include improvement in our understanding and decrease in ambiguity, allow reproducibility in future studies, and facilitate clear dialogue between investigators and clinicians (Elkoundi and El Koraichi 2020; Hamilton 2020). Further investigations are required in veterinary medicine to determine the most reliable target for the local anesthetic injection, with anatomic variations of the vertebrae and surrounding musculature along the spine being taken into consideration. Volume recommendations and the optimal number of injections (i.e. multisite versus single injection) also need further investigation so as to maximize ESPB efficacy while minimizing the risk of complications.

In the human literature, volumes used for ESPBs in pediatric patients vary between 0.2 and 0.5 ml kg^{-1} (De Cassai et al. 2019a). A wider range of 0.2–1 ml kg^{-1} per injection, with a dose range of 1–2.8 mg kg^{-1} of bupivacaine or levobupivacaine has been used in dogs and cats (Ferreira et al. 2019; Portela et al. 2020, 2021; Zannin et al. 2020; Alza Salvatierra et al. 2021; Bartholomew and Ferreira 2021; Medina-Serra et al. 2021b; Rodriguez Mulet et al. 2021; Cavalcanti et al. 2022; Ferré et al. 2022; Sambugaro et al. 2022). Studies directly comparing different volumes (0.3 versus 0.6 ml kg^{-1} and 0.5 versus 1.0 ml kg^{-1}) in dog cadavers could not find significant differences in nerve staining between groups (Ferreira et al. 2019; Portela et al. 2020). There are no clinical studies assessing the impact of different volumes in live animals and further studies assessing the optimum volume are warranted. One important aspect of ESPBs is that different regions of the body (i.e. thoracic versus lumbar) have anatomical differences that could play a role in the distribution of the injectate. In humans, lumbar ESPBs seem to require higher volumes of injectate for similar vertebral level spread when compared to thoracic ESPBs. For example, De Cassai et al. (2020) found that a median of 5 ml was required to cover one vertebral level in the lumbar region, compared to 3.3–3.5 ml in the thoracic region.

No studies to date have investigated the use of adjuvants for ESPBs in veterinary species. A case report in a dog with intractable abdominal pain due to pancreatitis used ESPBs as part of a multimodal analgesic approach (Bartholomew and Ferreira 2021). In that report, three ESPB injections were performed over the course of four days, with one injection being made with a bupivacaine liposomal injectable suspension combined with bupivacaine in an attempt to increase its duration of effect. Only a mild increase in duration was noted (38 hours versus 24 hours) and the dog appeared to experience a subjectively less profound analgesic effect.

Although the remainder of this chapter will primarily focus on the traditional parasagittal approach for performing ESPBs due to more information being available in the human and veterinary literature, the transverse approach will be also considered where appropriate.

PATIENT SELECTION
INDICATIONS FOR THE BLOCK

Depending on which level of the spine they are performed on, ESPBs have several applications in the human literature, including treating painful medical conditions and providing analgesia for surgical procedures involving the thorax, spine, abdomen, upper limb, neck, lower limb, and pelvis (De Cassai et al. 2020; Saadawi et al. 2021; Campbell and Chin 2022). In veterinary medicine, studies to date have been limited in scope, focusing primarily on ESPBs for procedures involving the spine (Zannin et al. 2020; Alza Salvatierra et al. 2021; Portela et al. 2021; Rodriguez Mulet et al. 2021; Chiavaccinia et al. 2022; Rodriguez et al. 2022; Viilmann et al. 2022). Two publications (a case report and a retrospective study) have reported on the use of ESPBs as part of multimodal analgesic approaches for treating pain associated with pancreatitis and thoracotomies (Bartholomew and Ferreira 2021; Ferré et al. 2022).

As would be expected, the location along the spine that is used as the injection target will differ depending on the intended area to be blocked. The anesthetist should be familiar with the anatomical differences between the thoracic and lumbar vertebrae since modifications to the described technique may be indicated.

CONTRAINDICATIONS

- Infection, neoplasia, or other lesions at or around the intended imaging and/or puncture site.

- Previous surgery or other anatomical abnormalities are relative contraindications as these factors could potentially affect the performance and efficacy of the block, predispose the patient to epidural spread, and/or potentially increase the risk of intravascular injection (Tulgar et al. 2020b; Sambugaro et al. 2022).

- Large (>30–40 kg) or obese patients can pose technical challenges when performing ESPBs because anatomic landmarks may be difficult to visualize using standard linear transducers that only scan to a depth of ~6 cm.

POTENTIAL SIDE EFFECTS AND COMPLICATIONS

- Local anesthetic systemic toxicity (LAST) due to high volume of local anesthetic required for appropriate spread

- Cardiovascular instability

- Hind limb weakness and/or motor blockade (due to local anesthetic spread to lumbar plexus and/or epidural spread), more likely for lumbar ESPB, especially when the transverse approach is performed

- Pneumothorax

- Visceral (thoracic or abdominal) damage

- Hematoma

- Infection

GENERAL CONSIDERATIONS
CLINICAL ANATOMY

The ESM are part of the epaxial muscle group and, at the level of the thorax, include the ***mm. spinalis thoracis, longissimus thoracis,*** and ***iliocostalis thoracis*** (Hermanson 2020b). The organization of these muscles is complex and there are significant variations reported in the literature. In this chapter, the organization described will follow the *Nomina Anatomica Veterinaria* (International Committee on Veterinary Gross Anatomical Nomenclature 2017).

There are several anatomical differences between the thoracic and lumbar regions that should be taken into consideration for the ESPB. For example, when compared with thoracic vertebrae, lumbar vertebrae have longer bodies, shorter spinal processes with a slight cranial inclination, longer transverse processes that are directed both cranial and slightly ventral, accessory processes that are well developed on the L1–4 vertebrae and absent on the L5–6 vertebrae, and all the cranial articular processes possess mamillary processes (Hermanson 2020a) (Figure 17.1).

The ESM group in the lumbar area is formed by the **m. iliocostalis lumborum**, which is much thicker than at the thoracic level and lies in close contact with the transverse processes, and the **m. longissimus lumborum**, which is located medial to the **m. iliocostalis lumborum** and lateral to

the spinal processes (Hermanson 2020b) (Figure 17.2). The **m. longissimus lumborum** is covered by a dense aponeurosis that acts as a retinaculum for the **m. longissimus lumborum**, **m. multifidus**, and **m. sacrocaudalis dorsalis lateralis** (Medina-Serra et al. 2021b). There is no **m. spinalis** in the lumbar area (Hermanson 2020b). The lumbar portion of the **m. multifidus** is larger compared to its thoracic component and arises from the articular processes and runs laterally to the spinal processes, immediately ventral to the supraspinous ligament (Hermanson 2020b). Some authors consider the **m. multifidus** to be part of the ESM group (Tulgar et al. 2020b; Medina-Serra et al. 2021b); however, the *Nomina Anatomica Veterinaria* (International Committee on Veterinary Gross Anatomical Nomenclature 2017), does not (Hermanson 2020b).

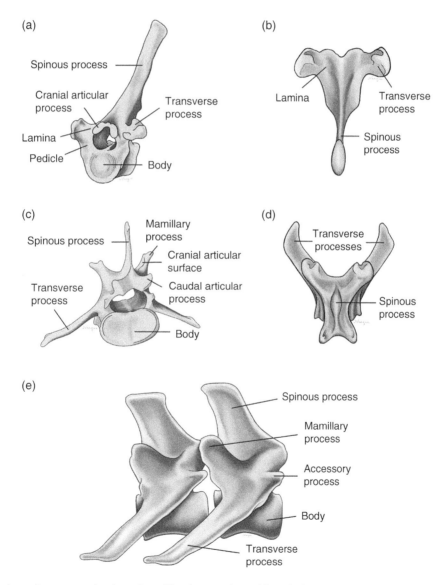

FIGURE 17.1 Illustrations of representative thoracic and lumbar vertebrae. (a) Sixth thoracic vertebra, cranio–lateral view. (b) Sixth thoracic vertebra, dorsal view. (c) Fourth lumbar vertebrae, caudo–lateral view. (d) Fourth lumbar vertebrae, dorsal view. (e) Third and fourth lumbar vertebrae, lateral view.

The *m. sacrocaudalis dorsalis lateralis* is not part of the ESM complex but may be visualized during lumbar ESPBs. This muscle lies between the *m. longissimus lumborum* (laterally) and the *m. multifidus* (medially) in the caudal portion of the lumbar region (Hermanson 2020b) (Figure 17.2). The deep layer of the thoracolumbar fascia covers the transverse processes within the lumbar area and, together with the intertransverse connective tissue, completely separates the epaxial (i.e. muscles that lie dorsal to the transverse processes) and hypaxial muscle groups (i.e. muscles that lie ventral to the transverse processes) (Medina-Serra et al. 2021b).

The hypaxial muscles of interest for the lumbar ESPB are the *m. psoas minor*, *m. psoas major*, and *m. quadratus lumborum*. The *m. quadratus lumborum* is the most dorsal of the lumbar hypaxial muscles and is positioned directly ventral to the bodies of the last three thoracic vertebrae (and last ribs) and all of the lumbar vertebrae, extending laterally under the transverse processes of the lumbar vertebrae (Hermanson 2020b). The *m. psoas major* lies ventral to the *m. quadratus lumborum* and dorsal to the *m. psoas minor*, with its origin on the transverse processes of L2–3 where it lies medial to the *m. quadratus lumborum*, before moving to a more ventro–lateral position as it approaches L4–7 (Hermanson 2020b). The *m. psoas minor* runs ventral to the *m. psoas major* and *m. quadratus lumborum*, arising from the last thoracic vertebra and extending to the level of L4–5 (Hermanson 2020b).

As it exits the spinal canal, each **spinal nerve** divides into three or four primary branches, which include a **meningeal branch**, a **communicating branch** (or ramus communicans), a **dorsal primary branch** (or dorsal ramus), and a **ventral primary branch** (or ventral ramus) (Figure 17.3).

The **meningeal branch** is the most proximal branch and is located just peripheral to the spinal ganglion (or dorsal root ganglion) (Hermanson 2020c). The **meningeal branch** consists of afferent (sensory) axons and postganglionic sympathetic axons that supply the dura mater, the dorsal longitudinal ligament, and blood vessels in the vertebral canal (Hermanson 2020c). There is controversy in the literature about the true existence of the **meningeal branch** in animals with one study that assessed the innervation of the thoracolumbar vertebral column in dogs reportedly not able to find this branch on gross dissections (Forsythe and Ghoshal 1984). The **ramus communicans**, also referred to as the "visceral branch", communicates with the sympathetic trunk (Figure 17.3) and carries visceral afferent and efferent axons to and from visceral structures (Hermanson 2020c).

The **dorsal branches** of each **spinal nerve**, more commonly referred as the "dorsal rami," are similar across the thoracic and lumbar regions. They typically divide into a **medial branch**, which arborizes in the *m. longissimus* and give off terminal branches to the *m. multifidus*, supplying the *mm. multifidus, rotatores, longissimus, spinalis*, and *semispinalis*, as well as the vertebrae, ligaments and dura mater, and a **lateral branch,** which runs through the *mm. longissimus* and *iliocostalis*, supplying the *m. iliocostalis* and eventually the skin of the dorso–lateral aspect of the trunk (Hermanson 2020c). The exception to this arrangement

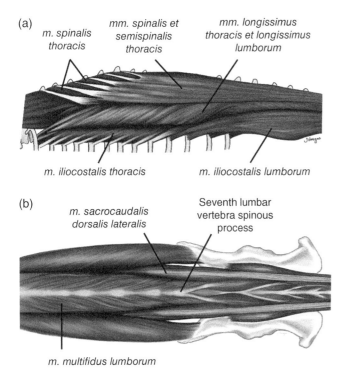

(a)
m. spinalis thoracis
mm. spinalis et semispinalis thoracis
mm. longissimus thoracis et longissimus lumborum

m. iliocostalis thoracis
m. iliocostalis lumborum

(b)
m. sacrocaudalis dorsalis lateralis
Seventh lumbar vertebra spinous process

m. multifidus lumborum

FIGURE 17.2 Illustration of the superficial epaxial muscles. (a) Thoracolumbar area, lateral view. (b) Lumbocaudal area, dorsal view.

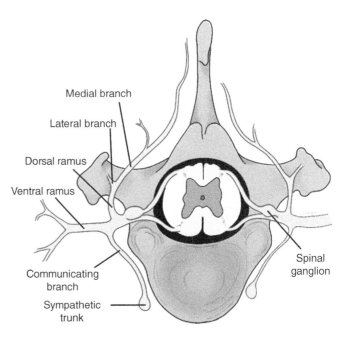

Medial branch
Lateral branch
Dorsal ramus
Ventral ramus
Spinal ganglion
Communicating branch
Sympathetic trunk

FIGURE 17.3 Illustration of a generalized spinal nerve and its branches.

is for the last three or four lumbar segments, where obvious separation of the **medial** and **lateral branches** does not occur (Hermanson 2020c).

Further division of the dorsal ramus into an **intermediate branch** that innervates the *m. longissimus* has also been reported in the thoracolumbar region of dogs, but its existence is not consistent (Forsythe and Ghoshal 1984). Additionally, the **lateral branches** of the **thoracic** and **lumbar dorsal rami** provide **cutaneous branches** (Hermanson 2020c). **Cutaneous branches** of the **caudal lumbar spinal nerves** innervate the skin of the gluteal region and over the tensor fascia lata (**cranial clunial nerves**).

Unlike the **dorsal branches**, the **ventral branches** of each **spinal nerve**, more commonly referred to as the "ventral rami," differ between the thoracic and lumbar regions. The **ventral rami** of the **thoracic spinal nerves**, more commonly known as the "**intercostal nerves**" (Figure 17.3), divide into **medial** and **lateral branches** that supply the hypaxial muscles of the body wall and give off **cutaneous branches** that supply the skin of the lateral and ventral aspects of the body wall (Hermanson 2020c). The **ventral rami** of **lumbar spinal nerves** are typically referred to as the "**lumbar nerves**," and the last five ventral rami and all ventral rami of the sacral nerves join to form the lumbosacral plexus, which is the origin of the pelvic limb nerves.

The first two lumbar ventral rami (**cranial** and **caudal iliohypogastric nerves**) run caudolaterally towards the abdominal wall, in series with the **caudal thoracic nerves** (Hermanson 2020c). Both nerves give off muscular branches to the *mm. quadratus lumborum* and *psoas minor*. The lumbar plexus is a term restricted to the interconnected third, fourth, and fifth lumbar nerves; however, contributions from the second and sixth lumbar nerves are common. All of these nerves penetrate the *m. psoas major*.

EXPECTED DISTRIBUTION OF ANESTHESIA

Based on the relatively consistent staining of the dorsal rami and their lateral and medial branches in animal cadavers, the distribution of anesthesia from an ESPB would be expected to be limited to the dorso–lateral aspect of the trunk. As a result, most of the clinical studies in veterinary medicine have been focused on procedures involving this area of the body.

Most cadaveric studies in veterinary medicine use single-point injections and document spread that is limited to the **dorsal rami** of the **spinal nerves** or, more specifically, to the **lateral** and/or **medial branches** of the **dorsal rami**. However, one study also showed staining of two contiguous **spinal nerves** (1 out of 16 injections) and staining of a **ventral ramus** (1/16 injections) (Ferreira et al. 2019) and another study showed epidural spread (2/17 injections) (Medina-Serra et al. 2021b).

After a single-point injection, the local anesthetic is expected to spread cranio–caudally and block multiple vertebral levels (Chin and El-Boghdadly 2021), as has been demonstrated after single-level ESPB injections in dog cadavers (Ferreira et al. 2019; Portela et al. 2020; Medina-Serra et al. 2021b; Cavalcanti et al. 2022). Different anatomical levels (i.e. thoracic versus lumbar), techniques (i.e. transverse versus parasagittal), and outcome assessment (i.e. staining of **dorsal rami** versus specific **lateral** and/or **medial branches** of the **dorsal rami**) make direct comparisons between studies difficult, however, the overall number of contiguous vertebral segments stained following single-level ESPB injections in dog cadavers would be expected to be between two and five (median values) (Ferreira et al. 2019; Portela et al. 2020; Medina-Serra et al. 2021b; Cavalcanti et al. 2022). The only exception to the direction of the spread was reported in a cadaveric study in dogs, where a preferential cranial spread was noted when the ESPB injection (using the mamillary process as landmark) was performed using a transverse approach at the level of T12 (Cavalcanti et al. 2022). This had not been previously noted when the injection was performed at T5, T9, or L4 (Ferreira et al. 2019; Portela et al. 2020; Medina-Serra et al. 2021b). Based on these findings, those authors suggested that ESPB at the thoracolumbar region be performed at least one spinal segment caudal to the affected vertebral level (Cavalcanti et al. 2022).

There are a few descriptions of multisite ESPB injections being performed in veterinary medicine (Tulgar et al. 2018a; D'Anselme et al. 2022). While no direct comparisons have been made between single versus multisite ESPB injections to date, Tulgar et al. (2018a) suggested that multiple injection sites may improve postoperative analgesia in humans.

LOCAL ANESTHETIC: DOSE, VOLUME, AND CONCENTRATION

The local anesthetic is deposited within a fascial plane, relying on a large volume of local anesthetic for appropriate distribution. Therefore, the doses of local anesthetics used for ESPBs are close to the maximum recommended limit and commonly require dilution to meet the reported desired volumes. Any local anesthetic can be used; although a long-lasting one (e.g. bupivacaine, ropivacaine, and levobupivacaine) is recommended.

For a typical single-site ESPB in the thoracic region, a volume of 0.3–0.5 ml kg^{-1} per injection site is recommended. The use of unilateral versus bilateral ESPBs may also factor into what volume and/or concentration of local anesthetic to use. The use of a lower concentration of local anesthetic allows for a higher volume to be used while keeping the total dose of local anesthetic within the maximum recommended dose for the particular drug. The possible disadvantages of using a lower concentration of drug are a decrease in efficacy or quality of analgesia and decrease in duration of effects.

Altıparmak et al. (2019) performed ESPBs in humans with the same volume (20 ml) but with two different concentrations of bupivacaine (0.375% and 0.25%) and produced effective analgesia after mastectomy surgeries. However, the blocks that used 0.375% bupivacaine resulted in significantly reduced postoperative opioid consumption and lower pain scores compared to the blocks that used the 0.25% solution. In dogs undergoing hemilaminectomies, there was no difference in the overall requirement for rescue analgesia when a lower concentration of local anesthetic was used; however, the duration of analgesia was shorter (Portela et al. 2021; Viilmann et al. 2022). It is difficult to compare the results of these two studies because of their retrospective nature and the lack of standardization. Further studies are required to fully assess the impact of concentration of the local anesthetic on the efficacy and duration of ESPBs in veterinary medicine.

PATIENT PREPARATION AND POSITIONING

The patient should be positioned in sternal recumbency with the elbows flexed. The area over the dorsum should be clipped and aseptically prepared as it would be for surgery (Figure 17.4).

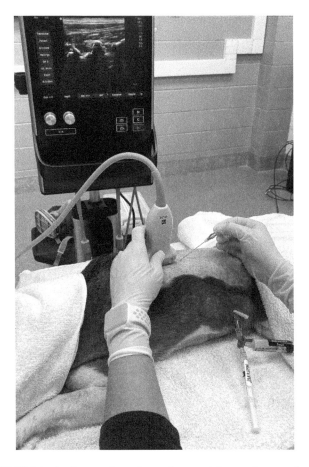

FIGURE 17.4 Image of a canine patient receiving an ultrasound-guided ESP block. The dog has been positioned in sternal recumbency with hair over the dorsum clipped and the skin surgically prepared. The US transducer is positioned in a parasagittal orientation, just lateral to the dorsal midline and the needle is being inserted on caudo-to-cranial trajectory using an in-plane needle technique.

STEP-BY-STEP PERFORMANCE

SURFACE ANATOMY AND LANDMARKS TO BE USED

A high frequency (15–6 MHz) linear array transducer should be positioned in a parasagittal orientation just lateral to dorsal midline (Figure 17.4). The vertebral level to be blocked will depend on the goal of the block; generally, the target vertebra should be the same as the spinal nerve supplying the area of desired effect (Chin and El-Boghdadly 2021). For example, for hemilaminectomies, the vertebra immediately cranial or caudal to the intervertebral space involved in the surgery is usually selected as the target (Zannin et al. 2020; Portela et al. 2021; Rodriguez Mulet et al. 2021; Sambugaro et al. 2022). For thoracotomies, most cases have used T5 as the target, but T5–T9 have also been selected (Ferré et al. 2022). A case report of using an ESPB as part of a multimodal analgesic approach for a dog with pancreatitis used T7 as the target (Bartholomew and Ferreira 2021). Although using palpation to initially identify bony anatomic landmarks (i.e. spinous processes and/or ribs) can be helpful, this is not always reliable for correctly identifying the target vertebra (Ferreira et al. 2018, 2019). Once a general impression has been made through the use of palpation, the use of US can confirm key landmarks and count spinous processes and/or ribs in order to identify the correct location to perform the block.

For the thoracolumbar and lumbar area, a transverse approach has been described in dogs (Medina-Serra et al. 2021b; Cavalcanti et al. 2022). As mentioned earlier, when using this approach for hemilaminectomies in the thoracolumbar area, those authors suggest that the target vertebra for the ESPB should be at least one spinal segment caudal to the affected vertebral level due to a preferential cranial spread in this area using the transverse approach (Cavalcanti et al. 2022).

ULTRASOUND ANATOMY

Once the target vertebra is identified and the transducer is positioned in a parasagittal orientation just lateral to dorsal midline; the transducer should be tilted medially and laterally to identify the different acoustic shadows that are associated with the lamina, transverse process, and rib (Figure 17.5). The transverse process is wider and more square-shaped, whereas the rib is rounder and thinner. This way, the anesthetist can scan through the transition between the different parts of the vertebrae and ribs and ensure that the optimal final position over the target transverse process is identified and it is positioned in the center of the US screen (Figures 17.5 and 17.6). The needle tip will need to be located between the transverse process and the ESM. The appearance of the other muscles superficial to the erector muscle group will vary depending on which vertebral level is being imaged.

As mentioned earlier, the anatomy of the lumbar spine differs from the anatomy of the thoracic region. Despite the

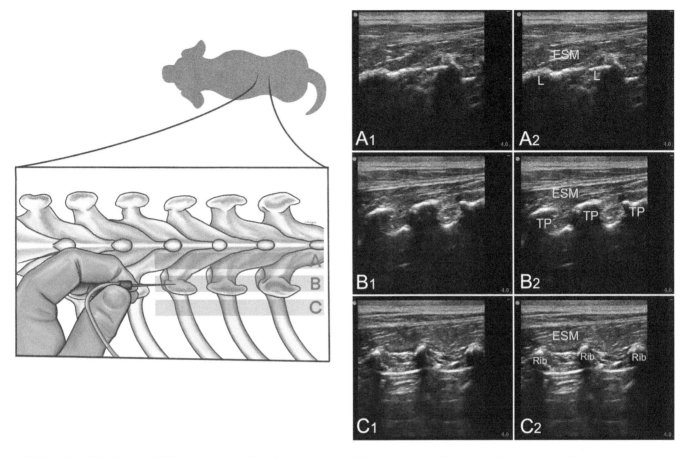

FIGURE 17.5   (A1, B1, and C1) Sonoanatomy of the relevant structures that are imaged using a parasagittal ultrasound transducer orientation to perform an ESP block, as the US transducer is moved from medial to lateral. (A2, B2, and C2) Same images, with labels. ESM, erector spinae muscles; L, laminae; TP, transverse processes.

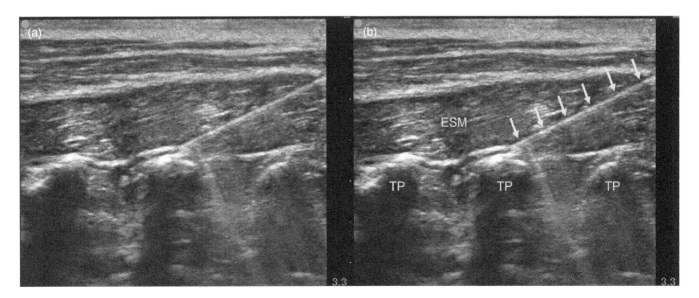

FIGURE 17.6   (a) Ultrasound image of a needle (solid arrows) at the target location for performing an ESP block. The needle tip is located on the dorsal aspect of a transverse process (TP), between the TP and the erector spinae muscles (ESM). (b) Same image, with labels.

anatomical differences, the classic site of injection for human lumbar ESPB is similar to the thoracic ESPB, which is at the tip of the transverse process deep to the ESM (Harbell et al. 2020; Tulgar et al. 2020b; Campbell and Chin 2022). The injection site at this level, however, is deeper and more lateral than thoracic ESPBs due to anatomical differences, and overall this approach is considered to be more challenging to perform due to worse sonographic visualization of landmarks and injectate spread (Kose et al. 2018; Tulgar et al. 2020b). In veterinary medicine, a transverse approach (i.e. US transducer is positioned on a transverse plane instead of parasagittal) has been reported and involves different landmarks than those used in humans (Medina-Serra et al. 2021b, Cavalcanti et al. 2022). For this transverse approach, the transducer is positioned at the level of the vertebral spinous process perpendicular to the spine. The transducer is then moved cranio–caudally until the accessory process of the lumbar vertebra and the mammillary processes of the next lumbar vertebra are visualized in the US screen. The site of injection is between the accessory process and the lateral aspect of the mammillary process of the next vertebra, which is more superficial and medial compared to the approach described for traditional thoracic ESPBs in dogs.

NEEDLE INSERTION TECHNIQUE

A short-bevel needle, Tuohy, or spinal needle (5–10 cm, 1.5–3.5 in. depending on the size of the patient) can be used. The use of an echogenic needle may facilitate its visualization during the performance of ESPBs since the needle insertion angle may be very steep or acute in relation to the US transducer surface, making needle visualization challenging. The direction of the needle when performing an ESPB using a parasagittal approach (cranio–caudal or caudo–cranial direction) varies between studies in the literature (Ferreira et al. 2019; Otero et al. 2020; Portela et al. 2020; Cavalcanti et al. 2022). Orientation does not seem to influence injectate spread in a study assessing thoracic ESPBs in pigs (Otero et al. 2020). Those investigators showed that regardless of needle direction (i.e. cranio–caudal or caudo–cranial), the median number of stained **medial** and **lateral branches** of the **dorsal rami** and the vertebral level range was similar (T5–T10 and T5–T9, respectively).

Using the most commonly described thoracic ESPB parasagittal approach, the needle should be advanced in-plane from a position either cranial or caudal to the transducer until it contacts the dorsal or dorso–lateral aspect of the tip of the transverse process (Ferreira et al. 2019; Otero et al. 2020; Portela et al. 2020) (Figure 17.6). In the case of performing a lumbar ESPB, an in-plane transverse approach uses a latero–medial trajectory for the needle until the tip of the needle contacts the lateral aspect of the mammillary process of the target vertebra, dorsal to the accessory process of the preceding vertebra (Cavalcanti et al. 2022).

EXPECTED MOTOR RESPONSES FROM NERVE STIMULATION

EXPECTED MOTOR RESPONSES FROM NERVE STIMULATION

The ESPB does not target any specific nerve or plexus; therefore, nerve stimulation is not used for this block.

ADMINISTRATION OF LOCAL ANESTHETIC – WHAT TO LOOK FOR, WHAT TO FEEL FOR, AND DECISION POINTS

The author finds it easier to have the needle attached to a prefilled T-connector extension before needle insertion. Test injections with a small volume (approximately 0.5 ml) can be used to help identify the correct plane. Having an assistant available to perform test injections is helpful so there is no risk of moving the tip of the needle. If saline is used as test injectate (hydrodissection), a stopcock can be added to the T-connector extension (Figure 17.7) to facilitate switching between syringes (i.e. saline and local anesthetic) and avoiding accidental insertion of air into the system which would negatively affect the quality of the US image.

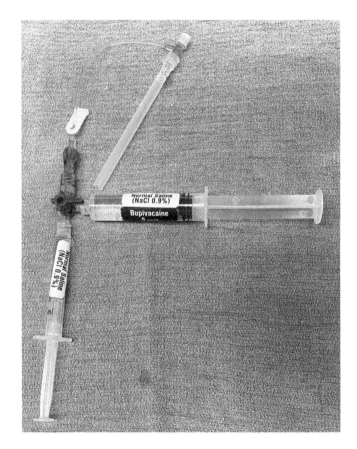

FIGURE 17.7 Needle attached to a T-connector. A stopcock is located between the T-connector and syringes (filled with saline and local anesthetic) to facilitate switching between solutions during test injections and local anesthetic administration.

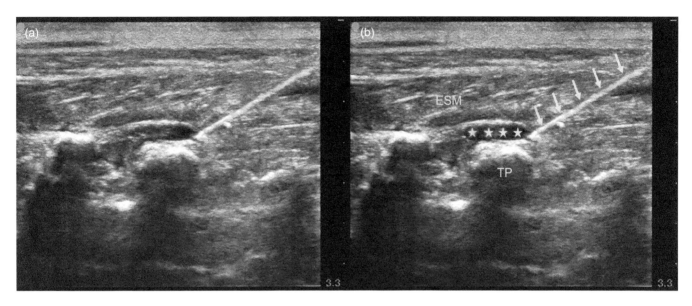

FIGURE 17.8 (a) Ultrasound image of ESP block being performed. The needle (arrows) is in the target plane. Hydrodissection is used to confirm that the injection is being made in the correct fascial plane, with cranial-caudal spread of the local anesthetic solution (stars) being observed between the erector spinae muscles (ESM) and transverse process (TP). (b) Same image, with labels.

Following confirmation of linear cranial–caudal spread of injectate between the ESM group and transverse process using the test dose(s), the total volume of local anesthetic can be slowly administered (Figure 17.8). In case of the transverse approach, injectate should be visualized separating *m. longissimus lumborum* from the mammillary process at the injection level.

BLOCK EFFECTS (SENSORY, MOTOR, ETC.) AND PATIENT MANAGEMENT

The ESPB sensory blockade coverage depends on the spinal level of the injection, with the literature suggesting that clinical efficacy and extent of sensory blockade can vary at different areas of the body (De Cassai et al. 2019a; Tulgar and Balaban 2019; Byrne and Smith 2020; Kendall et al. 2020; Ferré et al. 2022). In veterinary species, clinical studies/reports focus on using ESPBs to desensitize the spine and associated soft tissues to facilitate spinal surgical procedures (Zannin et al. 2020; Alza Salvatierra et al. 2021; Portela et al. 2021; Rodriguez Mulet et al. 2021; Chiavaccinia et al. 2022; Rodriguez et al. 2022; Viilmann et al. 2022). Sensory blockade following thoracotomy and the provision of visceral analgesia for pancreatitis do not exclude other yet unknown, block effects (Bartholomew and Ferreira 2021; Ferré et al. 2022). It is promising, however, that several studies in humans using ESPBs following a variety of procedures or pain conditions have demonstrated lower opioid consumption, decreased postoperative nausea and vomiting, and improved postoperative pain control and recovery quality (De Cassai et al. 2019a; Kendall et al. 2020; Bartholomew and Ferreira 2021; Ma

et al. 2021; Portela et al. 2021; Rizkalla et al. 2021; Rodriguez Mulet et al. 2021; Saadawi et al. 2021; Ferré et al. 2022; Jiao et al. 2022; Koo et al. 2022; Viilmann et al. 2022). Until further clinical studies are performed, the current recommendation is to employ ESPBs as part of a multimodal analgesic approach (Tulgar et al. 2018b; Bartholomew and Ferreira 2021; Portela et al. 2021; Ferré et al. 2022) and not as the sole analgesic/anesthetic protocol.

Regarding the use of ESPB for spinal surgery specifically, the use of both unilateral (Alza Salvatierra et al. 2021; Portela et al. 2021; Rodriguez Mulet et al. 2021) or bilateral blocks (Singh et al. 2020; Zannin et al. 2020; Chiavaccinia et al. 2022; Oezel et al. 2022; Rodriguez et al. 2022; Viilmann et al. 2022) have been reported in the literature. Cutaneous nerves and nerves in the vertebral canal can cross midline or communicate across midline (Forsythe and Ghoshal 1984; Capek et al. 2015), which would justify the use of bilateral ESPBs for these procedures. However, the use of bilateral blocks can increase the total dose of local anesthetic used or decrease the concentration of the local anesthetic (because the drug may need to be diluted to achieve reasonable volumes to provide appropriate coverage/spread). The latter could potentially result in decreased efficacy of the block and/or duration of the beneficial clinical effects. However, this is a speculation, and studies directly comparing the use of unilateral versus bilateral ESPBs for spinal procedures are warranted to determine the effects of both approaches in efficacy and duration of clinical effects, as well as potential incidence of LAST if total doses exceeding the maximum local anesthetic recommendations are selected for bilateral blocks.

COMPLICATIONS AND HOW TO AVOID THEM

In the human literature, ESPBs demonstrate an excellent safety profile and are associated with minimal risk of complications (De Cassai et al. 2021b; Oezel et al. 2022). Some of the reported potential complications include pneumothorax, lower extremity weakness, and motor block due to spread of local anesthetic to either the lumbar plexus or epidural space, LAST, and priapism (De Cassai et al. 2019a; Tulgar et al. 2019a, 2020b; Saadawi et al. 2021). Three cases of sinus arrest have been reported in healthy dogs following ESPBs (Sambugaro et al. 2022; Viilmann et al. 2022). In those cases, the blocks were performed at L1, T13, and T13 with reported doses of 2.37, 2.62, and 2.4 mg kg^{-1} of levobupivacaine, respectively. One of these cases, the dog had history of a previous hemilaminectomy surgery (Sambugaro et al. 2022), which as mentioned earlier could be considered a relative contraindication. Though all the dogs survived, aggressive intervention including the use of atropine, epinephrine, ephedrine, and intralipid was required (Sambugaro et al. 2022; Viilmann et al. 2022). Those authors suspect these events were due to LAST or potential epidural spread (Sambugaro et al. 2022; Viilmann et al. 2022). A case of severe hypotension and bradycardia was successfully treated with ephedrine boluses in a human following a single point ESPB performed at T8 (Coviello et al. 2021). The authors of that report hypothesized that the hemodynamic instability was due to epidural spread of the local anesthetic because the resultant extensive and long-lasting sensory block was bilateral (despite the unilateral injection). In that case, the authors suggested that several factors contributed to epidural spread, including the block being performed with patient in lateral recumbency, high intrabdominal pressure from CO$_2$ insufflation for laparoscopy, and the use of an out-of-plane, and transverse approach (Coviello et al. 2021).

Suspected epidural spread following ESPBs has been reported in humans, dogs, cows, and horses (Chin and El-Boghdadly 2021; Delgado et al. 2021; Medina-Serra et al. 2021b; D'Anselme et al. 2022). While this could contribute to analgesia (Adhikary et al. 2018; Schwartzmann et al. 2018), the large volume/dose of local anesthetic could result in extensive motor blockade (Selvi and Tulgar 2018) and hemodynamic instability from sympathetic blockade (Coviello et al. 2021; Sambugaro et al. 2022).

ESPBs utilize large volumes/doses of local anesthetics so veterinary clinicians should always remain attentive for signs of LAST following performance of a block. Since veterinary patients are often anesthetized when the blocks are performed, many of the early signs of systemic toxicity may be missed or misidentified as "normal/expected" general anesthesia complications. Calculating the dose of local anesthetic for an ESPB using lean body weight, keeping the total dose selected within the maximum recommended range, and diluting the local anesthetic as needed to obtain the desired volume, is advisable.

Other potential complications include infection, hematoma, visceral (thoracic or abdominal) puncture, and epidural injection. As with any regional anesthetic technique, aseptic technique should be performed to avoid infections. Additionally, US guidance with good visualization of landmarks, use of in-plane needle technique with constant needle tip visualization, and negative aspiration before drug administration is essential to minimize the chances of inadvertent intravascular drug administration, potential hematoma formation, thoracic/abdominal visceral damage, pneumothorax, and/or epidural injections. Hydrodissection with small volumes of saline can be helpful to identify the correct fascial plane, confirm the location of the needle tip, and maximize the use of local anesthetic in the correct fascial plane.

COMMON MISTAKES AND HOW TO AVOID THEM

Identification of the correct target vertebra is a crucial first step when performing a successful ESPB. Use of US guidance (i.e. imaging and counting the spinous processes and/or ribs) should be used for that purpose since the sole use of anatomic landmarks by palpation has been shown to be unreliable (Ferreira et al. 2018, 2019). Additionally, clear identification of the transverse process is mandatory. Making sure to identify the different parts of the target vertebra (e.g. transverse process, lamina, spinous process, mammillary process, etc.) and rib is essential.

Injection of the local anesthetic too superficially into the ESM or too deeply into the intercostal muscles may lead to limited spread and block failure. Hydrodissection to identify the correct plane by visualizing linear cranio–caudal spread of the injectate between the ESM group and the transverse process while performing the parasagittal approach before administering the full volume/dose of local anesthetic is imperative. For the transverse approach, the injectate should be visualized separating ***m. longissimus lumborum*** from the mammillary process.

HOW TO TALK TO CLIENTS/PROFESSIONAL COLLEAGUES

- The ESPB is a relatively simple technique associated with an excellent safety profile.

- This block is used as part of a multimodal pain management approach and can significantly decrease opioid consumption during the intra- and postoperative period.

- The primary use of ESPBs in veterinary species so far is for the provision of analgesia for surgeries or painful conditions of the spine. Successful blockade can be expected to provide analgesia for 12–48 hours, depending on the local anesthetic that is used.

Adhikary SD, Bernard S, Lopez H et al. (2018) Erector spinae plane block versus retrolaminar block: a magnetic resonance imaging and anatomical study. Reg Anesth Pain Med 43, 1–7.

Aksu C, Gürkan Y (2019). Aksu approach for lumbar erector spinae plane block for pediatric surgeries. J Clin Anesth 54, 74–75.

Altıparmak B, Korkmaz Toker M, Uysal Aİ et al. (2019). Comparison of the efficacy of erector spinae plane block performed with different concentrations of bupivacaine on postoperative analgesia after mastectomy surgery: ramdomized, prospective, double blinded trial. BMC Anesthesiol 19, 31.

Alza Salvatierra DN, Herrera Linares ME, Motta L et al. (2021) Ultrasoundguided erector spinae interfascial plane block for spinal surgery in three cats. JFMS Open Rep 7, 1–6.

Bartholomew KJ, Ferreira TH (2021) Ultrasound-guided erector spinae plane block as part of a multimodal analgesic approach in a dog with acute pancreatitis. Vet Anaesth Analg 48, 629–632.

Byrne K, Smith C (2020) Human volunteer study examining the sensory changes of the thorax after an erector spinae plane block. Reg Anesth Pain Med 45, 761–762.

Campbell S, Chin K (2022) Erector spinae block: beyond the torso. Curr Opin Anaesthesiol 35, 600–604.

Capek S, Tubbs RS, Spinner RJ (2015) Do cutaneous nerves cross the midline? Clin Anat 28, 96–100.

Cavalcanti M, Teixeira JG, Medina-Serra R et al. (2022) Erector spinae plane block at the thoracolumbar spine: a canine cadaveric study. Vet Anaesth Analg 49, 656–663.

Chiavaccinia L, Cavalcanti M, De Gasperi D et al. (2022). Clinical efficacy of ultrasound-guided bilateral erector spinae plane block for standing lumbar spinous osteotomy in a horse. Vet Anaesth Analg 49, 518–519.

Chin K, El-Boghdadly K (2021) Mechanisms of action of the erector spinae plane (ESP) block: a narrative review. Can J Anesth 68, 387–408.

Choi Y-J, Kwon H-J, Jehoon O et al. (2019). Influence of injectate volume on paravertebral spread in erector spinae plane block: an endoscopic and anatomical evaluation. PLoS One 14, e0224487.

Coviello A, Golino L, Maresca A et al. (2021) Erector spinae plane block in laparoscopic nephrectomy as a cause of involuntary hemodynamic instability: a case report. Clin Case Rep 9, e04026.

D'Anselme O, Hartnack A, Andrade JSS et al. (2022) Description of an ultrasound-guided erector spinae plane block and comparison to a blind proximal paravertebral nerve block in cows: a cadaveric study. Animals 12, 2191.

Dautzenberg KHW, Zegers MJ, Bleeker CP et al. (2019) Unpredictable injectate spread of the erector spinae plane block in human cadavers. Anesth Analg 129, e163–e166.

De Cassai A, Andreatta G, Bonvicini D et al. (2020) Injectate spread in ESP block: a review of anatomical investigations. J Clin Anesth 61, 109669.

De Cassai A, Bonanno C, Padrini R et al. (2021a) Pharmacokinetics of lidocaine after bilateral ESP block. Reg Anesth Pain Med 46, 86–89.

De Cassai A, Bonvicini D, Correale C et al. (2019a) Erector spinae plane block: a systematic qualitative review. Minerva Anestesiol 85, 308–319.

De Cassai A, Geraldini F, Carere A et al. (2021b). Complications rate estimation after thoracic erector spinae plane block. J Cardiothorac Vasc Anesth 35, 3142–3143.

De Cassai A, Sgarabotto C, Dal Cin S (2019b) Old approach for a new indication: shamrock sign for ESP block. Reg Anesth Pain Med 44, 256–256.

De Lara González SJ, Pomés J, Prats-Galino A et al. (2019) Anatomical description of anaesthetic spread after deep erector spinae block at L-4. Rev Esp Anestesiol Reanim 66, 409–416.

Delgado OBD, Louro LF, Rocchigiani G et al. (2021) Ultrasound-guided erector spinae plane block in horses: a cadaver study. Vet Anaesth Analg 48, 577–584.

Elkoundi A, El Koraichi A (2020) Erector spinae plane block dilemma. Reg Anesth Pain Med 45, 842–843.

Ferré BMI, Drozdzynska M, Vettorato E (2022) Ultrasound-guided bilateral erector spinae plane block in dogs undergoing sternotomies anaesthetised with propofol-dexmedetomidine continuous infusion. Vet Res Commun 46, 1331–1337.

Ferreira TH, St James M, Schroeder CA et al. (2019) Description of an ultrasound-guided erector spinae plane block and the spread of dye in dog cadavers. Vet Anaesth Analg 46, 516–522.

Ferreira TH, Teixeira LBC, Schroeder CA et al. (2018) Description of an ultrasound-guided thoracic paravertebral block technique and the spread of dye in dog cadavers. Vet Anaesth Analg 45, 811–819.

Forero M, Adhikary SD, Lopez H et al. (2016) The erector spinae plane block: a novel analgesic technique in thoracic neuropathic pain. Reg Anesth Pain Med 41, 621–627.

Forsythe WB, Ghoshal NG (1984) Innervation of the canine thoracolumbar vertebral column. Anat Rec 208, 57–63.

Goel VK, Chandramohan M, Murugan C et al. (2021) Clinical efficacy of ultrasound guided bilateral erector spinae block for single-level lumbar fusion surgery: a prospective, randomized, case-control study. Spine J 21, 1873–1880.

Gürkan Y, Aksu C, Kuş A et al. (2020) Erector spinae plane block and thoracic paravertebral block for breast surgery compared to IV-morphine: a randomized controlled trial. J Clin Anesth 59, 84–88.

Hamilton DL (2020). The erector spinae plane block: time for clarity over anatomical nomenclature. J Clin Anesth 62, 109699.

Harbell MW, Seamans DP, Koyyalamudi V et al. (2020). Evaluating the extent of lumbar erector spinae plane block: an anatomical study. Reg Anesth Pain Med 45, 640–644.

Hermanson JW (2020a) The skeleton. In: Miller and Evans' Anatomy of the Dog. Hermanson JW, de Lahunta A, Evans HE (eds.) Elsevier, USA. pp. 86–175.

Hermanson JW (2020b) The muscular system. In: Miller and Evans' Anatomy of the Dog. Hermanson JW, de Lahunta A, Evans HE (eds.) Elsevier, USA. pp. 207–318.

Hermanson JW (2020c). The spinal nerves. In: Miller and Evans' Anatomy of the Dog. Hermanson JW, de Lahunta A, Evans HE (eds.) Elsevier, USA. pp. 704–756.

International Committee on Veterinary Gross Anatomical Nomenclature (2017) Nomina Anatomica Veterinaria, 6th edition. International Committee on Veterinary Gross Anatomical Nomenclature.

Ivanusic J, Konishi Y, Barrington MJ (2018) A cadaveric study investigating the mechanism of action of erector spinae blockade. Reg Anesth Pain Med 43, 567–571.

Jiao B, Chen H, Chen M et al. (2022) Opioid-sparing effects of ultrasound-guided erector spinae plane block for adult patients undergoing surgery: a systematic review and meta-analysis. Pain Pract 22, 391–404.

Kanna RM, Ramachandran K, Subramanian JB et al. (2023) Peri-operative analgesic efficacy and safety of erector spinae plane block in posterior cervical spine surgery – a double blinded, randomized controlled study. Spine J 23, 6–13.

Kendall MC, Alves L, Traill LL et al. (2020) The effect of ultrasound-guided erector spinae plane block on postsurgical pain: a meta-analysis of randomized controlled trials. BMC Anesthesiol 20, 99.

Koo C-H, Lee H-T, Na H-S et al. (2022) Efficacy of erector spinae plane block for analgesia in thoracic surgery: a systematic review and meta-analysis. J Cardiothorac Vasc Anesth 36, 1387–1395.

Kose HC, Kose SG, Thomas DT (2018) Lumbar versus thoracic erector spinae plane block – similar nomenclature, different mechanism of action. J Clin Anesth 48, 1.

Ma J, Bi Y, Zhang Y et al. (2021) Erector spinae plane block for postoperative analgesia in spine surgery: a systematic review and meta-analysis. Eur Spine J 30, 3137–3149.

Medina-Serra R, Cavalcanti M, Portela DA et al. (2021a) Transversal approach to the canine lumbar erector spinae plane block: returning to the dissecting room. Vet Anaesth Analg 48, 811–813.

Medina-Serra R, Foster A, Plested M et al. (2021b) Lumbar erector spinae plane block: an anatomical and dye distribution evaluation of two ultrasound-guided approaches in canine cadavers. Vet Anaesth Analg 48, 125–133.

Nagaraja P, Ragavendran S, Singh NG et al. (2018) Comparison of continuous thoracic epidural analgesia with bilateral erector spinae plane block for perioperative pain management in cardiac surgery. Ann Card Anaesth 21, 323–327.

Oezel L, Hughes AP, Onyekwere I et al. (2022) Procedure-specific complications associated with ultrasound-guided erector spinae plane block for lumbar spine surgery: a retrospective analysis of 342 consecutive cases. J Pain Res 15, 655–661.

Otero PE, Fuensalida SE, Russo PC et al. (2020) Mechanism of action of the erector spinae plane block: distribution of dye in a porcine model. Reg Anesth Pain Med 45, 198–203.

Portela DA, Castro D, Romano M et al. (2020) Ultrasound-guided erector spinae plane block in canine cadavers: relevant anatomy and injectate distribution. Vet Anaesth Analg 47, 229–237.

Portela DA, Romano M, Zamora GA et al. (2021) The effect of erector spinae plane block on perioperative analgesic consumption and complications in dogs undergoing hemilaminectomy surgery: a retrospective cohort study. Vet Anaesth Analg 48, 116–124.

Rizkalla JM, Holderread B, Awad M et al. (2021) The erector spinae plane block for analgesia after lumbar spine surgery: a systematic review. J Orthop 24, 145–150.

Rodriguez A, Medina-Serra R, Lynch N et al. (2022) Erector spinae plane block as part of a multimodal analgesic approach in an anaesthetised horse undergoing dorsal spinous process ostectomy and desmotomy. Vet Rec Case Rep 10, e345.

Rodriguez Mulet A, Medina-Serra R, Veres-Nyéki K et al. (2021) Transversal approach for the lumbar erector spine plane block in a dog undergoing dorsal hemilaminectomy. Vet Anaesth Analg 48, 625–627.

Saadawi M, Layera S, Aliste J et al. (2021) Erector spinae plane block: a narrative review with systematic analysis of the evidence pertaining to clinical indications and alternative truncal blocks. J Clin Anesth 68, 110063.

Sambugaro B, Campbella N, Drozdzynska MJ (2022) Two cases of sinus arrest following erector spinae plane block in dogs. Vet Anaesth Analg 49, 510–511.

Schwartzmann A, Peng P, Maciel MA et al. (2018) Mechanism of the erector spinae plane block: insights from a magnetic resonance imaging study. Can J Anesth 65, 1165–1166.

Selvi O, Tulgar S (2018) Ultrasound guided erector spinae plane block as a cause of unintended motor block. Rev Esp Anestesiol Reanim 65, 589–592.

Singh S, Choudhary NK, Lalin D et al. (2020) Bilateral ultrasound-guided erector spinae plane block for postoperative analgesia in lumbar spine surgery: a randomized control trial. J Neurosurg Anesthesiol 32, 330–334.

Tulgar S, Ahiskalioglu A, Thomas DT et al. (2020a) Should erector spinae plane block applications be standardized or should we revise nomenclature? Reg Anesth Pain Med 45, 318–319.

Tulgar S, Aydin ME, Ahiskalioglu A et al. (2020b) Anesthetic techniques: focus on lumbar erector spinae plane block. Local Reg Anesth 13, 121–133.

Tulgar S, Balaban O (2019) Spread of local anesthetic in erector spine plane block at thoracic and lumbar levels. Reg Anesth Pain Med 44, 134–135.

Tulgar S, Selvi O, Ozer Z (2018a) Clinical experience of ultrasound-guided single and bi-level erector spinae plane block for postoperative analgesia in patients undergoing thoracotomy. J Clin Anesth 50, 22–23.

Tulgar S, Selvi O, Senturk O et al. (2018b) Clinical experiences of ultrasound-guided lumbar erector spinae plane block for hip joint and proximal femur surgeries. J Clin Anesth 47, 5–6.

Tulgar S, Selvi O, Senturk O et al. (2019a) Ultrasound-guided erector spinae plane block: indications, complications, and effects on acute and chronic pain based on a single-center experience. Cureus 11, e3815

Tulgar S, Unal OK, Thomas DT et al. (2019b) A novel modification to ultrasound guided lumbar erector spinae plane block: Tulgar approach. J Clin Anesth 56, 30–31.

Vidal E, Giménez H, Forero M et al. (2018) Erector spinae plane block: a cadaver study to determine its mechanism of action. Rev Esp Anestesiol Reanim 65, 514–519.

Viilmann I, Drozdzynska M, Vettorato E (2022) Analgesic efficacy of a bilateral erector spinae plane block versus a fentanyl constant rate infusion in dogs undergoing hemilaminectomy: a retrospective cohort study. BMC Vet Res 18, 423.

Yang H-M, Choi YJ, Kwon H-J et al. (2018) Comparison of injectate spread and nerve involvement between retrolaminar and erector spinae plane blocks in the thoracic region: a cadaveric study. Anaesthesia 73, 1244–1250.

Yao Y, Fu S, Dai S et al. (2020) Impact of ultrasound-guided erector spinae plane block on postoperative quality of recovery in video-assisted thoracic surgery: a prospective, randomized, controlled trial. J Clin Anesth 63, 109783.

Zannin D, Isaka LJ, Pereira RH et al. (2020) Opioid-free total intravenous anesthesia with bilateral ultrasound-guided erector spinae plane block for perioperative pain control in a dog undergoing dorsal hemilaminectomy. Vet Anaesth Analg 47, 728–730.

Zhang J, Xu X, Sun H (2020) How current researches are redefining our view of ESP block? J Clin Anesth 60, 41.

Zhao H, Xin L, Feng Y (2020) The effect of preoperative erector spinae plane vs. paravertebral blocks on patient-controlled oxycodone consumption after video-assisted thoracic surgery: a prospective randomized, blinded, non-inferiority study. J Clin Anesth 62, 109737.

Ultrasound-Guided Quadratus Lumborum Block

Marta Garbin

BLOCK AT A GLANCE

What is it used for?

- To supplement anesthesia for abdominal surgeries (e.g. exploratory laparotomy, ovariectomy and ovario-hysterectomy, cholecystectomy and cholelithiasis removal, and nephrectomy).

- To provide pain management for patients with severe abdominal pain (i.e. gallstones and pancreatitis).

Landmarks/transducer position

- The ultrasound transducer is typically positioned either caudal and parallel to the last rib, transverse to the lumbar musculature or caudal to the last rib and longitudinal to the lumbar musculature.

- Regardless of the technique used, the final needle tip position will be within the **m. quadratus lumborum** fascial plane, deep to the **thoracolumbar fascia**.

- Various techniques for performing Quadratus Lumborum blocks (QLBs) have been described. Depending on the technique that is used to perform the block, the final needle tip position will be between the **m. quadratus lumborum** and the **m. psoas** ("transmuscular-QLB"); the **m. quadratus lumborum** ventrally, the epaxial muscles dorsally, and the **thoracolumbar fascia** dorsolaterally ("lateral-QLB"); or the **m. quadratus lumborum** and the body of the first or second lumbar vertebra ("dorsal-QLB").

- Using the transmuscular-QLB, the needle can be advanced along either a ventral-to-dorsal trajectory or on a dorsal-to-ventral trajectory. Using the dorsal-QLB, the needle is advanced along a ventral-to-dorsal trajectory. Using the lateral-QLB, the needle is advanced along a ventral-to-dorsal trajectory or a caudal-to-dorsal trajectory, depending on which side of the transducer the needle enters the patient.

Landmarks/transducer position:

- Different techniques for performing Quadratus Lumborum blocks (QLB) have been described – "Transmuscular-QLB," "Dorsal-QLB," and "Lateral-QLB."

  ○ Transmuscular-QLB:

    ■ The ultrasound transducer is positioned caudal and parallel to the last rib, transverse to the lumbar musculature.

    ■ The final needle tip position is between the **m. quadratus lumborum** and the **mm. psoas**.

    ■ The needle can be advanced along either a ventral-to-dorsal trajectory (*ventral* approach) or on a dorsal-to-ventral trajectory (*dorsal* approach).

  ○ Dorsal-QLB:

    ■ The ultrasound transducer is positioned caudal and parallel to the last rib, transverse to the lumbar musculature.

    ■ The final needle tip position is between the body of the first or second lumbar vertebra and the dorsal aspect of the **m. quadratus lumborum**.

    ■ The needle can be advanced along either a ventral-to-dorsal trajectory (*ventral* approach) or on a dorsal-to-ventral trajectory (*dorsal* approach).

  ○ Lateral-QLB:

    ■ The ultrasound transducer is positioned either caudal and parallel to the last rib, transverse to the lumbar musculature (*ventral* approach) or caudal to the last rib and longitudinal to the lumbar musculature (*longitudinal* approach).

    ■ The final needle tip position is between the lateral aspect of the **m. quadratus lumborum** and the **m. psoas**.

    ■ The needle can be advanced along either a ventral-to-dorsal trajectory (*ventral* approach) or on a dorsal-to-ventral trajectory (*longitudinal* approach).

Small Animal Regional Anesthesia and Analgesia, Second Edition. Edited by Matt Read, Luis Campoy, and Berit Fischer.
© 2024 John Wiley & Sons, Inc. Published 2024 by John Wiley & Sons, Inc.

What equipment and personnel are required?

- 20–22 Ga, 63–100 mm spinal or echogenic needle (or similar)
- Syringe of drug(s)
- Ultrasound machine
- High frequency (15–6 MHz) linear array transducer +/− protective sleeve
- Gloves
- Coupling agent (e.g. alcohol)
- Assistant to perform the injection

When do I perform the block?

- Prior to surgery, after the abdomen and puncture sites are clipped, and surgical skin preparation is complete. Final skin preparation will still be needed prior to surgery.

What volume of local anesthetic is used?

- 0.3-0.6 ml kg^{-1}

Goal

- During the injection, the local anesthetic should spread within the quadratus lumborum fascial plane, creating an anechoic pocket between the **m. quadratus lumborum** and the surrounding structures.

Complexity level:

- Advanced

Clinical pearl:

- Using ultrasound, the **m. quadratus lumborum** is relatively easy to identify mid-way between the last rib and the ilium, where its diameter usually appears to be the largest.
- "Pops" or "clicks" can be felt when encountering fascial planes.
- Small aliquots of injectate can be used to verify the correct needle tip location.

WHAT DO WE ALREADY KNOW?

An injection of local anesthetic in the fascial plain surrounding the **m. quadratus lumborum** (QL), aims to block the **ventral rami** of the caudal **thoracic** and **lumbar spinal nerves** (Elsharkawy et al. 2019), providing somatic and, potentially, visceral analgesia of the abdomen. In humans, QL blocks (QLBs) have been shown to be effective in contributing to postoperative pain management after a wide range of abdominal surgeries. Different approaches that provide sensory analgesia from the mid-thoracic to the upper-lumbar dermatomes have been described (Elsharkawy et al. 2019).

To date, three techniques to perform the QLB have been described in animals, with the terminology that is used relating to the final position and orientation of the ultrasound transducer, and/or the final position of the needle tip (Figure 18.1). These different techniques will be referred to here based on the final position of the needle tip relative to the QL muscle and the distribution of the local anesthetic in the fascial plane between the **m. quadratus lumborum** and **m. psoas** ("*transmuscular-QLB*"), the QL muscle medially, the epaxial muscles dorsally, and the thoracolumbar fascia dorsolaterally ("*lateral-QLB*"), or the QL muscle and the body of the first or second lumbar vertebra ("*dorsal-QLB*").

Various nomenclatures have been proposed to describe the different approaches to the QLBs. This author proposes the following terminology when referring to this block:

- **Ventral approach to the QLB** –The transducer is positioned caudal to the last rib in a transverse orientation, relative to the hypaxial muscles, and the needle is advanced along a ventrolateral-to-dorsomedial trajectory.

- **Dorsal approach to the QLB** – The transducer is positioned caudal to the last rib in a transverse orientation, relative to the hypaxial muscles, and the needle is advanced along a dorsolateral-to-ventromedial trajectory.

- **Longitudinal approach to the QLB** – The transducer is positioned caudal to the last rib in a longitudinal orientation to the vertebral column and the needle is advanced along a caudolateral-to-craniomedial trajectory.

In veterinary medicine, studies to date have mainly involved the use of canine cadavers. The first canine cadaveric investigation evaluated the spread of either 0.15 or 0.3 ml kg^{-1} of a dye-lidocaine solution, following a *ventral* approach to the transmuscular-QLB (Garbin et al. 2020a). Compared with the low volume, the high volume resulted in more consistent staining of the ventral branches of the T13–L3 spinal nerves and the lumbar sympathetic trunk, suggesting that the distribution of local anesthetics could be volume-dependent. Viscasillas et al. (2021b) described the use of a *dorsal* approach for performing the transmuscular-QLB in nine canine cadavers and found that based on anatomical dissection, 0.2 ml kg^{-1} of a mixture of iomeprol and methylene blue stained the ventral branches of spinal nerves from T13 to L4, similar to the high volume solution that was reported by Garbin et al. (2020a). Advanced imaging using computed tomography (CT) showed a median (range) distribution of 5 (3–6) vertebral spaces, with contrast reaching the T13 vertebra.

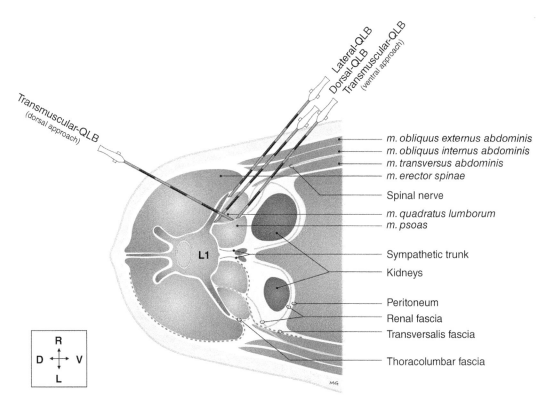

FIGURE 18.1 Schematic illustration of a cross section at the level of the first lumbar vertebra (L1) showing the relevant abdominal musculature and fascial layers surrounding the ***m. quadratus lumborum***. The different needle trajectories (and terminology) used to perform QLBs
in dogs are shown.

Dos-Santos et al. (2021, 2022) investigated the use of the
transmuscular-QLB in cat cadavers and showed that the distribution of 0.4 ml kg^{-1} of dye was similar to the previously
reported canine investigation by Garbin et al. (2020a). In that
study, a ropivacaine–dye–iohexol solution was distributed on
the ventral rami of the spinal nerves between the first three
lumbar vertebrae (6/8), and on the sympathetic trunk from
the T13 to L3 vertebrae (7/8). Dos-Santos et al. (2022) also
demonstrated that the *ventral* approach of the transmuscular-
QLB resulted in more consistent injectate distribution to the
ventral branches of the lumbar nerves (10/14), compared to
the *dorsal* approach (6/14), as well as significantly improving
needle visualization using ultrasound. In both canine and
feline cadavers, no epidural migration of injectate was
observed following either the *ventral* or the *dorsal* approaches
to the transmuscular-QLB.

A *ventral* approach to the dorsal-QLB has also been
investigated in canine cadavers. Marchina-Gonçalves et al.
(2022) demonstrated that a high volume of injectate
(0.6 ml kg^{-1}) resulted in 100% staining of the sympathetic
trunk from the T10 to L4 vertebrae, and the ventral branches
of the first three lumbar spinal nerves but failed to dye the
spinal nerves cranial to the T13 vertebra. Using a similar
approach, Alaman et al. (2022) compared the spread of 0.3
and 0.5 ml kg^{-1} of methylene blue and found that the high
volume consistently stained the ventral branches of the

T13–L3 spinal nerves and the sympathetic trunk from the
T11–L3 vertebrae. Given the different volumes and composi-
tions of injectate solutions used, a comparison of the results
from these different studies should be interpreted cautiously
(De Miguel Garcia et al. 2020). Unlike the previously mentioned studies that investigated transmuscular-QLBs, both of
the studies that used *ventral* approaches to perform dorsal-
QLBs in dogs demonstrated that epidural migration is a possible complication – 1/12 injections by Marchina-Gonçalves
et al. (2022) and 5/20 injections by Alaman et al. (2022)
resulted in epidural spread.

Using 0.3 ml kg^{-1} of a dye-lidocaine solution in eight
canine cadavers, Garbin et al. (2020b) investigated the use of a
lateral-QLB technique and compared *ventral* and *longitudinal*
approaches to the target site. The *longitudinal* approach
resulted in less consistent dye staining of the thoracolumbar
nerve ventral branches than the *ventral* approach (median
(range) 3 (0–4) versus 4 (3–5)), and an incidence of staining
the sympathetic trunk (1/8 versus 6/8), and its further use was
therefore not recommended. Overall, the *ventral* approach for
performing the lateral-QLB resulted in a greater degree of
cranial spread to the thoracic paravertebral space (T11) and
staining of the thoracic spinal nerves than the previously
reported transmuscular-QLB (Garbin et al. 2020a) and dorsal-
QLB (Alaman et al. 2022), when equivalent volumes of injectate were used (0.3 ml kg^{-1}).

The results of these studies suggest that different approaches to performing QLBs may result in different distributions of local anesthetic solutions and subsequent dermatomal coverage. Based on the results of these cadaveric studies, it is reasonable to conclude that QLBs will provide somatic analgesia for the mid-caudal abdomen, and they might provide visceral analgesia to structures in the cranial and mid-abdomen.

To date, only one clinical study has assessed the analgesic efficacy of QLBs in live patients (Viscasillas et al. 2021a). The authors of that study investigated the local anesthetic spread and resulting analgesia following the performance of a transmuscular-QLB (*dorsal* approach) using $0.4\,ml\,kg^{-1}$ of a 0.25% bupivacaine/iohexol solution in dogs undergoing ovariohysterectomies. Using CT imaging, they showed that the injectate spanned a median (range) of 3 (2–5) vertebrae, demonstrating that the spread of the injectate along the QL plane, following transmuscular-QLB, is similar in live dogs and canine cadavers. Postoperatively, pain scores in the dogs were <4/24 (using the Glasgow Pain Scale – Short Form) in the first four hours, suggesting that the duration of the block was approximately six hours. Those authors concluded that the transmuscular-QLB provided intraoperative analgesia for abdominal surgery that extended into the recovery period. To date, a single case report suggested that the use of a *ventral* approach for transmuscular-QLB in a cat provided effective analgesia for a cystotomy (Argus et al. 2020).

As the data in veterinary medicine are still very limited, further studies are needed to assess the analgesic efficacy of the described approaches to QLBs in dogs and cats.

PATIENT SELECTION
INDICATIONS FOR THE BLOCK

The QLB should be considered for any abdominal surgery, as stand-alone or as part of a multimodal analgesic approach. The analgesic efficacy of transmuscular-QLB has been reported for ovariohysterectomy in dogs and exploratory laparotomy for cystotomy in a cat. Lateral-QLB has been successfully used by the author to provide perioperative analgesia in cases of cholecystectomy, cholelithiasis removal, and nephrectomy in dogs.

Given the QLB potential for blocking the sympathetic trunk, it may also serve as a valid analgesic adjuvant for visceral pain (i.e. pancreatitis and gallstones).

CONTRAINDICATIONS

- Skin infection or other lesions at the intended puncture site.

- The QLB may be technically challenging in animals of extreme size. Very small patients may have an increased risk of peritoneal perforation, given the thinness of the thoracolumbar fascia and the musculature. In very large breeds, the interfascial plane between *m. quadratus lumborum* and *m. psoas* may be deeper than 6 cm, and

therefore, difficult to visualize sonographically, using a high-frequency transducer.

- Previous spinal surgery in the proximity of the QLB puncture site could affect the distribution of the local anesthetic, leading to block failure or epidural migration of the drug solution if the integrity of the fascial plane is compromised.

POTENTIAL SIDE EFFECTS AND COMPLICATIONS

- There is a risk of perforation of the peritoneum and puncture of intraabdominal organs (e.g. kidneys, liver, and spleen). The needle tip should be maintained in the field of view while it is being advanced through the skin, the abdominal wall and/or the epaxial muscles.

- Migration of the local anesthetic into the epidural space. Amongst the various cadaveric studies that have been reported in dogs, the dorsal-QLB has been shown to result in occasional epidural spread. This potential risk should be considered when the type of QLB is chosen.

- Injection outside the target interfascial plane (e.g. into the QL muscle) will result in block failure and lack of analgesic effect.

- Transient femoral nerve palsy and weakness of the hindlimbs have been reported in humans. Currently, there are no data available in animals related to this observation.

- The risk of intravascular injection is low, given the lack of large vessels in the area of the target injection site. However, as is good practice, an aspiration test should always be performed before injecting any local anesthetic.

- Local anesthetic systemic toxicity should be considered when performing bilateral QLB with a high-volume local anesthetic. The local anesthetic should be properly diluted to ensure that the maximum recommended dose is not exceeded.

GENERAL CONSIDERATIONS
CLINICAL ANATOMY

The *m. quadratus lumborum* lies ventral to the bodies of the last three thoracic and all of the lumbar vertebrae, ending caudally on the medial surface of the wing of the ilium. Thoracic and cranial abdominal portions of the *m. quadratus lumborum* is formed by distinct bundles that are attached to the proximal portions of the last two ribs, the bodies, or the transverse processes of the vertebrae. Caudal to the first lumbar vertebra, the medioventral aspect of the QL muscle is covered by the *m. psoas minor*, and caudal to the fourth lumbar vertebra, by the *m. psoas major*, with some individual variability. The lateral aspect of the *m. quadratus lumborum* is in contact with the aponeurosis of the *m. transversus abdominis* dorsally, and the peritoneum or the perirenal fat ventrally.

The **m. quadratus lumborum** is surrounded by the ventral layer of the thoracolumbar fascia and is covered ventrally by the endothoracic fascia (in the thorax) and the transversalis fascia (in the abdomen) (Figure 18.1).

The ventral branches of the last two thoracic and the first three lumbar spinal nerves, involved in the innervation of the abdominal wall, exit from the vertebral foramen and run in the subserous endothoracic fascia at its origin. With some individual variations, these nerves run between the bundles of the **m. quadratus lumborum,** or between the **m. quadratus lumborum** and **m. psoas**, then pass through the aponeurosis of origin of the **m. transversus abdominis,** or between the **m. transversus abdominis** and the **m. obliquus internus abdominis**. The **rami communicantes** exit the spinal nerves shortly after emerging from the intervertebral foramina and run between the vertebral body and the dorsal aspect of the **m. quadratus lumborum** and **m. psoas**, and connect with the sympathetic trunk. The sympathetic trunk, which is involved in the visceral innervation of the abdomen, runs medioventral to the hypaxial muscles, and dorsal to the transversalis fascia (Figure 18.1).

EXPECTED DISTRIBUTION OF ANESTHESIA

Based on reported clinical and cadaveric studies, successful QLBs should consistently provide somatic and visceral analgesia of the L1–L3 spinal nerves, with frequent extension to the T13 spinal nerve cranially, and the L4 spinal nerve caudally. Therefore, the cranial portion of the abdominal wall that is innervated by the T9–T12 spinal nerves might not be covered by a QLB. Based on CT scans, the QLB may occasionally extend caudally to L5–L7 (Viscasillas et al. 2021b), but the clinical significance of blocking this area is currently unknown.

LOCAL ANESTHETIC: DOSE, VOLUME, AND CONCENTRATION

Long-acting local anesthetics (e.g. bupivacaine, ropivacaine, and levobupivacaine) are usually administered for QLBs. The coadministration of an adjuvant (e.g. dexmedetomidine, dexamethasone, and buprenorphine) has not been investigated to date. Bupivacaine liposome injectable suspension has been administered as part of QLBs in humans, but its safety and efficacy have not been assessed for this block in animals.

A volume of 0.4 ml kg^{-1} of bupivacaine 0.25% per side (the block must be performed bilaterally) has been used clinically in dogs without complications (Viscasillas et al. 2021a), and a dose of 0.3 ml kg^{-1} of ropivacaine 0.75% per side has been successfully administered in a cat (Argus et al. 2020). Although the optimal clinical dose and concentration are still unknown, it appears reasonable to use diluted local anesthetics (e.g. bupivacaine 0.25–0.125% or ropivacaine 0.5–0.2%) to administer 0.3–0.6 ml kg^{-1} per injection site, so as to not exceed the recommended maximum dose for the particular local anesthetic. The author most commonly uses 0.5 ml kg^{-1} bupivacaine 0.2% per injection (i.e. on each side).

PATIENT PREPARATION AND POSITIONING

The patient should be positioned in lateral recumbency with the side to be blocked uppermost. The abdomen should be clipped free of hair with wider dorsal margins than would normally be required for surgery (Figure 18.2). Standard surgical preparation of the skin over the injection site should be performed. A wider clipping area is necessary to perform the *dorsal* approach compared to the transmuscular-QLB.

All QLB techniques can be performed with the anesthetist positioned beside the patient, with the ultrasound machine

(a)
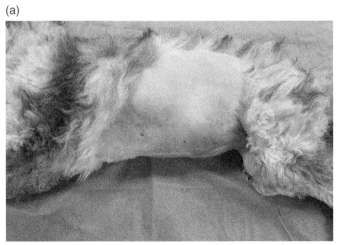
(b)
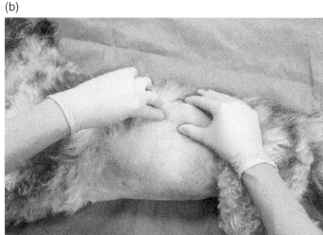

FIGURE 18.2 Patient positioning to perform the QLB. (a) A dog is positioned in right lateral recumbency. (b) Major relevant anatomic landmarks (i.e. the last rib and the lumbar musculature) should be palpated and identified.

aligned with the visual axis. The *dorsal* approach to the transmuscular-QLB may be facilitated if the operator stands caudal to the patient.

STEP-BY-STEP PERFORMANCE

SURFACE ANATOMY AND LANDMARKS TO BE USED

To perform transmuscular- or dorsal-QLBs, and the *ventral* approach to the lateral-QLB, the ultrasound transducer should be positioned transverse to the hypaxial musculature, caudal and parallel to the proximal aspect of the last rib, with the transducer marker oriented dorsally (Figure 18.3).

To perform the *longitudinal* approach to the lateral-QLB, the ultrasound transducer should be positioned parallel to the spinal musculature in a parasagittal plane, just caudal to the last rib (approximately at the level of the transverse processes of the lumbar vertebrae), with the transducer marker oriented cranially (Figure 18.4).

ULTRASOUND ANATOMY

Transverse View

Once in position, the transducer should be tilted slightly cranially to visualize the following landmarks – transverse processes of L1 (in dogs) or L2 (in cats), epaxial muscles, **m. quadratus lumborum,** and **m. psoas**, and the thoracolumbar fascia (Figure 18.5).

The transverse processes of the lumbar vertebrae are identified as hyperechoic structures with an acoustic shadow underneath. The epaxial muscles are visualized dorsally and laterally to the transverse processes. The thoracolumbar fascia is visualized as a hyperechoic linear structure surrounding the epaxial muscles and attaching to the transverse processes.

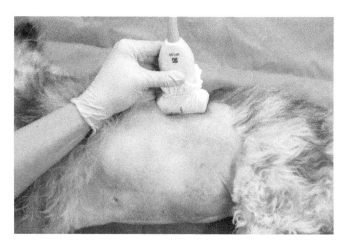

FIGURE 18.4   Ultrasound transducer positioning to perform the *longitudinal* approach to the **lateral-QLB**. The transducer is oriented parallel to the vertebral column, caudal to the last rib, with the transducer marker oriented cranially.

The **m. quadratus lumborum** is located ventral to the transverse processes, has a rounded cross-section and is usually hypoechoic compared with the epaxial muscles and **m. psoas**. The **m. psoas** is located ventromedial to the **m. quadratus lumborum**. Lastly, the interfascial plane between **m. quadratus lumborum** and **m. psoas** should be identified as a thin hyperechoic line.

Longitudinal View

Once in position, the transducer should slide along the short axis to scan the spinal musculature, and then be tilted dorsally until the transverse processes of L1 and L2 are identified between the epaxial musculature (dorsally) and the **m. quadratus lumborum** (ventrally) (Figure 18.6).

(a)

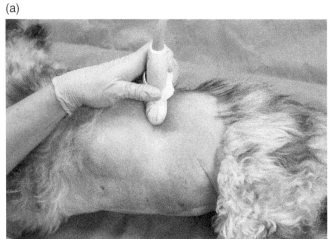

(b)

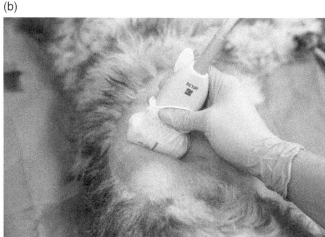

FIGURE 18.3   Ultrasound transducer positioning to perform the QLB. Generally, the transducer is positioned transverse to the spinal musculature, caudal and parallel to the last rib with the transducer marker oriented dorsally. (a) Ventral view to perform the *ventral* approach to the **transmuscular-QLB**, **lateral-QLB** and **dorsal-QLB**. (b) Caudal view to perform the *dorsal* approach to the **transmuscular-QLB**.

(a) 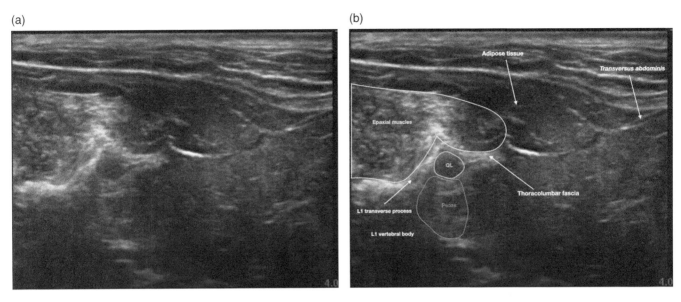 (b)

FIGURE 18.5   (a) Sonoanatomy of the lumbar musculature and landmarks to perform *ventral* or *dorsal* approaches to the **transmuscular-QLB**, **lateral-QLB** and **dorsal-QLB**. (b) Same images, with superimposed schematic drawing identifying anatomical landmarks.

(a) 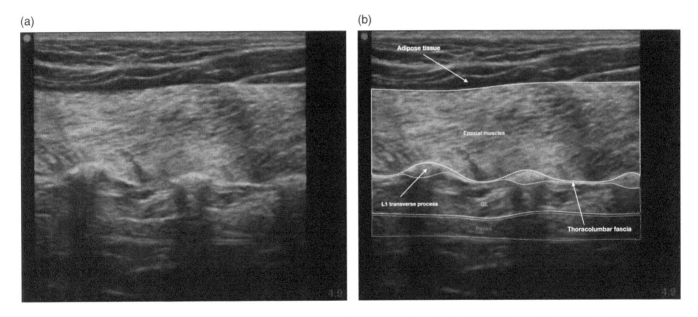 (b)

FIGURE 18.6   (a) Sonoanatomy of the lumbar musculature and landmarks to perform the *longitudinal* approach to the **lateral-QLB**. (b) Same image, with superimposed schematic drawing identifying anatomical landmarks.

NEEDLE INSERTION TECHNIQUE

Regardless of the technique and/or approach being used, the needle should be carefully advanced towards the target fascial plane using an in-plane needle technique, while always maintaining the tip of the needle in the field of view. Once the needle is in its final position, a standard aspiration test should be performed to verify that the tip of the needle is not in an intravascular location and a small aliquot of injectate should be injected to observe for the hydrodissection of the target

plane before administering the full volume of the local anesthetic.

TRANSMUSCULAR-QLB

Ventral approach – The needle should be introduced with an angle of 30° on a ventrolateral-to-dorsomedial trajectory, passing through the ***mm. obliquus externus abdominis*** and ***obliquus internus abdominis***, the aponeurosis of insertion of the ***m. transversus abdominis***, and the belly of the *m. quadratus lumborum* until the neuronal fascia between the *m. quadratus lumborum* and the *m. psoas* is reached (Garbin et al. 2020a) (Figures 18.7 and 18.8).

    Dorsal approach – The needle should be inserted at a 45° angle on a dorsolateral-to-ventromedial trajectory through the epaxial muscles, the thoracolumbar fascia, and the *m. quadratus lumborum,* until it reaches the fascial plane between the *m. quadratus lumborum* and *m. psoas* (Viscasillas et al. 2021b) (Figures 18.9 and 18.10).

DORSAL-QLB:

Ventral approach – The needle should be introduced and advanced similar to the *ventral* approach to the transmuscular-QLB, until its tip is visualized either between the dorsal aspect of *m. quadratus lumborum* and the vertebral body of L1 (caudal to its point of insertion on the transverse process of the L1 vertebra) (Alaman et al. 2022), or between the *m. psoas* and the ventral body of the L1 vertebra (Marchina-Gonçalves et al. 2022) (Figures 18.7 and 18.11).

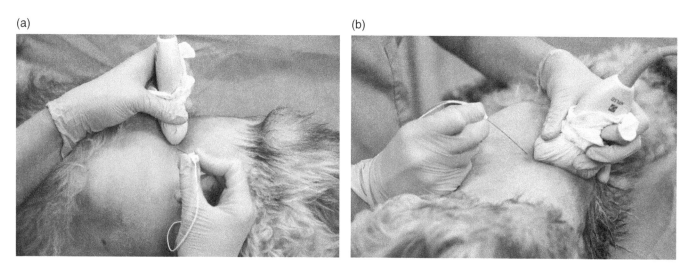

FIGURE 18.7 Ultrasound transducer position and needle insertion to perform the *ventral* approach to the **transmuscular-QLB**, **lateral-QLB** and **dorsal-QLB**, with a ventral view (a) and a caudal view (b). The needle is introduced in-plane, at about 30° angle, on a ventrolateral-to-dorsomedial trajectory.

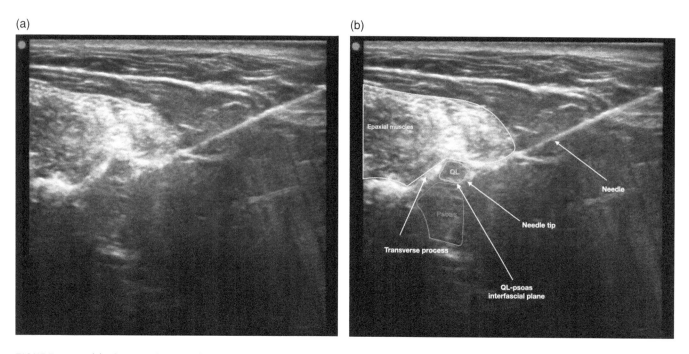

FIGURE 18.8 (a) Ultrasound image of the lumbar musculature and landmarks to perform the *ventral* approach to the **transmuscular-QLB**. (b) Same image, with superimposed schematic drawing identifying anatomical landmarks.

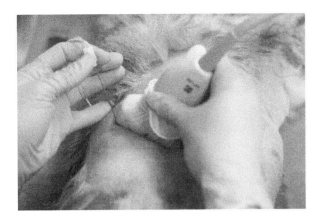

FIGURE 18.9   Caudal view of ultrasound transducer position and needle insertion to perform the *dorsal* approach to the **transmuscular-QLB**. The needle is introduced in-plane at a 45° angle on a dorsolateral-to-ventromedial trajectory.

LATERAL-QLB:

Ventral approach – The needle should be introduced at an angle of ~ 30° on a ventrolateral-to-dorsomedial trajectory, passing through the ***mm. obliquus externus abdominis*** and ***obliquus internus abdominis***, the epaxial muscles, the thoracolumbar fascia, and the aponeurosis of insertion of the ***m. transversus abdominis***. The needle tip should reach the lateral aspect of the ***m. quadratus lumborum***, ventral to the transverse process of L1 (Garbin et al. 2020b) (Figures 18.7 and 18.12).

    Longitudinal approach – The needle should be introduced in-plane on a caudolateral-to-craniomedial trajectory, and the local anesthetic injected between ***m. quadratus lumborum*** and epaxial muscles, medial to the thoracolumbar fascia and ventral to the transverse process of the L1 vertebra (Garbin et al. 2020b) (Figures 18.13 and 18.14). This approach has a poor success rate because landmarks may be difficult to

(a) (b)

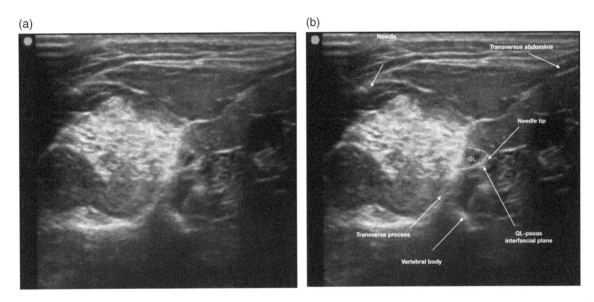

FIGURE 18.10   (a) Ultrasound image of the lumbar musculature and landmarks to perform the *dorsal* approach to the **transmuscular-QLB**. (b) Same image, with superimposed schematic drawing identifying anatomical landmarks.

(a) (b)

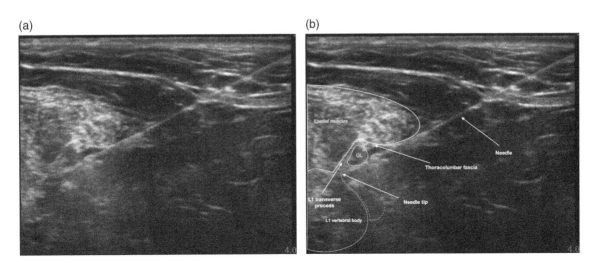

FIGURE 18.11   (a) Ultrasound image of the lumbar musculature and landmarks to perform the *ventral* approach to the **dorsal-QLB**. (b) Same image, with superimposed schematic drawing identifying anatomical landmarks.

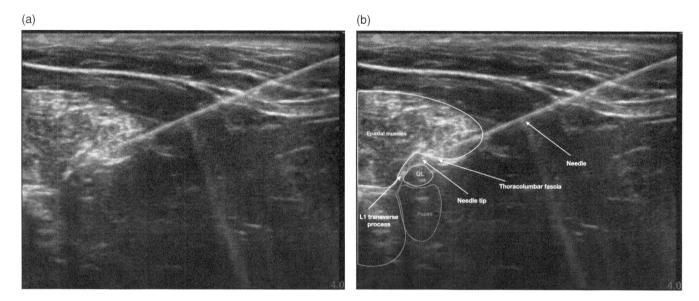

FIGURE 18.12   (a) Ultrasound image of the lumbar musculature and landmarks to perform the *ventral* approach to the **lateral-QLB**. (b) Same image, with superimposed schematic drawing identifying anatomical landmarks.

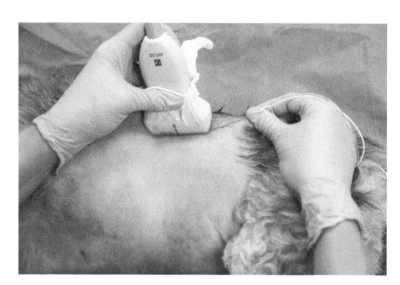

FIGURE 18.13   Ultrasound transducer position and needle insertion to perform the *longitudinal* approach to the **lateral-QLB**. The needle is introduced in-plane on a caudolateral-to-craniomedial trajectory.

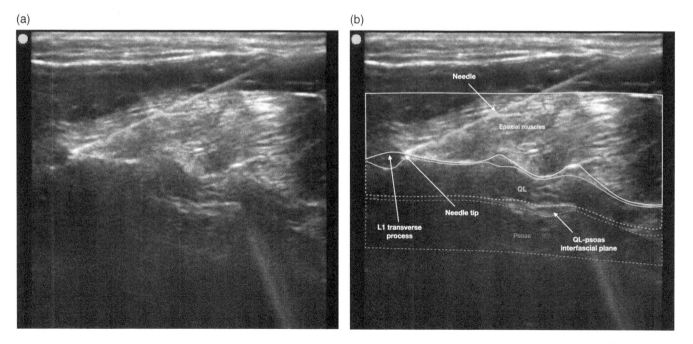

FIGURE 18.14   (a) Ultrasound image of the lumbar musculature and landmarks to perform the *longitudinal* approach to the **lateral-QLB**. (b) Same image, with superimposed schematic drawing identifying anatomical landmarks.

identify, and hydrodissection may not be observed. For these reasons, it is not recommended.

This block does not involve the use of nerve stimulation.

During needle advancement using the *ventral* approaches to the QLBs, it is common to feel two distinctive "pops" that correspond with the needle passing through – (1) the aponeurosis of the *m. transversus abdominis,* and (2) the interfascial plane between *m. quadratus lumborum* and *m. psoas* (transmuscular-QLB), or the thoracolumbar fascia surrounding the epaxial muscles (lateral-QLB).

Depending on the QLB technique, the initial injection of local anesthetic should result in the formation of an anechoic pocket between – (1) the *m. quadratus lumborum* and *m. psoas* (transmuscular-QLB), (2) the *m. quadratus lumborum* and the transverse process of the L1 vertebra (lateral-QLB), or (3) the *m. quadratus lumborum*, the transverse process, and vertebral body of the L1 vertebra (dorsal-QLB). Eventually, an injection of the local anesthetic solution, regardless of the technique being employed, will result in hydrodissection of the *m. quadratus lumborum*

and *m. psoas*, together with the ventral deflection of the thoracolumbar fascia (Figure 18.15).

After performing the block on one side, the patient should be re-positioned in the opposite recumbency because the block needs to be repeated on the other side of the patient.

Regardless of the approach being used, the QLB should result in dermatomal analgesia on the mid-caudal abdominal wall from T13 to L3. The analgesic distribution above T13, and visceral analgesia, are theoretically possible but need to be confirmed by further clinical investigations. For this reason, it is recommended to employ QLBs as part of a multimodal analgesia plan, at least when the cranial abdomen is involved.

COMPLICATIONS AND HOW TO AVOID THEM

Puncture and injury of the vital structures adjacent to the *m. quadratus lumborum* is possible. The right kidney lies at the level of the L2 vertebra and is separated by the *m. quadratus lumborum* by perirenal fat and the thoracolumbar fascia. On the left hemiabdomen, the stomach, liver, and spleen lie nearby. Careful ultrasound scanning should be performed prior to needle insertion to understand the relative anatomy of the *m. quadratus lumborum* and surrounding structures. QLBs are **advanced**-level blocks and should not be performed unless the operator has a thorough understanding and appreciation of the local anatomy.

(a)

(b)

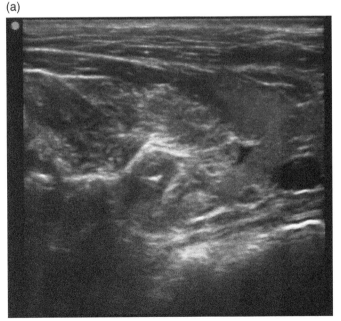
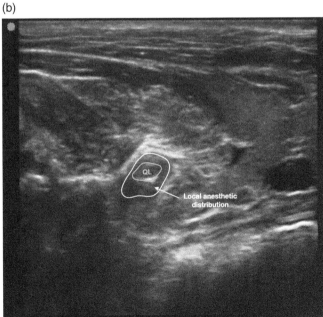

FIGURE 18.15   (a) Ultrasound image of the lumbar musculature after performing a QLB. The image shows the distribution of the local anesthetic along the *m. quadratus lumborum*. (b) Same image, with superimposed schematic drawing identifying the local anesthetic distribution surrounding the *m. quadratus lumborum*.

Epidural migration of local anesthetic is a possible complication that has been observed in cadavers post dorsal-QLB. Transient respiratory arrest and hypotension were observed after bilateral transmuscular-QLB with 0.22 ml kg⁻¹ bupivacaine 0.5% in a dog with a recent history of T12–T13 mini-hemilaminectomy (Herrera-Linare and Martínez 2022). When the vertebral canal and the dura mater have been exposed in proximity to the injection point of the QLB, epidural migration of local anesthetic is possible. The anesthetist should be aware of this risk before performing a QLB.

COMMON MISTAKES AND HOW TO AVOID THEM

Poor visualization of the needle may lead to the injection of local anesthetic outside the target plane.

The steep needle angle necessary to perform the *dorsal* approach to the transmuscular-QLB in relation to the transducer will result in poor needle visualization. Needle visualization may be improved by employing an echogenic needle and gently moving the needle "in-and-out" slightly, resulting in the deflection of the adjacent tissues.

Due to the complexity of the anatomical structures, misplacement of local anesthetic is possible. When performing dorsal-QLB and lateral-QLB, the local anesthetic might be injected superficially into the thoracolumbar fascia, leading to anesthetic spread within the erector spinae fascial plane. When performing transmuscular-QLB, intramuscular injection is also possible. A test injection should be performed to observe the hydrodissection to ensure adequate needle location.

HOW TO TALK TO CLIENTS/PROFESSIONAL COLLEAGUES

- For an experienced clinician, the bilateral QLB should take less than five minutes to perform.

- Depending on the local anesthetic used, a bilateral QLB will provide abdominal analgesia for up to six hours.

- The need for additional pain medications in the postoperative period should be assessed using a validated pain scale and examination of the patient.

- After receiving QLBs, patients should be able to walk immediately following recovery from anesthesia, can eat four to six hours post-recovery, and should be able to void.

REFERENCES

Alaman M, Bonastre C, de Blas I et al. (2022) Description of a novel ultrasound-guided approach for a dorsal quadratus lumborum block: a canine cadaver study. Vet Anaesth Analg 49, 118–125.

Argus APV, Freitag FAV, Bassetto JE et al. (2020) Quadratus lumbar block for intraoperative and postoperative analgesia in a cat. Vet Anaesth Analg 47, 415–417.

De Miguel Garcia C, Whyte M, St James M et al. (2020) Effect of contrast and local anesthetic on dye spread following transversus abdominis plane injection in dog cadavers. Vet Anaesth Analg 47, 391–395.

Dos-Santos JD, Ginja M, Alves-Pimenta S et al. (2021) A description of an ultrasound-guided technique for a quadratus lumborum block in the cat: a cadaver study. Vet Anaesth Analg 48, 804–808.

Dos-Santos JD, Ginja M, Alves-Pimenta S et al. (2022) Comparison of dorsoventral and ventrodorsal approaches for the ultrasound-guided quadratus lumborum block in cats: a cadaver study. Vet Anaesth Analg (in press) https://doi.org/10.1016/j.vaa.2022.05.003

Elsharkawy H, El-Boghdadly K, Barrington M (2019) Quadratus lumborum block: anatomical concepts, mechanisms, and techniques. Anesthesiology 130, 322–335.

Garbin M, Portela DA, Bertolizio G et al. (2020a) Description of ultrasoundguided quadratus lumborum block technique and evaluation of injectate spread in canine cadavers. Vet Anaesth Analg 47, 249–258.

Garbin M, Portela DA, Bertolizio G et al. (2020b) A novel ultrasoundguided lateral quadratus lumborum block in dogs: a comparative cadaveric study of two approaches. Vet Anaesth Analg 47, 810–818.

Herrera-Linare ME, Martínez M (2022) Transient respiratory arrest after quadratus lumborum block in a dog. Vet Rec Case Rep 10, e448.

Marchina-Gonçalves A, Gil F, Laredo FG et al. (2022) Evaluation of highvolume injections using a modified dorsal quadratus lumborum block approach in canine cadavers. Animals 12, 18.

Viscasillas J, Sanchis-Mora S, Burillo P et al. (2021a) Evaluation of quadratus lumborum block as part of an opioid-free anaesthesia for canine ovariohysterectomy. Animals 11, 3424.

Viscasillas J, Terrado J, Marti-Scharfhausen R et al. (2021b) A modified approach for the ultrasound-guided quadratus lumborum block in dogs: a cadaveric study. Animals 11, 2945.

Ultrasound-Guided Transversus Abdominis Plane (TAP) Block

Marta Romano

BLOCK AT A GLANCE

What is it used for?

- The transversus abdominis plane (TAP) block is used to provide analgesia for procedures involving the abdominal wall, including mastectomy, celiotomy, and abdominal wall wound repair.

- The TAP block does not provide visceral analgesia; therefore, it should be combined with systemic analgesics in patients undergoing intra-abdominal surgery.

Landmarks/transducer position:

- **Lateral TAP block** – The ultrasound (US) transducer is placed between the iliac crest and the last rib, on the lateral aspect of the abdominal wall. It can be oriented either parallel (parasagittal) or perpendicular (transverse) to the longitudinal axis of the patient. To ensure sufficient distribution of the local anesthetic, two injections for each side of the lateral abdomen should be performed, one injection immediately caudal to the last rib ("retrocostal TAP"), and the second injection cranial to the iliac crest ("pre-iliac TAP"). Alternatively, one single injection halfway between these two points can be performed.

- **Subcostal TAP block** – The US transducer is positioned with an oblique orientation immediately caudal to the costal arch. The subcostal TAP block can be combined with one or two lateral abdominal TAP injections.

- **Longitudinal approach** – One single longitudinal injection, starting halfway between the umbilicus and the cranial aspect of the wing of the ilium. The needle should be progressively advanced in a cranial direction as hydrodissection is taking place.

What equipment and personnel are required?

- Quincke spinal needle (20 or 22G, 3.5 in. for dogs larger than 8–10 kg; 22G or 25G 2.5 or 1.5 in. for cats or dogs smaller than 8–10 kg) with T connector.

- Alternatively, a 21G 100 mm (or similar) blunt atraumatic needle may be used.

- Syringe of drug(s)

- Ultrasound machine

- High frequency (e.g. 15–6 MHz) linear array transducer +/− protective sleeve

- Gloves

- Coupling agent (e.g. alcohol)

- +/− Assistant to help perform the injections

When do I perform the block?

- Prior to surgery, after the ventral abdomen is clipped and skin preparation is complete. Final skin preparation will still be needed before surgery.

- The TAP block can also be performed postoperatively or as part of a multimodal analgesic plan in patients with chronic pain.

What volume of local anesthetic is used?

- Approximately 1 ml kg^{-1} total volume (may dilute the local anesthetic in cases where the maximum recommended dose of the LA will not allow for this volume to be used). Divide the total volume into appropriate aliquots depending on the technique(s) used.

Goal

- To place local anesthetic within the intermuscular fascial plane between the **m. transversus abdominis** and the

Small Animal Regional Anesthesia and Analgesia, Second Edition. Edited by Matt Read, Luis Campoy, and Berit Fischer.
© 2024 John Wiley & Sons, Inc. Published 2024 by John Wiley & Sons, Inc.

m. obliquus internus abdominis ("retrocostal" and "pre-iliac" TAP blocks), or between the *m. transversus abdominis* and the *m. rectus abdominis* ("subcostal" TAP block), producing blockade of the spinal nerves that innervate the abdominal wall (T9–T13, L1–L3).

Complexity level

- Basic for most patients, intermediate for small patients or cachectic animals.

Clinical pearl

- Successful TAP block requires adequate visualization and correct identification of the target planes.

WHAT DO WE ALREADY KNOW?

In humans, TAP blocks are used as effective components of multimodal analgesia for a variety of major abdominal surgical procedures (Børglum et al. 2011), including cesarean section (McDonnell et al. 2008), open prostatectomy (O'Donnell et al. 2006), large bowel resection (McDonnell et al. 2007), hysterectomy (Carney et al. 2008), appendectomy (Niraj et al. 2009), laparoscopic cholecystectomy (El-Dawlatly et al. 2009) and abdominoplasty (Sforza et al. 2011).

Based on the successful use of TAP blocks in humans, interest in TAP blocks in animals has followed. An anatomical study that investigated the distribution of the thoracolumbar nerves in the TAP of canine cadavers showed that the ventral branches of the T10, T11, T12, T13 (**costoabdominal nerve**), L1 (**cranial iliohypogastric nerve**), L2 (**caudal iliohypogastric nerve**), and L3 (**ilioinguinal nerve**) spinal nerves were located in the TAP in 100% of the subjects that were evaluated (Figure 19.1). Branches of T9 were present within the TAP in 95% of the examined cadavers, while branches of T7 and T8 were present in 20% and 60% of the subjects, respectively. Communicant branches were identified among T7–L3 nerves in this study (Castañeda-Herrera et al. 2017).

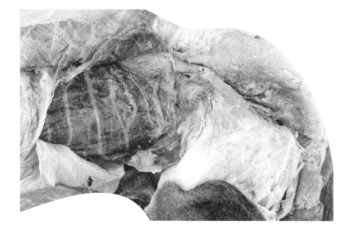

FIGURE 19.1   Innervation of the canine abdominal wall. The ventral branches of spinal nerves T9–T13 and L1–L3 contribute to the innervation of the abdominal wall. Occasionally, branches of T7 and T8 may also be present in the TAP.

The first anatomical description of a TAP block in canine cadavers was published by Schroeder et al. (2011) and showed that approximately 1 ml kg⁻¹ of a dye solution, injected as a single injection in the fascial plane between the *m. transversus abdominis* and the *m. obliquus internus abdominis* on the *lateral* aspect of each hemiabdomen, produced consistent staining of spinal nerves T13 and L1 (100% of the injections), and T12 and L2 in 80% and 90% of injections, respectively. The large volume injected in this study failed to reliably stain the branches of T11 and L3, with successful staining occurring in only 20% and 30% of the injections, respectively. These findings suggest that the injected solution tends to pool at the injection site when a single, large-volume TAP injection is performed. A more recent study (Zoff et al. 2017) investigating the tomographic spread of a single TAP injection of either 0.5 or 1 ml kg⁻¹ of a contrast solution showed similar results, suggesting that injection of smaller volumes at multiple sites (rather than a larger volume at a single injection) are necessary to maximize the distribution of local anesthetic across multiple dermatomes.

In contrast to these findings, one study showed the number of stained nerves increased when a greater volume of injectate was used (Bruggink et al. 2012). This finding was also supported in a more recent study where a single TAP injection of 0.3 ml kg⁻¹ of colorant solution successfully stained a similar number of nerves as a single 1 ml kg⁻¹ injection or two 0.3 ml kg⁻¹ injection performed in the *lateral* abdomen (Freitag et al. 2021). Based on these conflicting findings, further studies in clinical patients are needed to determine the most effective dosing regimen for TAP injections in live animals.

A variation on the original approach to performing a TAP block, the *subcostal* TAP block, was first described in humans with the objective of providing analgesia for surgical procedures of the cranial abdomen (Hebbard 2008). This approach involves positioning the US transducer parallel to the costal margin (i.e. oblique to the sagittal plane) (Figure 19.2) and injecting into the fascial plane between the *m. rectus abdominis* and *m. transversus abdominis*. A similar approach has been described in a cadaveric study in dogs (Drozdzynska et al. 2017). In that study, the authors performed three subcostal injections of a dye solution for each hemiabdomen, using approximately 1 ml kg⁻¹ for each side. This approach produced staining of T10, T11, and T12 in 95%, 100%, and 95% of the cases, T9 and T13 in 72% and 61% of the cases, and L1 and L2 in only 33% and 11% of the cases, respectively. This suggests that, in a clinical setting, this approach should be combined with a caudal TAP block to ensure desensitization of the entire abdomen.

A pilot study in canine cadavers examined two *lateral* TAP injections (0.3 ml kg⁻¹) – one performed at the level of the thirteenth rib and the other just cranial to the tuber coxae (Figure 19.3). This resulted in good stain distribution of the branches caudal to T13, however, T12 was rarely stained and T11 never became stained, suggesting that two *lateral* TAP injections of local anesthetics may be insufficient at providing regional anesthesia of the cranial abdomen

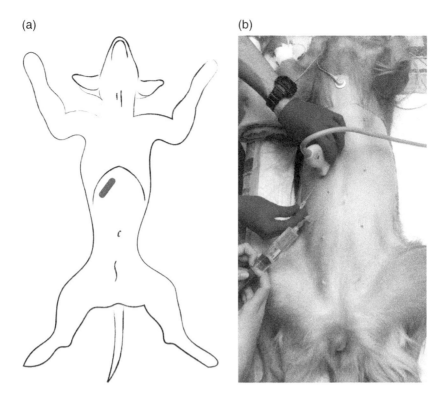

FIGURE 19.2 (a) Ultrasound transducer position for a "*subcostal*" TAP block. This approach is used to provide analgesia to the cranial abdomen. The transducer should be positioned immediately caudal to the costal arch, with an oblique orientation. (b) Performance of a "*subcostal*" TAP block in a dog. An assistant is handling the syringe and performing the injection.

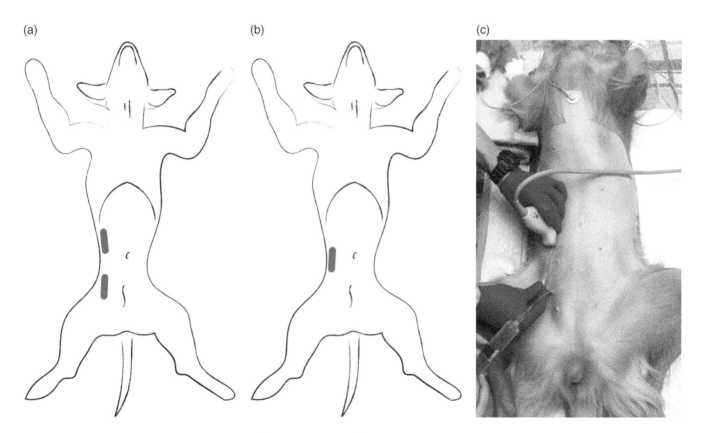

FIGURE 19.3 (a) Ultrasound transducer position for lateral abdominal "*retrocostal*" and "*pre-iliac*" TAP blocks. The transducer may be oriented transversally or longitudinally. Two injections may be performed to maximize local anesthetic distribution, one immediately caudal to the last rib ("*retrocostal*" TAP block) and one immediately cranial to the iliac crest ("*pre-iliac*" TAP block). (b) Alternatively, one mid-abdominal injection can be performed. (c) Performance of a mid-abdominal TAP injection in a dog. An assistant is handling the syringe and performing the injection.

(Johnson et al. 2018). Another study compared two *lateral abdominal* TAP injections versus one *lateral* and one *subcostal* injection in canine cadavers and showed a broader spread of the colorant solution when the latter technique was used with a volume of 0.25 ml kg^{-1} per location (Romano et al. 2021). In that study, the combination of *lateral* and *subcostal* TAP injections only resulted in adequate staining of T13 in 62.5% of injections.

In cat cadavers, three smaller volume (0.16 ml kg^{-1}) TAP injections (i.e. one each of *subcostal*, *retrocostal*, and *pre-iliac*) provided a better stain distribution compared with two larger-volume (0.25 ml kg^{-1}) TAP injections (*subcostal* and *pre-iliac* locations only) (Otero et al. 2021). These findings suggest that the former approach might provide a broader area of desensitization when performed in live animals (Otero et al. 2021).

Two studies have identified a potential source of error when performing *lateral* abdominal TAP injections (Romano et al. 2021; Otero et al. 2021). If injections are performed too close to midline, the injections could be located superficial to the aponeurosis of the **m. obliquus internus abdominis**, potentially contributing to block failure. To prevent this, prior to performing these injections, the transducer should ideally be positioned lateral to where the **m. obliquus internus abdominis** can be clearly identified (Figure 19.4). Those authors refer to the area of the abdominal wall immediately lateral to the **m. rectus abdominis** and medial to the **m. obliquus internus abdominis** as a "transitional area" that should be avoided when performing TAP injections since it may easily lead to errors in performing the injection (Otero et al. 2021).

TAP blocks have also been investigated in other species. A combination of *subcostal* and *lateral* TAP injections has

been described in New Zealand white rabbit cadavers and was found to have a better injectate distribution when compared to a single TAP injection (Di Bella et al. 2021).

Veterinary clinical studies evaluating the efficacy of the TAP block alone or as part of a multimodal analgesic approach are sparse. Currently, these include a case report in a lynx undergoing exploratory laparotomy (Schroeder et al. 2010), a retrospective study describing the combined use of unilateral TAP blocks and **intercostal nerve** blocks in dogs undergoing radical mastectomy (Portela et al. 2014), and a prospective study comparing bilateral TAP injections of either a combination of lidocaine and bupivacaine or saline as part of a multimodal analgesic protocol in cats undergoing ovariectomy (Skouropoulou et al. 2018). The latter study identified significantly reduced pain scores and opioid consumption for up to 24 hours postoperatively in the treatment group versus control. This is similar to results reported in human studies, with analgesia reportedly lasting up to 36 hours post-block following bupivacaine or ropivacaine injection (McDonnel et al. 2008; Bharti et al. 2011). Additionally, human studies have shown that TAP blocks are effective for decreasing severe pain associated with abdominal surgery and that patients receiving TAP blocks as part of their multimodal analgesic plans had reduced postoperative pain scores, reduced opioid consumption, and lower sedation scores compared to those given a saline control (Bharti et al. 2011; Børglum et al. 2011). The administration of a TAP block to dogs undergoing ovariohysterectomy, with either a combination of bupivacaine-dexmedetomidine or bupivacaine liposome injectable suspension provided better postoperative analgesia compared to a control group that received systemic analgesics only

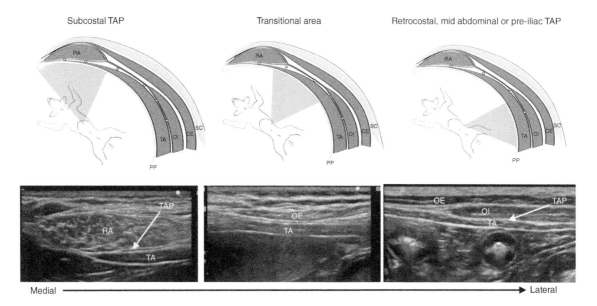

FIGURE 19.4   Representation and ultrasound pictures showing the anatomy of the abdominal wall muscles as the transducer is moved from medial to lateral. The "transitional area" should be avoided when performing TAP injections as the aponeurosis of the **m. obliquus internus abdominis** is located between the **m. obliquus externus abdominis** and the **m. transversus abdominis**, making it impossible to ensure the correct location of the injection. Retrocostal, mid-abdominal, or pre-iliac injections should be performed more laterally, where the **m. obliquus internus abdominis** can be clearly visualized. OE, **m. obliquus externus abdominis**; OI, **m. obliquus internus abdominis**; PP, parietal peritoneum; RA, **m. rectus abdominis**; SC, subcutaneous tissue; TA, **m. transversus abdominis**.

(Campoy et al. 2022). However, the use bupivacaine liposome injectable suspension did not prolong the duration of analgesia in this study compared to the injection of bupivacaine combined with dexmedetomidine.

Since TAP blocks result in desensitization of the spinal nerves that innervate the abdominal wall and the underlying parietal peritoneum, they are considered to only be effective for treating or preventing somatic pain associated with the abdominal body wall. Some evidence suggests, however, that they may also reduce visceral pain. For example, a study in humans described the use of TAP blocks to treat pain associated with acute-on-chronic pancreatitis, with patients reporting almost immediate alleviation of all components of pain, including referred pain radiating to the mid-back, and poorly localized aching considered to be visceral in origin (Smith et al. 2014). The analgesic effect lasted 7–10 days as determined by follow-up. Whether this effect is attributable to a systemic effect of the local anesthetic, or if the overlap and mutual influence of somatic and visceral afferents in the dorsal horn of the spinal cord play a role, remains speculative (Kato et al. 2009; Todd 2010).

The use of TAP catheters is well-described in humans as a safe and effective way to provide prolonged postoperative analgesia following abdominal surgery (Maeda et al. 2015; Yoshida et al. 2016). A report described the use of epidural catheters placed bilaterally in the TAP in three dogs suffering from severe abdominal pain caused by either pancreatitis or abdominal surgery (Freitag et al. 2018). In that report, commercial epidural catheters were placed in the TAP bilaterally using a Tuohy needle with the US transducer positioned on the lateral aspect of the abdomen, midway between the iliac crest and the caudal aspect of the last rib. After placement, the catheters were secured to the skin with suture and protected with a semiocclusive dressing. Injections of bupivacaine (0.3 ml kg^{-1} of 0.5% per side) were performed through the catheters every six hours and resulted in significantly reduced pain scores in the patients. The catheters did not become dislodged and were able to be kept in place longer than five days in one of the dogs.

Complications associated with TAP blocks have been reported. Visceral organ damage following a blind TAP block (i.e. not performed using US) has been described in humans (Farooq and Carey 2008). Although US guidance can minimize this risk, intra-abdominal puncture can still occur if the needle tip is not continuously visualized while performing the block (Lancaster and Chadwick 2010). In a canine cadaver study, inadvertent intra-abdominal puncture occurred in 23% of cases, highlighting the importance of continuous needle visualization during advancement (Zoff et al. 2017).

Clinical signs of local anesthetic neurotoxicity, including seizures, have been reported in pregnant women following TAP blocks for cesarean section (Griffiths et al. 2013; Weiss et al. 2014). In one of these studies, the measured plasma concentrations of ropivacaine were consistent with those commonly associated with systemic toxicity (Griffiths et al. 2013). Cardiac arrest due to local anesthetic overdose has also been reported in a woman following administration of both peritoneal infiltration and a TAP block, due to miscommunication between the surgeon and the anesthesiologist (Scherrer et al. 2013). Because of the relatively large volume of local anesthetic solution that is needed for a successful TAP block, the immediate availability of lipid emulsion and other emergency drugs, along with close monitoring for signs of local anesthetic toxicity is recommended (Sakai et al. 2010). A study evaluating the safety of up to 2.5 mg kg^{-1} bupivacaine TAP injections in cats showed that plasma concentrations remained below toxic levels with no adverse events being observed with this dosing regimen (Garbin et al. 2022).

Incorrect deposition of the local anesthetic solution between the ***m. transversus abdominis*** and the transversalis fascia, resulting in transient **femoral nerve** dysfunction, has been reported in humans following blind TAP blocks (Manatakis et al. 2013).

The parietal peritoneum may act as a reflective boundary under some circumstances and may lead to an artifact on the US screen that is known as "mirroring artifact" (Figure 19.5). When this occurs, the US image shows the abdominal wall fascial planes mirrored deep to the highly reflective peritoneum. This artifact is more likely to occur in the presence of pneumoperitoneum (e.g. when TAP blocks are performed postoperatively when air may be present in the abdomen following exploratory laparotomy) and may render image interpretation more challenging, leading to inadvertent intrabdominal needle advancement (Romano et al. 2020).

PATIENT SELECTION

INDICATIONS FOR THE BLOCK

A successful TAP block provides desensitization of the T9–L2 dermatomes, providing sensory desensitization of the abdominal wall including the skin, muscles, and underlying parietal peritoneum. As such, this approach can be used as part of a multimodal analgesic plan for intra-abdominal surgery, mastectomy of the abdominal and inguinal mammary glands, and for abdominal wall wounds.

CONTRAINDICATIONS

- Skin infection or neoplasia at the puncture site.

- In small patients, the target layer may be smaller than the bevel of the needle, making the execution of this block extremely challenging. The total volume of local anesthetic, even following dilution, is also very small which may make it challenging to inject a test dose to confirm correct positioning of the needle while still having enough volume remaining to successfully perform the block (especially at more than one site). "Small patient size" is a relative contraindication and the feasibility of performing TAP blocks in patients weighting less than 3 kg depends on the skill of the operator, the availability of small needles (i.e. 25G), and a small linear transducer (e.g. 25 mm).

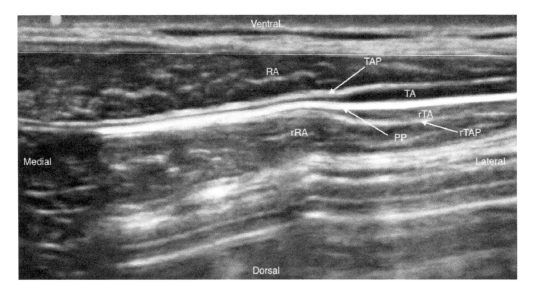

FIGURE 19.5   Mirroring artifact during performance of a postoperative TAP block. Note that the parietal peritoneum is acting as a reflective boundary and that the abdominal muscles are reflected deep to it. PP, parietal peritoneum; RA, *m. rectus abdominis*; rRA, reflected *m. rectus abdominis*; rTA, reflected *m. transversus abdominis*; rTAP, reflected TAP; TA, *m. transversus abdominis*; TAP, transversus abdominis plane.

POTENTIAL SIDE EFFECTS AND COMPLICATIONS

Local Anesthetic Toxicity

Effective TAP blockade can only be achieved when relatively large volumes of local anesthetic are injected in the transversus abdominis plane, which carries the potential of causing local anesthetic systemic toxicity (LAST) (Kato et al. 2009; Griffiths et al. 2013). For this reason, dilution of the local anesthetic solution is recommended when performing this block so the total administered dose of local anesthetic is not greater than the maximum recommended dose for the patient. Particular care should be taken if additional peripheral nerve blocks are planned for the patient, or in pregnant animals that are considered at higher risk of developing LAST due to the increased availability of free drug (Santos et al. 1989; Tsen et al. 1999) and their increased susceptibility to the neurotoxic effects of local anesthetics (Santos and DeArmas 2001).

Branches of the deep circumflex iliac artery provide vascularization to the TAP (Castañeda-Herrera et al. 2017). For this reason, extravascular positioning of the tip of the needle should always be confirmed via a negative aspiration test prior to administration of the local anesthetic solution. Visualization of the local anesthetic in the target plane during injection provides confidence that the solution is not being administered intravascularly.

Accidental Intra-Abdominal Needle Advancement or Organ Puncture

While performing this block, the entire needle (but particularly its tip) should be visualized at all times. If needle visualization is temporarily lost, it is imperative that the transducer be adjusted to obtain a good image before advancing the needle further. As long as the tip of the needle is able to be continuously visualized, the risk of inadvertent abdominal puncture will be minimized. Extra care should be taken in small-sized or cachectic patients whose body walls are especially thin and difficult to image using US. Introducing the needle in-plane with a minimal angle (i.e. almost parallel to the surface of the transducer as it contacts the skin) will provide the best image and help to reduce the risk of accidentally advancing it into the abdominal cavity.

Nerve Damage

Because the target nerves are too small to be visualized by US, nerve damage can potentially occur. Intrafascicular placement of the tip of the needle is associated with high resistance to injection and can result in neurologic injury (Hadzic et al. 2004). As with any other block, if high resistance to the injection is detected while performing a TAP block, administration of the local anesthetic should be immediately discontinued and the needle repositioned. Having said this, based on the body size of dogs and cats and the size of the target nerves within the TAP, it is unlikely that intrafascicular needle placement will occur.

GENERAL CONSIDERATIONS

CLINICAL ANATOMY

The innervation of the abdominal wall is comprised of the ventral branches of the T9–T13 and L1–L3 spinal nerves (Figure 19.1). The T9–T12 **intercostal nerves** and the **costoabdominal nerve** (T13) innervate the cranial and middle aspects of the abdominal wall. The **cranial** and **caudal ilio-hypogastric nerves** (L1 and L2, respectively) innervate the lateral and ventro–caudal aspects of the abdominal wall. The **ilioinguinal nerve** (L3) innervates the inguinal region but its area of innervation does not extend to the ventral midline.

The abdominal wall (from superficial to deep) is generally comprised of the *m. obliquus externus abdominis*, the *m. obliquus internus abdominis*, and the *m. transversus abdominis*. The parietal peritoneum is adhered to the *m. transversus abdominis* via the transversalis fascia. On the ventromedial aspect of the abdomen, the *m. rectus abdominis* is located superficial to the *m. transversus abdominis*.

The nerves that participate in the innervation of the abdominal wall (i.e. T9–T13 and L1–L3) run in the fascial plane between the *m. obliquus internus abdominis* and the *m. transversus abdominis* (Figure 19.6) on the lateral aspect of the abdominal wall or in the fascial plane between the *m. rectus abdominis* and the *m. transversus abdominis* as they approach the ventral midline (Figure 19.7).

When performing *lateral* abdominal TAP injections, care should be taken to clearly identify the *m. obliquus internus abdominis* to ensure that the injection is performed in the correct fascial plane. To do this, start on midline and move the transducer laterally. The *m. rectus abdominis* will initially be visible (Figure 19.8), followed by a "transition zone" immediately lateral to the *m. rectus abdominis*, where the aponeurosis of the *m. obliquus internus abdominis* is visible, but not the muscle itself (Figure 19.4). Lateral to this

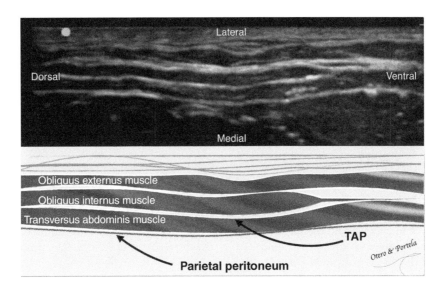

FIGURE 19.6 Ultrasound anatomy and representation of the lateral abdominal wall. Source: With permission of Pablo Otero and Diego Portela.

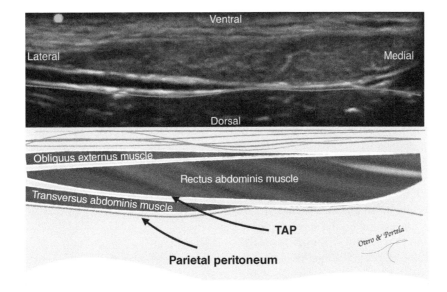

FIGURE 19.7 Ultrasound anatomy and representation of the subcostal TAP. Source: With permission of Pablo Otero and Diego Portela.

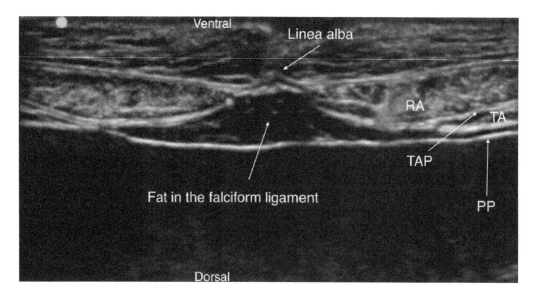

FIGURE 19.8 Ultrasound anatomy when the transducer is positioned transversally over the ventral midline. Identification of the TA at this level can be used to follow the target fascia by slowly moving the transducer laterally until it is positioned adequately to perform the selected approach. PP, parietal peritoneum; RA, *m. rectus abdominis*; TA, *m. transversus abdominis*. Source: With permission of Pablo Otero and Diego Portela.

area, the *m. obliquus internus abdominis* will be identifiable as a thick, triangular-shaped muscle (Figure 19.6).

Performing an injection in the "transition zone" may result in a failed block as the local anesthetic might be deposited superficial to the aponeurosis of the *m. obliquus internus abdominis* and not be in contact with the target nerves between the *m. obliquus internus abdominis* and the *m. transversus abdominis*. To be performed correctly, the injection should be made between the *m. obliquus internus abdominis* and the *m. transversus abdominis* (Castañeda-Herrera et al. 2017).

EXPECTED DISTRIBUTION OF ANESTHESIA

The abdominal skin may not be desensitized unless the local anesthetic migrates proximal to the point where the lateral cutaneous branches cross the abdominal wall and run superficial to the *m. obliquus externus abdominis*. Multiple TAP injections may need to be performed in order to desensitize the entire abdominal wall, while a single injection is only expected to desensitize a portion of it.

The T9–L2 dermatomes need to be blocked bilaterally to ensure analgesia to the entire abdominal wall, including the ventral midline. This might be achieved by combining *subcostal* and *lateral* abdominal TAP blocks bilaterally (two- or three-point TAP blocks, depending on the species) (Otero et al. 2021; Romano et al. 2021). With this approach, the *subcostal* TAP block would be expected to target the T10–T12 dermatomes, while the *lateral* TAP block would extend the resulting anesthesia to the T13–L2 dermatomes (Figures 19.2 and 19.3b).

Alternatively, bilateral *lateral* abdominal TAP injections can be performed (Figure 19.3a). The expected distribution of anesthesia with *lateral* abdominal TAP injections, however, is limited to the dermatomes caudal to T12 (Romano et al. 2021). Therefore, this approach is considered less effective in providing analgesia to the cranial abdomen compared to the *subcostal* TAP block, although specific studies comparing the two techniques in live animals undergoing abdominal surgery are lacking.

Lateral TAP injections can be performed in conjunction with **intercostal nerve** blocks to extend analgesia further cranially. This approach has been successfully used to provide analgesia in dogs undergoing radical mastectomy (Portela et al. 2014). For unilateral mastectomies, a TAP block can be performed on a single side, if the surgical margins are not expected to extend across the ventral midline.

Advancing (aka "chasing") the needle within the local anesthetic pocket in the interfascial plane, while the injection is being performed (often referred to as "hydrodissection"), may increase the area of distribution of the injected solution over multiple dermatomes, potentially resulting in a larger area of desensitization from a single needle puncture.

LOCAL ANESTHETIC: DOSE, VOLUME, AND CONCENTRATION

Long-acting local anesthetic solutions (e.g. bupivacaine or ropivacaine) or bupivacaine liposome injectable suspension are usually recommended for this block due to their prolonged duration of effect. Based on anatomical studies using dye solutions in cadavers, the recommended injected volume for TAP blocks is 0.25–0.35 ml kg^{-1} per injection site. Therefore, for a four-point approach to desensitize the entire abdominal wall and the ventral midline (i.e. *subcostal* and *lateral* injections made bilaterally), the local anesthetic should be diluted to a final concentration of 0.125–0.25%, not to exceed the maximum recommended dose for each species (e.g. not more than 2–3 mg kg^{-1} bupivacaine). For example, the author routinely uses a total volume of 1–1.2 ml kg^{-1} bupivacaine (0.25%) for a four-point TAP block (i.e. 0.25–0.3 ml kg^{-1} per injection site), using a total of 3 mg kg^{-1} bupivacaine. The use of bupivacaine liposome injectable suspension did not prolong the duration of analgesia when compared to a combination of bupivacaine and dexmedetomidine in dogs undergoing abdominal surgery (Campoy et al. 2022).

PATIENT PREPARATION AND POSITIONING

The block may be performed with the animal positioned in either dorsal or lateral recumbency. The former is preferred as the patient will usually already be in this position for clipping and preparation of the surgical field for abdominal surgery. Aseptic skin preparation should be performed prior to injection.

STEP-BY-STEP PERFORMANCE
SURFACE ANATOMY AND LANDMARKS TO BE USED

Lateral abdominal ("retrocostal" location) – The injection point is on the lateral aspect of the abdomen, immediately caudal to the last rib. The transducer should be oriented either transversally or parasagittally (Figure 19.3). This approach may be combined with a lateral abdominal "pre-iliac" and/or a "subcostal" TAP block (Figure 19.2), depending on the desired dermatomes to be blocked.

Lateral abdominal ("pre-iliac" location) – The injection point is on the lateral aspect of the abdomen, immediately cranial to the iliac crest. The transducer should be oriented either transversally or parasagittally (Figure 19.3). This approach may be combined with a lateral abdominal "retrocostal" and/or a "subcostal" TAP block (Figure 19.2), depending on the desired dermatomes to be blocked.

In general, *lateral* abdominal TAP injections can be performed anywhere between the retrocostal and pre-iliac injection points (Figure 19.3). Alternatively, bilateral injections using a single *longitudinal* needle approach on each side of the abdomen (i.e. with cephalad advancement of the needle during hydrodissection) can be performed. Drawing an imaginary line perpendicular to midline at the level of the umbilicus, and a second line parallel to midline extending from the wing of the ilium to the level of the umbilicus, the puncture site would be found equidistant between where these two points cross and the most cranial point of the wing of the ilium (Figure 19.3).

Subcostal approach: The injection point is immediately caudal and parallel to the costal arch (Figure 19.2). This approach may be combined with any of the above-listed lateral abdominal approaches, depending on the desired dermatomes to be blocked.

ULTRASOUND ANATOMY

With the US transducer located abaxial to midline in a longitudinal direction, the three layers of the abdominal wall should be readily visible. Usually, a depth of approximately 2 cm and the highest resolution setting are adequate to optimize the image.

The peritoneum should be identified first and will be visible as a hyperechoic line with abdominal organs deep to it (Figure 19.6). Superficial to the peritoneum, the **m. transversus abdominis** will appear as a variably hypoechoic structure with a thin hyperechoic line superficial to it. This line represents the interface between the fascial surfaces of the **m. transversus abdominis** and the **m. obliquus internus abdominis**. If this thin hyperechoic line is visualized during the patient's respiratory cycle, the two muscles will be seen to slide along each other on this line. When performing a TAP block, the target nerves will not be able to be directly visualized with US. However, as with other interfascial blocks, if a local anesthetic solution is injected within the fascial plane between the target muscle layers where the nerves are embedded, perineural distribution of the administered solution should occur.

Lateral abdominal TAP block – The easiest way to correctly identify the target plane is to position the transducer on midline and slowly move it laterally (Figure 19.8). Initially, the **m. rectus abdominis** will be visible immediately superficial to the **m. transversus abdominis**. As the transducer is moved further laterally, the **m. rectus abdominis** disappears and the **m. obliquus externus abdominis** will be visible immediately superficial to the **m. transversus abdominis** (Figure 19.4). This anatomical location, referred to by some authors as the "transition zone," should be avoided for TAP injections since the landmarks are often not clearly visible or able to be differentiated (Otero et al. 2021). At this location, the thin aponeurosis of the **m. obliquus internus abdominis**, located between the **m. obliquus externus abdominis** and the **m. transversus abdominis**, might prevent the local anesthetic from distributing around the target nerves if the solution is deposited superficial to it. This aponeurosis cannot be clearly visualized with an US, rendering this particular area unsuitable for TAP injection. The **m. obliquus internus abdominis** becomes more clearly visible as a triangular-shaped muscle when moving the transducer further laterally (Figure 19.6), so *lateral* TAP injections should be performed where this muscle can be more clearly visualized and the correct fascial plane identified prior to drug administration (Figure 19.6).

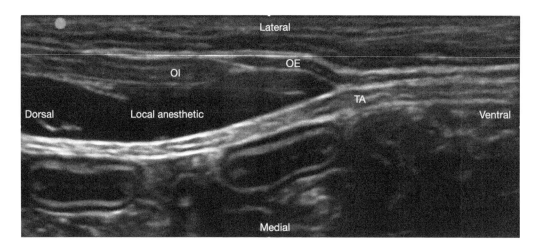

FIGURE 19.9 Deposition of local anesthetic during a lateral abdominal TAP. Note the hydrodissection of the TAP that results in separation of the IO and TA muscles. OE, *m. obliquus externus abdominis*; OI, *m. obliquus internus abdominis*; TA, *m. transversus abdominis*.

Subcostal TAP block – The transducer is placed immediately caudal to the costal arch, close to midline (Figure 19.2). The **m. rectus abdominis** will be visible superficial to the **m. transversus abdominis** (Figure 19.7). The target injection site is the fascial plane between these two muscles.

NEEDLE INSERTION TECHNIQUE

The needle should be inserted in-plane, as parallel to the surface of the US transducer as possible to minimize the risk of inadvertent intra-abdominal puncture (Figures 19.2b and 19.3c). The needle should be slowly advanced toward the target plane while maintaining continuous visualization of the needle tip. The different layers of abdominal wall muscle and fasciae will offer some resistance to advancing the needle so, as the needle is slowly advanced, it may deform the abdominal wall slightly instead of piercing these layers (especially if a blunt needle is being used). A distinct "click" or "pop" might be perceived as the needle is advanced through the more superficial muscle into the target plane. This might also be seen on the US as the fascial layers are penetrated. The final position of the bevel of the needle should be immediately deep to the superficial hyperechoic surface of the **m. transversus abdominis** (i.e. deep to its superficial fascia).

EXPECTED MOTOR RESPONSES FROM NERVE STIMULATION

This block does not involve the use of nerve stimulation.

ADMINISTRATION OF LOCAL ANESTHETIC – WHAT TO LOOK FOR, WHAT TO FEEL FOR, AND DECISION POINTS

Before administering the planned volume of local anesthetic solution at a given location, a small test dose should be injected to confirm that the tip of the needle is correctly positioned

within the target space. As this dose is slowly being injected, hydrodissection along the muscle plane and separation of the two muscles should be observed, making more room for the needle between them (Figures 19.9 and 19.10). These test injections can be made as several small boluses (e.g. "tap, tap, tap" on the syringe plunger) or as a slow push. Slight resistance to injection may be appreciated by the person making the injections as the surface of the muscle and the fascia dissect away from the belly of the muscle and open up the potential space between them.

If, during injection, there is not a clean dissection between the two muscles along the thin hyperechoic line that represents the fascial plane and the local anesthetic solution appears within one of the muscles (Figure 19.11), stop the injection and reposition the needle. If the entire volume of local anesthetic for that particular injection site is administered intramuscularly, the block will fail in that location and the patient may experience stimulation during the surgical procedure.

BLOCK EFFECTS AND PATIENT MANAGEMENT

Clinical experience with the TAP block suggests that is a reasonable complement to a multimodal analgesic plan for animals undergoing abdominal surgery and it can reduce the requirement of intra- and postoperative opioids and other injectable analgesics. Further studies aimed at examining the TAP block for specific surgical procedures and evaluating its effects on intraoperative nociception and postoperative pain scores are warranted.

COMPLICATIONS AND HOW TO AVOID THEM

Intra-abdominal and visceral organ puncture may occur if the technique is not performed correctly. Small or cachectic patients with thin abdominal walls are at higher risk for this complication. To avoid this, the needle should be advanced

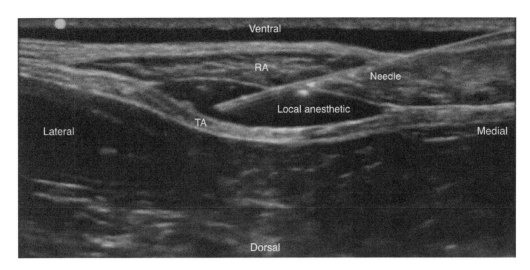

FIGURE 19.10   Deposition of local anesthetic during a "*subcostal*" TAP block. Note the hydrodissection of the TAP that results in separation of the RA and TA muscles. RA, *m. rectus abdominis*; TA, *m. transversus abdominis*.

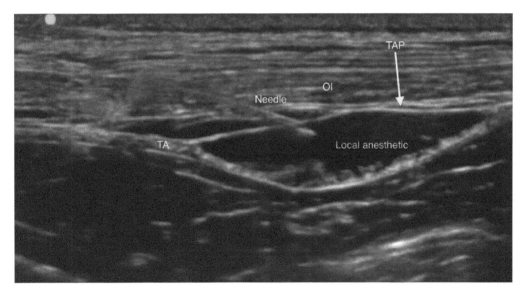

FIGURE 19.11   Inadvertent intramuscular injection during performance of a lateral abdominal TAP block. Note that the local anesthetic is being injected into the *m. transversus abdominis*, not the TAP. OI, *m. obliquus internus abdominis*; TA, *m. transversus abdominis*.

slowly, while the whole shaft, but particularly its tip, is under direct US visualization. The orientation of the needle should be as parallel as possible to the surface of the transducer and the abdominal wall, with only slight angulation. This allows for good visualization of the needle and reduces the risk of inadvertently advancing it into the abdomen. The target fascial plane offers some resistance to advancement of the tip of the needle. If resistance is encountered, gentle pressure should be applied while reducing the needle angulation, to minimize the risk of sudden and inadvertent advancement of the needle into the peritoneal cavity once the fascial layer is penetrated. Use of a blunt, atraumatic needle may reduce the risk of inadvertent intra-abdominal puncture.

Because of the relatively large volume of local anesthetic needed for TAP blocks, LAST is possible. This is even more likely if multiple blocks are being performed in the same patient. For this reason, dilution of the local anesthetic is recommended when performing TAP blocks, especially if two or three-point TAP injections are performed on each hemiabdomen. There are currently no reports of local anesthetic toxicity in association with TAP block in animals but seizures and cardiac arrest have been reported in humans (Scherrer et al. 2013; Weiss et al. 2014). Early recognition and prompt treatment are essential for successful management of local anesthetic toxicity.

When TAP blocks are performed following surgery, identification of the muscular layers and the target fascial plane may be more difficult due to the presence of air within the abdominal cavity.

The presence of enlarged mammary glands in pregnant patients makes the execution of this block challenging, especially if attempting a subcostal approach. The use of a combination of bilateral lateral TAP blocks and intercostal nerve blocks T9–T11 may be a better choice in this category of patients.

COMMON MISTAKES AND HOW TO AVOID THEM

- The most common reason for an unsuccessful block is that the injection was made either intramuscularly or within the incorrect fascial plane. This is more likely to occur when performing *lateral* TAP injections. As described above, since the **m. obliquus internus abdominis** is only present on the lateral aspect of the abdomen, an injection placed too close to midline may result in local anesthetic being deposited superficial to the aponeurosis of the **m. obliquus internus abdominis** rather than between the **m. transversus abdominus** and the **m. obliquus internus abdominis**, resulting in block failure (Figure 19.4).

- Administration of a small test dose of local anesthetic, when the tip of the needle is thought to be located in the target fascial plane, can be used to rule out intramuscular injection. If the injection is within the target plane, distinct separation of the **m. transversus abdominus** from the fascia present on its surface and the **m. obliquus internus abdominis or rectus abdominis** should be able to be visualized (Figures 19.6 and 19.8).

- Failure to correctly identify the TAP prior to injection may result in deposition of the local anesthetic solution in a different intermuscular plane. Identification of the TAP may be more challenging in some patients. Visualization of the **m. transversus abdominis** and the parietal peritoneum in proximity to the linea alba can be used to facilitate identification of the TAP when the target plane cannot be easily seen with the US, as described earlier in this chapter.

- Care should be taken to avoid performing *lateral* abdominal TAP injection in the "transition zone" where the **m. obliquus internus abdominis** is still not visible, as this might result in administration in the incorrect fascial plane.

- Insufficient distribution of the local anesthetic within the TAP may also result in block failure. For this reason, a large volume (i.e. 0.25–0.3 ml kg^{-1} per injection site) of local anesthetic solution is recommended when performing this block. Performing multiple injections (i.e. two- or three-point injections per hemiabdomen), helps to maximize the area of distribution of the injected solution. Alternatively, a longitudinal needle approach may be used with the needle being advanced during hydrodissection to cover a broader area within the fascial plane.

HOW TO TALK TO CLIENTS/PROFESSIONAL COLLEAGUES

The TAP block is a relatively simple technique that can contribute to providing multimodal anesthesia for abdominal surgeries or in animals suffering from abdominal pain. This block is safe when performed correctly under US guidance, and it does not cause motor dysfunction. Unlike infiltrative incisional local anesthetic techniques, since TAP block injections are made away from ventral midline, no edema will be encountered when a ventral midline incision is made. To date, no complications have been reported in association with TAP blocks in animals. A trained individual can perform a TAP block in less than 5 minutes and the analgesia is expected to last >24 hours.

TAP BLOCK – CATS

The execution of a TAP block in cats, and other small-sized patients, may be challenging. Availability of a high-frequency 25 mm linear US transducer and small needles (e.g. 25G spinal needle) are essential to successfully performing TAP blocks in cats. Although cats are said to be more sensitive to the toxic effects of local anesthetics than dogs, this statement is not supported by the scientific literature (Heavner and Amory 1981; de Jong et al. 1982; Seo et al. 1982; Chadwick 1985). A study evaluating the administration of bupivacaine TAP injections in healthy cats undergoing ovariohysterectomy identified plasmatic concentrations below toxic levels with doses of bupivacaine up to 2.5 mg kg^{-1} and no adverse cardiovascular effects were recorded with this dosing regimen (Garbin et al. 2022). It is advised, however, that the anesthetist use caution and not exceed the maximum recommended dose of the local anesthetic, as well as be able to quickly identify and treat local anesthetic toxicity should it occur. The "three-point" injection technique described previously (i.e. *subcostal*, *retrocostal*, and *pre-iliac*) provided better distribution of the injected solution compared to a two-point injection in cat cadavers (Otero et al. 2021).

TAP CATHETER PLACEMENT

Further studies evaluating the placement of TAP catheters with different approaches and how this relates to the distribution of the injected solution are warranted to determine the ideal position of TAP catheters to produce the most complete sensory block. Studies evaluating the likelihood of catheter displacement are also necessary. The use of a closed-tip multi-port catheter as opposed to a point-source catheter, such as an epidural catheter, may also be considered to provide a wider distribution of the injected solution.

Bharti N, Kumar P, Bala I et al. (2011) The efficacy of a novel approach to transversus abdominis plane block for postoperative analgesia after colorectal surgery. Anesth Analg 112, 1504–1508.

Børglum J, Maschmann C, Belhage B et al. (2011) Ultrasound-guided bilateral dual transversus abdominis plane block: a new four-point approach. Acta Anaesthesiol Scand 55, 658–663.

Bruggink SM, Schroeder KM, Baker-Herman TL et al. (2012) Weight-based volume of injection influences cranial to caudal spread of local anesthetic solution in ultrasound-guided transversus abdominis plane blocks in canine cadavers. Vet Surg 41, 455–457.

Campoy L, Martin-Flores M, Boesch JM et al. (2022) Transverse abdominis plane injection of bupivacaine with dexmedetomidine or a bupivacaine liposomal suspension yielded lower pain scores and requirement for rescue analgesia in a controlled, randomized trial in dogs undergoing elective ovariohysterectomy. Am J Vet Res. 83(9), ajvr.22.03.0037.

Carney J, McDonnell JG, Ochana A et al. (2008) The transversus abdominis plane block provides effective postoperative analgesia in patients undergoing total abdominal hysterectomy. Anesth Analg 107, 2056–2060.

Castañeda-Herrera FE, Buritica-Gaviria EF, Echeverry-Bonilla DF (2017) Anatomical evaluation of the thoracolumbar nerves related to the transversus abdominis plane block technique in the dog. Anat Histol Embriol 46, 373–377.

Chadwick HS (1985) Toxicity and resuscitation in lidocaine or bupivacaine-infused cats. Anesthesiology 63, 385–390.

de Jong RH, Ronfeld RA, DeRosa RA (1982) Cardiovascular effects of convulsant and supraconvulsant doses of amide local anesthetics. Anesth Analg 61, 3–9.

Di Bella C, Pennasilico L, Staffieri F et al. (2021) Ultrasound-guided lateral transversus abdominis plane (TAP) block in rabbits: a cadaveric study. Animals 11, 1953.

Drozdzynska M, Monticelli P, Neilson D et al. (2017). Ultrasound-guided subcostal oblique transversus abdominis plane block in canine cadavers. Vet Anaesth Analg 44, 183–186.

El-Dawlatly AA, Turkistani A, Kettner SC et al. (2009) Ultrasound-guided transversus abdominis plane block: description of a new technique and comparison with conventional systemic analgesia during laparoscopic cholecystectomy. Br J Anaesth 102, 763–767.

Farooq M, Carey M (2008) A case of liver trauma with a blunt regional anesthesia needle while performing transversus abdominis plane block. Reg Anesth Pain Med 33, 274–275.

Freitag FAV, Bozak VL, do Carmo MPW et al. (2018) Continuous transversus abdominis plane block for analgesia in three dogs with abdominal pain. Vet Anaesth Analg 45, 581–583.

Freitag FAV, Muehlbauer E, dos Santos AA et al. (2021) Evaluation of injection volumes for transversus abdominis plane block in dog cadavers: a preliminary trial. Vet Anaesth Analg 48, 142–146.

Garbin M, Benito J, Ruel HLM et al. (2022) Pharmacokinetics of bupivacaine following administration by an ultrasound-guided transversus abdominis plane block in cats undergoing ovariohysterectomy. Pharmaceutics 14, 1548.

Griffiths JD, Le NV, Grant S et al. (2013) Symptomatic local anaesthetic toxicity and plasma ropivacaine concentrations after transversus abdominis plane block for caesarean section. Br J Anaesth 110, 996–1000.

Hadzic A, Dilberovic F, Shah S et al. (2004) Combination of intraneural injection and high injection pressure leads to fascicular injury and neurologic deficits in dogs. Reg Anesth Pain Med 29, 417–423.

Heavner JE, Amory DW (1981) Lidocaine and pentylenetetrazol seizure thresholds in cats are not reduced after enflurane anesthesia. Anesthesiology 54, 403–408.

Hebbard P (2008) Subcostal transversus abdominis plane block under ultrasound guidance. Anesth Analg 106, 674–675.

Johnson EK, Bauquier SH, Carter, JE et al. (2018) Two-point ultrasound-guided transversus abdominis plane injection in canine cadavers – a pilot study. Vet Anaesth Analg 45, 871–875.

Kato N, Fujiwara Y, Harato M et al. (2009) Serum concentration of lidocaine after transversus abdominis plane block. J Anesth 23, 298–300.

Lancaster P, Chadwick M (2010) Liver trauma secondary to ultrasound-guided transversus abdominis plane block. Br J Anaesth 104, 509–510.

Manatakis DK, Stamos N, Agalianos C et al. (2013) Transient femoral nerve palsy complicating "blind" transversus abdominis plane block. Case Rep Anesthesiol 2013, 3.

McDonnell JG, O'Donnell B, Curley G et al. (2007) The analgesic efficacy of transversus abdominis plane block after abdominal surgery: a prospective randomized controlled trial. Anesth Analg 104, 193–197.

McDonnell JG, Curley G, Carney J et al. (2008) The analgesic efficacy of transversus abdominis plane block after cesarean delivery: a randomized controlled trial. Anesth Analg 106, 186–91.

Maeda A, Shibata SC, Kamibayashi T et al. (2015) Continuous subcostal oblique transversus abdominis plane block provides more effective analgesia than single-shot block after gynaecological laparotomy. Eur J Anesthesiol 32, 514–515.

Niraj G, Searle A, Mathews M et al. (2009) Analgesic efficacy of ultrasound-guided transversus abdominis plane block in patients undergoing open appendectomy. Br J Anesth 103, 601–605.

O'Donnell BD, McDonnell JG, McShane AJ (2006) The transversus abdominis plane (TAP) block in open retropubic prostatectomy. Reg Anesth Pain Med 31, 91.

Otero PE, Romano M, Zaccagnini AS (2021) Transversus abdominis plane block in cat cadavers: anatomical description and comparison of injectate spread using two- and three-point approaches. Vet Anaesth Analg 48, 432–441.

Portela DA, Romano M, Briganti A (2014) Retrospective clinical evaluation of ultrasound guided transverse abdominis plane block in dogs undergoing mastectomy. Vet Anaesth Analg 41, 319–324.

Romano M, Portela DA, Otero PE et al. (2020) Mirroring artefact during postoperative transversus abdominis plane (TAP) block in two dogs. Vet Anaesth Analg 47, 727–728.

Romano M, Portela DA, Thomson A et al. (2021) Comparison between two approaches for the transversus abdominis plane block in canine cadavers. Vet Anaesth Analg 48, 101–106.

Sakai T, Manabe W, Kamitani T et al. (2010) Ropivacaine-induced late-onset systemic toxicity after transversus abdominis plane block under general anesthesia: successful reversal with 20% lipid emulsion. Masui 59, 1502–1505.

Santos AC, Pedersen H, Harmon TW et al. (1989) Does pregnancy alter the systemic toxicity of local anesthetics? Anesthesiology 70, 991–995.

Santos AC, DeArmas PI (2001) Systemic toxicity of levobupivacaine, bupivacaine, and ropivacaine during continuous intravenous infusion to nonpregnant and pregnant ewes. Anesthesiology 95, 1256–1264.

Seo N, Oshima E, Stevens J et al. (1982) The tetraphasic action of lidocaine on CNS electrical activity and behavior in cats. Anesthesiology 57, 451–457.

Scherrer V, Compere V, Loisel C et al. (2013) Cardiac arrest from local anesthetic toxicity after a field block and transversus abdominis plane block: a consequence of miscommunication between the anesthesiologist and surgeon. A A Case Rep 1, 75–76

Schroeder CA, Schroeder KM, Johnson RA (2010) Transversus abdominis plane block for exploratory laparotomy in a canadian lynx (lynx canadensis). J Zoo Wildl Med 41, 338–341.

Schroeder CA, Snyder LBC, Tearney CC et al. (2011) Ultrasound-guided transversus abdominis plane block in the dog: an anatomical evaluation. Vet Anaesth Analg 38, 267–271.

Sforza M, Andjelkov K, Zaccheddu R et al. (2011) Transversus abdominis plane block anesthesia in abdominoplasties. Plast Reconstr Surg 128, 529–535.

Skouropoulou D, Lacitignola L, Centonze P et al. (2018) Perioperative analgesic effects of an ultrasound-guided transversus abdominis plane block with a mixture of bupivacaine and lidocaine in cats undergoing ovariectomy. Vet Anaesth Analg 45, 374–383.

Smith D, Hoang K, Gelbard W (2014) Treatment of acute flares of chronic pancreatitis pain with ultrasound guided transversus abdominis plane block: a novel application of a pain management technique in the acute care setting. Case Rep Emerg Med 2014, 759508.

Todd AJ (2010) Neuronal circuitry for pain processing in the dorsal horn. Nat Rev Neurosci 11, 823–836.

Tsen LC, Tarshis J, Denson DD et al. (1999) Measurements of maternal protein binding of bupivacaine throughout pregnancy. Anesth Analg 89, 965–968.

Weiss E, Jolly C, Dumoulin JL et al. (2014) Convulsions in 2 patients after bilateral ultrasound-guided transversus abdominis plane blocks for cesarean analgesia. Reg Anesth Pain Med 39, 248–251.

Yoshida T, Furutani K, Watanabe Y et al. (2016) Analgesic efficacy of bilateral continuous transversus abdominis plane blocks using an oblique subcostal approach in patients undergoing laparotomy for gynaecological cancer: a prospective, randomized, triple-blind, placebo-controlled study. Br J Anaesth 117, 812–820.

Zoff A, Laborda-Vidal P, Mortier J et al. (2017) Comparison of the spread of two different volumes of contrast medium when performing ultrasound-guided transversus abdominis plane injection in dog cadavers. J Small Anim Pract 58, 269–275.

Ultrasound-Guided Rectus Sheath Block

CHAPTER 20

Tatiana H. Ferreira

BLOCK AT A GLANCE

What is it used for?

- As part of a multimodal analgesic approach for procedures involving the abdominal midline including umbilical hernia repair, midline laparoscopic procedures, and laparotomies.

Landmarks/transducer position:

- The ultrasound (US) transducer should be positioned in a transverse orientation at midline just cranial to the umbilicus.

What equipment and personnel are required?

- 21–22G 40–60 mm (1.5–2.5 in.) blunt atraumatic or spinal (Quincke) needle depending on the size of the patient
- Ultrasound machine
- High frequency (15–6 MHz) linear array transducer
- Syringe with local anesthetic (± syringe with saline and stopcock – optional)
- +/− T-connector extension (recommended)
- Gloves
- Coupling agent (e.g. alcohol)
- +/− Assistant to help perform test injections and final drug administration

When do I perform the block?

- Prior to surgery, after the ventral abdomen is clipped and skin preparation is complete. Final skin preparation will still be needed prior to surgery. This block can be repeated in the sedated or anesthetized patient postoperatively if additional analgesia is needed.

What volume of local anesthetic is used?

- 0.5 ml kg^{-1} per side (total 1 ml kg^{-1}). Dilution of the local anesthetic may be required to achieve this volume without exceeding the maximum recommended dose for the local anesthetic.

Goal:

- During injection, the local anesthetic should initially be observed as a hypoechoic area causing clear separation of the fascia between the **m. rectus abdominis** and the internal rectus sheath (RS), with additional separation of the **m. rectus abdominis** and **m. transversus abdominus** laterally as the injection is continued.

Complexity level:

- Basic

Clinical pearl:

- This block **does not** provide visceral analgesia and should always be considered as part of a multimodal analgesic approach.

WHAT DO WE ALREADY KNOW?

The rectus sheath block (RSB) is a fascial plane block. US-guidance is used to identify the target muscle plane and confirm the spread (cranio–caudal) of the local anesthetic along the target fascial plane. The goal of the RSB is to desensitize the ventral branches of the spinal nerves that course along the surface of the **m. transversus abdominis,** ultimately piercing through the RS and the **m. rectus abdominis**.

In humans, the **m. rectus abdominis** and the umbilicus are innervated by the ventral branches of the sixth thoracic (T6) to the first lumbar (L1) spinal nerves and the ventral branch of T10, respectively (Rozen et al. 2008; Sakai-Tamura et al. 2020). The innervation of the ventral abdomen is not well described in veterinary medicine; anatomical variations and conflicting information are found in the literature.

The innervation of the abdominal wall of dogs may involve branches from T7 to L3, with branches of T10 likely innervating the umbilical area (Bailey et al. 1984; Castañeda-Herrera et al. 2017; Hermanson 2020).

US-guided RSB in humans was described in 2006 (Willschke et al. 2006). RSBs have been used in humans primarily for laparoscopic procedures (Bakshi et al. 2016; Hamid et al. 2021) and procedures involving midline incisions (Bashandy and Elkholy 2014), especially those involving the umbilicus (Gurnaney et al. 2011; Manassero et al. 2015). This results in relaxation of the abdominal wall intraoperatively and serves to provide adjunctive pain management intra- and postoperatively. RSBs have also been used for chronic abdominal wall pain management in humans, more specifically abdominal cutaneous nerve entrapment, iatrogenic peripheral nerve injury, and myofascial pain syndrome (Skinner and Lauder 2007).

US-guided RSBs have been recently described in veterinary medicine. To date, only cadaveric studies in dogs (St James et al. 2020), calves (Ferreira et al. 2022), and pigs (Ienello et al. 2022) have been published. The target fascial plane is located between the *m. rectus abdominis* and the internal RS. A single bilateral injection (0.5 ml kg^{-1}) just proximal to the umbilicus resulted in similar spread between species (most consistently staining the ventral branches of the T11–T13 spinal nerves). Lower injectate volumes (0.25 ml kg^{-1} per side) have been tested which resulted in more limited spread (St James et al. 2020; Ferreira et al. 2022). No information on duration of anesthesia/analgesia is available in veterinary medicine at this time. Duration of analgesia in humans is reported to be 6–12 hours following a single injection (Uppal et al. 2019; Hamid et al. 2021).

PATIENT SELECTION
INDICATIONS FOR THE BLOCK

RSBs may be indicated for any surgical procedure involving the abdominal midline (e.g. laparotomies or laparoscopies) and, more specifically, procedures involving the periumbilical area (e.g. herniorrhaphies).

CONTRAINDICATIONS

- Infection and/or neoplasia around the intended puncture site.

- Previous surgeries, injuries, or anatomical abnormalities affecting the landmarks for the RSB could pose a challenge to performing the technique and/or influence the efficacy of the block due to altered distribution of the injectate (Seidel et al. 2017).

- Small patient size (<2 kg), very young, or cachectic patients may present additional challenges due to their thin body wall and target muscle layer, which can make visualization difficult and predispose the patient to potential complications such as inadvertent puncture of the peritoneum.

POTENTIAL SIDE EFFECTS AND COMPLICATIONS

- Peritoneal perforation with potential damage to underlying abdominal viscera.

- Local anesthetic systemic toxicity (LAST) due to the high volume of local anesthetic required for appropriate spread.

- Although unlikely, puncture of cranial and caudal epigastric vessels located deep in the *m. rectus abdominis* is possible, with subsequent hemorrhage, hematoma formation, and/or inadvertent vascular injection.

- Infection.

GENERAL CONSIDERATIONS
CLINICAL ANATOMY

The *m. rectus abdominis* is a long, flat muscle that extends from the sternum to the pubis (Hermanson 2020) (Figure 20.1). The linea alba lies between the left and right *mm. rectus abdominis*. The *m. transversus abdominis* is the deepest abdominal muscle and lies along the lateral and ventral abdominal wall, overlapping with the *m. rectus abdominis* in the cranial quadrants and mid-abdominal wall sections (Hermanson 2020). The *mm. obliquus internus abdominis* and *obliquus externus abdominis* lie lateral to the *m. rectus abdominis* and superficial (ventral) to the *m. transversus abdominis*.

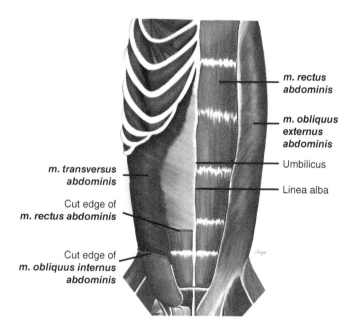

FIGURE 20.1 Illustration of the muscles of the canine abdominal wall. Note that on the left side, the *m. obliquus externus abdominis* was dissected out to expose the *m. obliquus internus abdominis* and the *m. transversus abdominis*. On this same side, the *mm. obliquus internus abdominis* and *rectus abdominis* were also partially dissected to further expose the *m. transversus abdominis*. See text for more details.

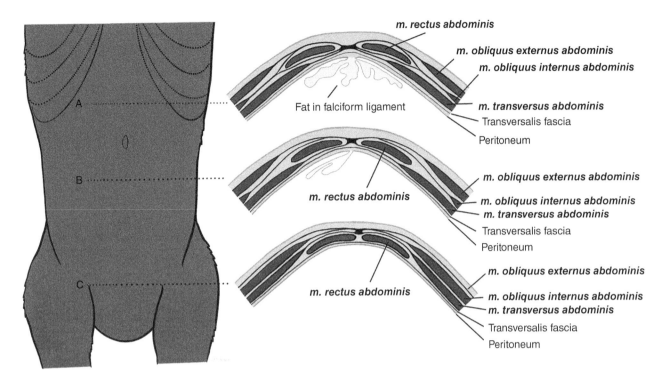

FIGURE 20.2   Illustration of the canine abdominal wall demonstrating the contributions of aponeuroses of different muscles and the transversalis fascia on the formation of the external and internal rectus sheath of dogs at different levels. (a) Cranial abdomen. (b) Mid-abdomen. (c) Caudal abdomen.

The **m. rectus abdominis** is covered by the internal and external RSs, which are formed by the aponeuroses of these abdominal muscles (Hermanson 2020). There are species variations regarding the contribution of different muscles' aponeuroses to the internal and external RS. The external RS (ventral) in dogs is formed by the aponeuroses of the **m. obliquus internus abdominis** and **m. obliquus externus abdominis**, with contribution from the aponeurosis of the **m. transversus abdominis** at the caudal abdominal wall section (Hermanson 2020) (Figure 20.2). The internal RS is an important landmark for the RSB and, in dogs, its composition varies depending on the location within the ventral abdominal wall (cranial-, mid-, or caudal abdomen). Cranially, the internal RS is formed by the aponeuroses of the **m. obliquus internus abdominis** and **m. transversus abdominis** and the transversalis fascia (Hermanson 2020). Mid-abdomen, it is formed by the aponeurosis of the **m. transversus abdominis** and transversalis fascia. In the caudal abdomen, the **m. rectus abdominis** is only covered by the transversalis fascia and peritoneum (Hermanson 2020).

The target branches of the T7–L3 **spinal nerves** (Bailey et al. 1984; Castañeda-Herrera et al. 2017; Hermanson 2020) course superficially on the **m. transversus abdominis** within the transversus abdominis plane (TAP) and pierce through the dorsal (deep) aspect of the **m. rectus abdominis** at its mid- to lateral border (Rozen et al. 2008; Castañeda-Herrera et al. 2017). However, some variations on the course of these nerves have been reported in the literature and could contribute to block failure. For example, in dogs, the ventral branches of T7, T8, and T9 were inconsistently observed traveling over the **m. transversus abdominis** and their course toward the **m. rectus abdominis** was variable (Castañeda-Herrera et al. 2017). Some of the ventral branches of spinal nerves, particularly the most cranial branches (T7–T9), may travel lateral to the costal cartilage and directly pierce the lateral margin of the **m. rectus abdominis** (Rozen et al. 2008; Hebbard et al. 2010; Castañeda-Herrera et al. 2017).

EXPECTED DISTRIBUTION OF ANESTHESIA

Based on cadaveric studies in dogs, calves, and pigs, the number of spinal nerve branches stained (i.e. >50% of the injections) following single-point bilateral injections (0.5 ml kg^{-1}) immediately cranial to the umbilicus varied between three and five (St James et al. 2020; Ferreira et al. 2022; Ienello et al. 2022). The specific nerves that were stained differed between species, with the most commonly stained branches in dogs being T11–T13 (St James et al. 2020). Based on this observation, it is unlikely that single-point bilateral injections will desensitize the entire ventral midline, with anesthesia of the cranial abdomen likely being limited. Instead, the potential area that would be desensitized would involve the periumbilical area and perhaps the areas caudal to it (St James et al. 2020).

LOCAL ANESTHETIC: DOSE, VOLUME, AND CONCENTRATION

Any local anesthetic (e.g. bupivacaine, ropivacaine, and levobupivacaine) can be used to perform RSBs, with or without the coadministration of an adjuvant (e.g. dexmedetomidine). In humans, the use of dexmedetomidine as an adjuvant in RSB resulted in more effective block and longer duration of analgesia (Xu et al. 2018). Future clinical studies may elucidate whether the use of adjuvants for RSBs in veterinary species is warranted.

Considering the relatively large volume of local anesthetic solution that is necessary to achieve the desired degree of spread, as well as the desire to minimize the potential for LAST, dilution of the local anesthetic will be required prior to injection. For example, if each injection (i.e. left and right sides) requires 0.5 ml kg^{-1} of injectate (i.e. 1 ml kg^{-1} total), if 0.5% bupivacaine is used and a maximum total dose of 2 mg kg^{-1} is not exceeded, dilution of the bupivacaine will be required to meet this volume requirement (i.e. combining 0.4 ml kg^{-1} bupivacaine with 0.6 ml kg^{-1} saline solution resulting in a final concentration of 2 mg ml^{-1} of bupivacaine). Dilution of local anesthetics can result in decreased efficacy and/or duration of effect following peripheral nerve blocks (Brockway et al. 1991; Moura et al. 2021; Gao et al. 2022). To the author's knowledge, no studies assessing the minimum effective dose of local anesthetics for peripheral nerve blocks or fascial blocks have been conducted in veterinary medicine. Further studies are needed to decide the ideal dose/volume of local anesthetic to be used for the RSB, not only in terms of local anesthetic spread to target nerves but also in terms of efficacy and duration of the block.

PATIENT PREPARATION AND POSITIONING

The patient should be positioned in dorsal recumbency (Figure 20.3). The ventral abdomen surrounding the umbilicus should be clipped free of hair and standard surgical preparation of the skin over the injection site should be performed.

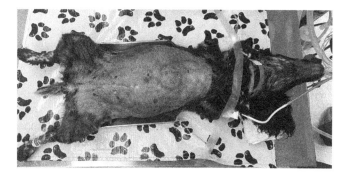

FIGURE 20.3 Positioning of a canine patient for ultrasound-guided rectus sheath blocks.

STEP-BY-STEP PERFORMANCE

SURFACE ANATOMY AND LANDMARKS TO BE USED

The US transducer should be positioned in a transverse orientation at midline just cranial to the umbilicus so a short-axis view of linea alba can be obtained (Figure 20.4).

ULTRASOUND ANATOMY

Once the linea alba is identified, the transducer should be glided laterally to identify the lateral border of the *m. rectus abdominis* and the medial border of the *m. transversus abdominis* (Figure 20.5). There can be some variability in the extent to which the *m. transversus abdominis* overlaps with the lateral corner of the *m. rectus abdominis* in dogs when the US transducer is positioned just cranial to the umbilicus (author's observation) (Figure 20.6). Deep to the *m. rectus abdominis* lies another important landmark, the internal RS. It will be identified as a hyperechoic line that gives the appearance of a "double line." This appearance is the result of the overlap of the internal RS, the transversalis fascia, and the peritoneum.

NEEDLE INSERTION TECHNIQUE

A short-bevel needle or spinal needle (40–60 mm depending on the size of the patient) attached to a prefilled T-connector extension set can be used (Figure 20.7). The needle is inserted

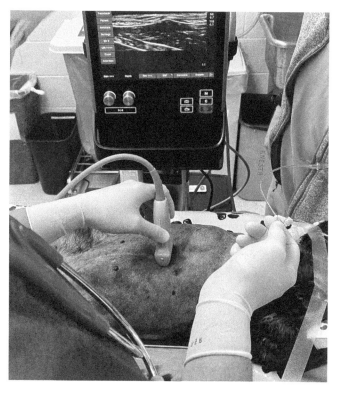

FIGURE 20.4 The ultrasound transducer is initially positioned on the patient's midline in the area of the umbilicus, allowing for identification of the relevant anatomical structures.

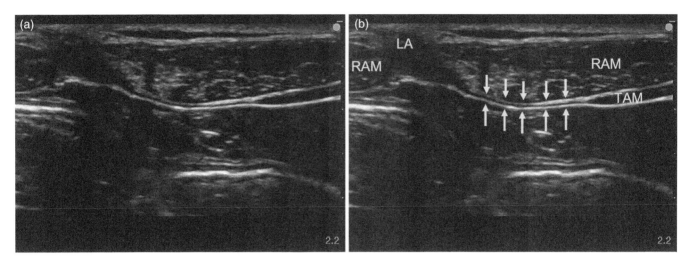

FIGURE 20.5   (a) Ultrasonographic image of the relevant anatomy prior to performance of an ultrasound-guided rectus sheath block. (b) Same image, with labels. Note the "double line" between the yellow arrows, representing the internal rectus sheath (including the transversalis fascia) and the peritoneum. LA, linea alba; RAM, *m. rectus abdominis*; TAM, *m. transversus abdominis* (TAM).

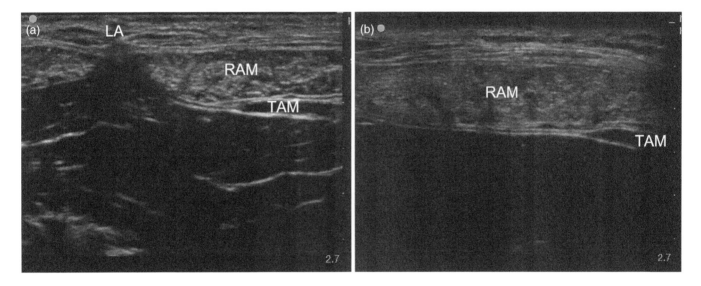

FIGURE 20.6   Ultrasonographic images from two different dogs taken at the same relative position on their abdomens to illustrate the observed variability in the extent of overlap between *mm. rectus abdominis* and *transversus abdominis* in different patients. (a) Image shows the *m. transversus abdominis* close to midline. (b) Image shows the *m. transversus abdominis* far away from midline. The LA does not appear in (b) because the *m. transversus abdominis* is so lateral that it cannot be captured in the same view. LA, linea alba; RAM, *m. rectus abdominis*; TAM, *m. transversus abdominis* (TAM).

in a lateral-to-medial orientation using an in-plane technique (St James et al. 2020; Ferreira et al. 2022) (Figure 20.8). Medial-to-lateral approaches have also been reported in people and pigs (Manassero et al. 2015; Go et al. 2016; Ienello et al. 2022), however, some authors recommend using a lateral-to-medial approach to avoid accidental puncture of the epigastric vessels (Seidel et al. 2017).

The needle should be advanced through the *m. rectus abdominis* and its tip positioned between the *m. rectus abdominis* and the internal RS ("double line"), medial to the medial border of the *m. transversus abdominis*.

EXPECTED MOTOR RESPONSES FROM NERVE STIMULATION

The RSB is a fascial plane technique where no specific nerves or plexus are targeted; therefore, nerve stimulation is not used.

ADMINISTRATION OF LOCAL ANESTHETIC – WHAT TO LOOK FOR, WHAT TO FEEL FOR, DECISION POINTS

Negative aspiration should be confirmed before injection. Having an assistant perform the negative aspiration test and the initial test injection is helpful as opposed to the anesthetist

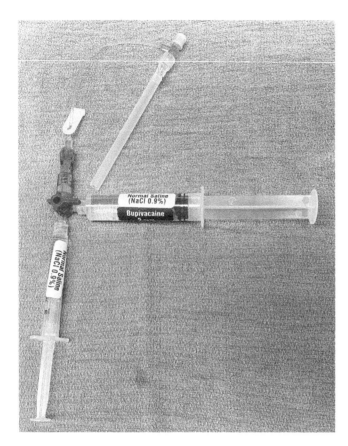

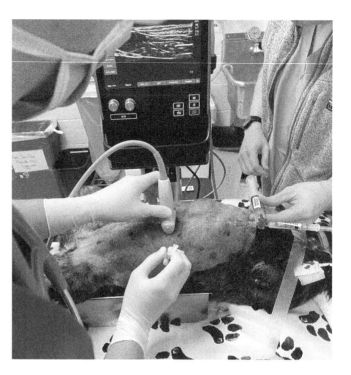

FIGURE 20.8 Performance of an ultrasound-guided rectus sheath block in a dog. The needle is being inserted on a lateral-to-medial trajectory using an in-plane technique. An assistant is available to assist with injections.

FIGURE 20.7 Needle attached to a T-connector. A stopcock is located between the T-connector and syringes (filled with saline and local anesthetic) to facilitate switching between injectates during test injections and final local anesthetic administration.

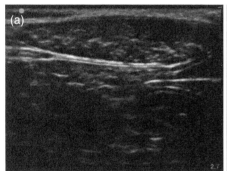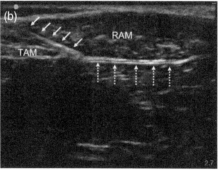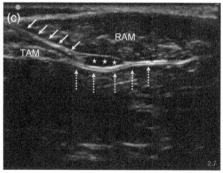

FIGURE 20.9 (a) Optimized ultrasonographic image prior to needle insertion. (b) The needle (solid arrows) has been advanced into the target plane between the RAM and the internal rectus sheath (represented by the "double line" – dashed arrows), medial to the medial edge of the TAM. (c) Ultrasonographic image showing hydrodissection to confirm correct needle placement. Note the clear separation of the RAM and internal rectus sheath (stars). RAM, *m. rectus abdominis*; TAM, *m. transversus abdominis* (TAM).

performing them and risking accidental movement of the needle tip either superficially toward the *m. rectus abdominis* or, more importantly, deeper toward the abdomen where accidental perforation of the internal RS could occur. A stopcock can be added to the T-connector extension to facilitate switching between syringes (saline and local anesthetic) and avoid accidental insertion of air into the system, which will negatively affect US image quality.

Test injections with a small volume of local anesthetic (approximately 0.5 ml) can be used to help identify the correct fascial plane (Figure 20.9). "Hydrodissection" to identify the correct fascial plane can also be performed with saline. Clear separation of the *m. rectus abdominis* and internal RS will initially be observed, with additional separation of the *m. rectus abdominis* and *m. transversus abdominis* further laterally as the injection is continued. This will confirm correct

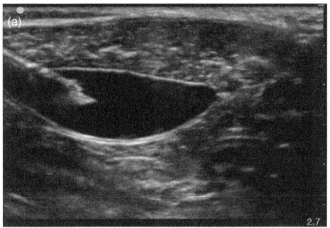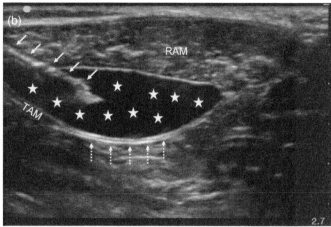

FIGURE 20.10   (a) Ultrasonographic image showing ideal dispersion of the local anesthetic. (b) Same image, with labels. Note the clear separation of the ***m. rectus abdominis*** and internal rectus sheath (represented by the "double line" – dashed arrows) with additional separation of the ***m. rectus abdominis*** and ***m. transversus abdominis*** laterally. Needle, solid arrows; local anesthetic, stars; RAM, ***m. rectus abdominis***; TAM, ***m. transversus abdominis*** (TAM).

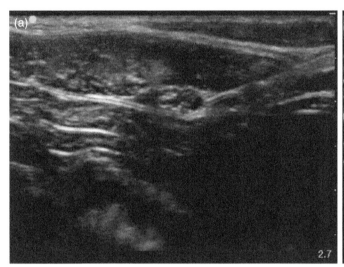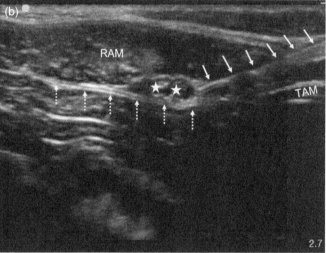

FIGURE 20.11   (a) Ultrasonographic image showing incorrect dispersion of the local anesthetic during a test injection. (b) Same image, with labels. Although the needle tip appears to be in the correct location, following the test injection, the local anesthetic has been injected within the ***m. rectus abdominis***, resulting in a mixed-, hyper-, and hypoechoic image. The needle tip should be repositioned before additional local anesthetic is administered. Needle, solid arrows; internal rectus sheath, dashed arrows; local anesthetic, stars; RAM, ***m. rectus abdominis***; TAM, ***m. transversus abdominis*** (TAM).

deposition of the local anesthetic in the target fascial plane (Figure 20.10). Improper distribution with local anesthetic spread within the ***m. rectus abdominis*** will produce a cloudy or mixed hyper- and hypoechoic image (Figure 20.11).

BLOCK EFFECTS (SENSORY, MOTOR, ETC.) AND PATIENT MANAGEMENT

A major limitation of the RSB is the lack of visceral analgesia, as it provides only somatic analgesia to the abdominal wall. To date, there are no clinical studies assessing this block in veterinary medicine, however, studies in people demonstrate that RSBs significantly decrease both opioid requirements

(intra- and postoperatively) and pain scores (postoperatively) for surgical procedures involving the umbilicus/midline (Gurnaney et al. 2011; Bashandy and Elkholy 2014; Hamill et al. 2015, 2016; Bakshi et al. 2016; Gupta et al. 2016; Kartalov et al. 2017; Cho et al. 2018; Maloney et al. 2018; Melesse et al. 2020). Nevertheless, RSBs have been associated with variable degrees of sensory blockade in the literature, potentially due to anatomical variations in distribution of nerves (in particular the cutaneous branches) and the spread of local anesthetic (Courreges et al. 1997; Hebbard et al. 2010; Manassero et al. 2015). This reaffirms that this block should not be used as the sole surgical anesthetic technique, even for procedures not involving viscera, such as umbilical hernia repairs

(Manassero et al. 2015), but should be part of a multimodal anesthetic/analgesic approach instead.

The use of RSB catheters has been associated with better outcomes than single-shot RSBs (Purdy et al. 2018; Uppal et al. 2019; Howle et al. 2022). Some studies in people show comparable efficacy between RSB catheters and epidurals (Tudor et al. 2015; Hausken et al. 2019; Gupta et al. 2020), demonstrating RSBs could be used as an alternative when epidurals are contraindicated. No studies describing the use of RSB catheters have been conducted in veterinary medicine to date.

COMPLICATIONS AND HOW TO AVOID THEM

RSBs are associated with a good safety profile in people. A recent meta-analysis in humans could not identify any reported local or systemic complications (Hamid et al. 2021). However, care should be taken to use appropriate doses of local anesthetic to avoid LAST. A systematic review assessing systemic concentrations of local anesthetic after RSB and the transversus abdominis plane (TAP) blocks in humans revealed that, even after using accepted local anesthetic doses for humans, these blocks can still result in plasma concentrations higher than the systemic toxicity thresholds (Rahiri et al. 2017). Nevertheless, in that study, the RSB was associated with slower systemic absorption, resulting in lower peak plasma concentration and delayed time to peak than the TAP block. This is likely due to the relatively avascular nature of the target fascial plane (Rahiri et al. 2017).

Despite the high local anesthetic concentrations in some cases, signs of toxicity in all instances were considered mild (e.g. tongue paresthesia, metallic taste, and slurred speech) with no seizures or cardiovascular instability observed. This allowed the authors to conclude that the risk of serious local anesthetic toxicity is low (Rahiri et al. 2017). Despite this, clinicians should always remain attentive for evidence of systemic toxicity, especially in veterinary medicine where our patients are typically anesthetized when blocks are being performed.

The cranial and caudal epigastric veins and arteries, which are located deep within the *m. rectus abdominis*, could potentially be punctured, leading to inadvertent vascular injection and/or hematoma formation (De Jose Maria et al. 2007; Chin et al. 2017; Uppal et al. 2019). These vessels are not commonly visualized during performance of RSBs in dogs and cats.

Due to the close proximity of the target fascial plane and the peritoneum, perforation of the peritoneum with potential visceral injury is possible (Sviggum et al. 2012). US guidance and use of an in-plane technique with constant needle tip visualization are essential to prevent this complication. Hydrodissection with small volumes of local anesthetic or saline can further minimize this risk. Failure to observe local anesthetic spread may indicate that the injection is being made intra-abdominally, below the hyper-

echoic "double line." In this situation, the injection should be discontinued and the needle redirected so the needle tip is in the proper fascial plane.

Additionally, injections caudal to the umbilicus can potentially be challenging and predispose the patient to complications (i.e. damage to viscera) because there is only a thin layer of transversalis fascia and peritoneum, not an internal aponeurotic covering the *m. rectus abdominis* at the caudal section of the abdomen.

COMMON MISTAKES AND HOW TO AVOID THEM

Local anesthetic can be injected into the incorrect location (i.e. into the *m. rectus abdominis* or intra-abdominally), potentially leading to limited spread and block failure. Hydrodissection to identify the correct plane as confirmed by clear separation of *m. rectus abdominis* and internal RS is, therefore, important prior to injecting the full volume/dose of local anesthetic (as described above).

Most of the time, the ventral branches of the nerves pierce the *m. rectus abdominis* on the deep aspect of the muscle at its mid- to lateral edge; thus, if the injection is performed too medially or too close to midline, the ventral branches may not be desensitized, leading to block failure. This has been observed in both calf cadavers (Ferreira et al. 2022) and humans (Seidel et al. 2017). Ensuring that the injection site is at the lateral aspect of the *m. rectus abdominis*, between it and the internal RS, and close to the medial edge of the *m. transversus abdominis* may improve success rates (Ferreira et al. 2022). Performing the block in this location has also been suggested in the human literature (Manassero et al. 2015; Seidel et al. 2017; Sakai-Tamura et al. 2020) and could potentially overcome an anatomical variation issue observed when the ventral branches pierce the *m. rectus abdominis* on its lateral margin instead of its deep aspect (Rozen et al. 2008; Hebbard et al. 2010; Castañeda-Herrera et al. 2017).

HOW TO TALK TO CLIENTS/PROFESSIONAL COLLEAGUES

- The RSB block is a simple technique and an experienced clinician can perform it in approximately two minutes.

- This block is associated with a good safety profile with minimal to no reported complications.

- The major limitation of the RSB is the lack of visceral analgesia; therefore, this block should always be used as part of a multimodal pain management approach.

- Currently, there is no information in the veterinary literature regarding the clinical use of RSBs; however, based on the human literature, bilateral single-point RSB injections should be expected to provide 6–12 hours of analgesia.

Bailey CS, Kitchell RL, Haghighi SS et al. (1984) Cutaneous innervation of the thorax and abdomen of the dog. Am J Vet Res 45, 1689–1698.

Bakshi SG, Mapari A, Shylasree TS (2016) Rectus Sheath block for postoperative analgesia in gynecological ONcology Surgery (RESONS): a randomized-controlled trial. Can J Anesth 63, 1335–1344.

Bashandy GMN, Elkholy AHH (2014) Reducing postoperative opioid consumption by adding an ultrasound-guided rectus sheath block to multimodal analgesia for abdominal cancer surgery with midline incision. Anesth Pain Med 4, e18263.

Brockway MS, Bannister J, McClure JH et al. (1991) Comparison of extradural ropivacaine and bupivacaine. Br J Anaesth 66, 31–37.

Castañeda-Herrera FE, Buriticá-Gaviria EF, Echeverry-Bonilla DF (2017) Anatomical evaluation of the thoracolumbar nerves related to the transversus abdominis plane block technique in the dog. Anat Histol Embryol 46, 373–377.

Chin KJ, McDonnell JG, Carvalho B et al. (2017) Essentials of our current understanding: abdominal wall blocks. Reg Anesth Pain Med 42, 133–183.

Cho S, Kim YJ, Jeong K et al. (2018) Ultrasound-guided bilateral rectus sheath block reduces early postoperative pain after laparoscopic gynecologic surgery: a randomized study. J Anesth 32, 189–197.

Courreges P, Poddevin F, Lecoutre D (1997) Paraumbilical block: a new concept for regional anaesthesia in children. Pediatr Anesth 7, 211–214.

De Jose Maria B, Götzens V, Mabrok M (2007) Ultrasound-guided umbilical nerve block in children: a brief description of a new approach. Pediatr Anesth 17, 44–50.

Ferreira TH, Schroeder CA, St James M et al. (2022) Description of an ultrasound-guided rectus sheath block injection technique and the spread of dye in calf cadavers. Vet Anaesth Analg 49, 203–209.

Gao W, Chen Y, Wang W et al. (2022) The 90% minimum effective volume and concentration of ropivacaine for ultrasound-guided median nerve block in children aged 1–3 years: a biased-coin design up-and-down sequential allocation trial. J Clin Anesth 79, 110754.

Go R, Huang YY, Weyker PD et al. (2016) Truncal blocks for perioperative pain management: a review of the literature and evolving techniques. Pain Manag 6, 455–468.

Gupta M, Naithani U, Singariya G et al. (2016) Comparison of 0.25% ropivacaine for intraperitoneal instillation v/s rectus sheath block for postoperative pain relief following laparoscopic cholecystectomy: a prospective study. J Clin Diagn Res 10, UC10–UC15.

Gupta N, Kumar A, Harish R et al. (2020) Comparison of postoperative analgesia and opioid requirement with thoracic epidural vs. continuous rectus sheath infusion in midline incision laparotomies under general anaesthesia – a prospective randomised controlled study. Indian J Anaesth 64, 750.

Gurnaney HG, Maxwell LG, Kraemer FW et al. (2011) Prospective randomized observer-blinded study comparing the analgesic efficacy of ultrasound-guided rectus sheath block and local anaesthetic infiltration for umbilical hernia repair. Br J Anaesth 107, 790–795.

Hamid HKS, Ahmed AY, Alhamo MA et al. (2021) Efficacy and safety profile of rectus sheath block in adult laparoscopic surgery: a meta-analysis. J Surg Res 261, 10–17.

Hamill JK, Liley A, Hill AG (2015) Rectus sheath block for laparoscopic appendicectomy: a randomized clinical trial. ANZ J Surg 85, 951–956.

Hamill JK, Rahiri JL, Liley A et al. (2016) Rectus sheath and transversus abdominis plane blocks in children: a systematic review and meta-analysis of randomized trials. Pediatr Anesth 26, 363–371.

Hausken J, Rydenfelt K, Horneland R et al. (2019) First experience with rectus sheath block for postoperative analgesia after pancreas transplant: a retrospective observational study. Transplant Proc 51, 479–484.

Hebbard PD, Barrington MJ, Vasey C (2010) Ultrasound-guided continuous oblique subcostal transversus abdominis plane blockade: description of anatomy and clinical technique. Reg Anesth Pain Med 35, 436–441.

Hermanson JW (2020) The muscular system. In: Miller and Evans' Anatomy of the Dog. Hermanson JW, de Lahunta A, Evans HE (eds.) Elsevier, St Louis, Missouri, pp. 207–318.

Howle R, Ng SC, Wong HY et al. (2022) Comparison of analgesic modalities for patients undergoing midline laparotomy: a systematic review and network meta-analysis. Can J Anesth 69, 140–176.

Ienello L, Kennedy M, Wendt-Hornickle E et al. (2022) Ultrasound-guided rectus sheath block injections in miniature swine cadavers: technique description and distribution of two injectate volumes. Vet Anaesth Analg 49, 210–218.

Kartalov A, Jankulovski N, Kuzmanovska B et al. (2017) The effect of rectus sheath block as a supplement of general anesthesia on postoperative analgesia in adult patient undergoing umbilical hernia repair. PRILOZI 38, 135–142.

Maloney C, Kallis M, El-Shafy IA et al. (2018) Ultrasound-guided bilateral rectus sheath block vs. conventional local analgesia in single port laparoscopic appendectomy for children with nonperforated appendicitis. J Pediatr Surg 53, 431–436.

Manassero A, Bossolasco M, Meineri M et al. (2015) Spread patterns and effectiveness for surgery after ultrasound-guided rectus sheath block in adult day-case patients scheduled for umbilical hernia repair. J Anaesthesiol Clin Pharmacol 31, 349.

Melesse DY, Chekol WB, Tawuye HY et al. (2020) Assessment of the analgesic effectiveness of rectus sheath block in patients who had emergency midline laparotomy: prospective observational cohort study. Int J Surg Open 24, 27–31.

Moura ECR, Oliveira CMB, da Cunha Leal P et al. (2021) Minimum effective analgesic concentration of ropivacaine in saphenous block guided by ultrasound for knee arthroscopic meniscectomy: randomized, double-blind study. J Pain Res 14, 53–59.

Purdy M, Kinnunen M, Kokki M et al. (2018) A prospective, randomized, open label, controlled study investigating the efficiency and safety of 3 different methods of rectus sheath block analgesia following midline laparotomy. Medicine (Baltimore) 97, e9968.

Rahiri J, Tuhoe J, Svirskis D et al. (2017) Systematic review of the systemic concentrations of local anaesthetic after transversus abdominis plane block and rectus sheath block. Br J Anaesth 118, 517–526.

Rozen WM, Tran TMN, Ashton MW et al. (2008) Refining the course of the thoracolumbar nerves: A new understanding of the innervation of the anterior abdominal wall. Clin Anat 21, 325–333.

Sakai-Tamura A, Murata H, Ogami-Takamura K et al. (2020) Course of the thoracic nerves around the umbilicus within the posterior layer of the rectus sheath: a cadaver study. J Anesth 34, 953–957.

Seidel R, Wree A, Schulze M (2017) Does the approach influence the success rate for ultrasound-guided rectus sheath blocks? An anatomical case series. Local Reg Anesth 10, 61–65.

Skinner AV, Lauder GR (2007) Rectus sheath block: successful use in the chronic pain management of pediatric abdominal wall pain. Pediatr Anesth 17, 1203–1211.

St James M, Ferreira TH, Schroeder CA et al. (2020) Ultrasound-guided rectus sheath block: an anatomic study in dog cadavers. Vet Anaesth Analg 47, 95–102.

Sviggum HP, Niesen AD, Sites BD et al. (2012) Trunk blocks 101: transversus abdominis plane, ilioinguinal-iliohypogastric, and rectus sheath blocks. Int Anesthesiol Clin 50, 74–92.

Tudor E, Yang W, Brown R et al. (2015) Rectus sheath catheters provide equivalent analgesia to epidurals following laparotomy for colorectal surgery. Ann R Coll Surg Engl 97, 530–533.

Uppal V, Sancheti S, Kalagara H (2019) Transversus abdominis plane (TAP) and rectus sheath blocks: a technical description and evidence review. Curr Anesthesiol Rep 9, 479–487.

Willschke H, Bösenberg A, Marhofer P et al. (2006) Ultrasonography-guided rectus sheath block in paediatric anaesthesia – a new approach to an old technique. Br J Anaesth 97, 244–249.

Xu L, Hu Z, Shen J et al. (2018) Efficacy of US-guided transversus abdominis plane block and rectus sheath block with ropivacaine and dexmedetomidine in elderly high-risk patients. Minerva Anestesiol 84, 18–24.

Ultrasound-Guided Femoral Nerve Block (Psoas Compartment Block)

CHAPTER 21

Stephan Mahler

What is it used for?

- To supplement anesthesia for surgeries involving the hip joint (e.g. femoral head ostectomy, acetabular fracture repair, hip luxation stabilization, total hip replacement, and arthroscopy) and the femur (e.g. fracture repair, corrective osteotomy) when used in combination with a **sciatic nerve** block.

Landmarks/transducer position:

- Position the dog in dorsal or lateral recumbency.

- The ultrasound (US) transducer should be placed on the ventral abdomen, perpendicular to the **m. iliopsoas**, just cranial to the inguinal nipple.

- The needle will be inserted in-plane through the skin from a lateral location and advanced into the **m. iliopsoas** towards the **femoral nerve**.

What equipment and personnel are required?

- 21- or 22G, 50–100 mm (or similar) blunt atraumatic needle

- Syringe of drug(s)

- Ultrasound machine

- High frequency (15–6 MHz) linear array transducer +/− protective sleeve

- Gloves

- Coupling agent (e.g. alcohol)

- Assistant to help position leg and perform the injection

When do I perform the block?

- Prior to surgery, after the limb is clipped and skin preparation is complete. Final skin preparation will still be needed prior to surgery.

What volume of local anesthetic is used?

- 0.1–0.2 ml kg^{-1}

Goal:

- During injection, the local anesthetic should spread around the **femoral nerve**, resulting in the separation of the **femoral nerve** from the surrounding muscle fibers.

Complexity level:

- Intermediate

Clinical pearl:

- The distribution of local anesthetic around the nerve (often referred to as the "doughnut" sign in people) may not always be obtained. This is because the injected solution does not accumulate in an interfascial plane like it does with some other blocks.

WHAT DO WE ALREADY KNOW?

After emerging from the spinal canal, the lumbar nerve roots that form the **femoral nerve** are found in the *psoas compartment*, an anatomical space formed dorsally, medially, and laterally by the bodies of the lumbar vertebrae and their transverse processes, and ventrally by the **m. psoas major**. Caudal to L6–L7, the **femoral nerve** travels within the **m. iliopsoas**. Mogicato et al. (2015) showed that, within the body of the **m. iliopsoas**, the **femoral nerve** is not located close to any major vascular structures since the external iliac vessels are located medial to the body of the **m. iliopsoas**. Based on this, the safest approach for a needle to be advanced towards the **femoral nerve** within the **m. iliopsoas** is from a lateral approach since not only are the vessels located away from the origin of the needle but also the medial fascia of the **m. iliopsoas** may act as a physical barrier to further needle advancement and protect the external iliac vessels from inadvertent needle puncture or trauma.

Mahler (2012) and Echeverry et al. (2012a) both described the ultrasonographic anatomy and approaches to the **femoral nerve** within the **m. iliopsoas** using a lateral approach. Using this technique, Echeverry et al. (2012b), Shimada et al. (2017), and O Cathasaigh et al. (2018) reported 100% success rates of achieving motor and sensory blockade of the **femoral nerve** using a total volume of 0.3 ml kg^{-1} of lidocaine 2%, 0.2–0.4 ml kg^{-1} bupivacaine 0.5%, and 0.15 ml kg^{-1} bupivacaine 0.5%, respectively. Using bupivacaine 0.5%, Shimada et al. (2017) showed that the onset time and duration of the sensory and motor blockades were approximately 15 minutes and 10 hours, respectively, and O Cathasaigh et al. (2018) reported the median (range) durations of motor and sensory blockade to be 11 (6–14) hours and 15 (10–18) hours, respectively. O Cathasaigh et al. (2018) also measured blood concentrations of bupivacaine following administration of the local anesthetic and reported that levels remained well below what would be associated with a systemic toxic dose.

Echeverry et al. (2012b) observed that injection of a dye solution within the **m. iliopsoas** led to cranial migration and distribution within the psoas compartment which resulted in additional staining of the **obturator nerve**. This technique was subsequently referred to by the authors as a "two-in-one" **femoral** and **obturator nerve** block. Graff et al. (2015) showed that distribution of local anesthetic solution to the **obturator nerve** was even better if the injection was performed more caudally (at the level of L7). In addition, Tayari et al. (2017) observed the **femoral** and **obturator nerves** in close proximity to each other by scanning the **m. iliopsoas** at the level of the L6–L7 vertebrae and then tilting the transducer caudally. This resulted in staining of both nerves in six out of six injections using a relatively small volume of dye (0.1 ml kg^{-1}).

The addition of an **obturator nerve** block has been an area of interest in human hip and knee joint surgeries since the **obturator nerve** provides some sensory innervation to these joints (Marhofer et al. 2010). In dogs, anatomical studies have established that the **obturator nerve** contributes to the innervation of the hip joint capsule (Huang et al. 2013) and, more inconsistently, to the stifle joint capsule (O'Connor and Woodbury 1982). The clinical utility and benefits of blocking the **obturator nerve** have been assessed in dogs undergoing tibial plateau leveling osteotomies (TPLOs) (Papadopoulos et al. 2022).

Blockade of the **femoral nerve** within the **m. iliopsoas** is most commonly performed in combination with a **sciatic nerve** block. Together, these blocks are used to supplement anesthesia for a variety of pelvic limb surgeries, with the majority of published research being focused on patients undergoing TPLOs (Tayari et al. 2017; Warrit et al. 2019). With the idea of providing prolonged analgesia postoperatively, Monticelli et al. (2016) evaluated the feasibility of performing US-guided lumbar plexus catheter placement in dog cadavers. Those authors showed that the **femoral** and **obturator nerves** could be stained in 14 and 12 of 14 cases, respectively, using a total dose of 0.4 ml kg^{-1} of dye. The clinical value of this technique has yet to be confirmed.

PATIENT SELECTION
INDICATIONS FOR THE BLOCK

A psoas compartment **femoral nerve** block is usually combined with a **sciatic nerve** block to achieve near-complete anesthesia of the pelvic limb. Depending on the technique that is used to block the **sciatic nerve**, a wide range of surgical procedures can be performed, including hip surgery, femoral fracture repair, and procedures involving the stifle joint and tibia (e.g. TPLO, TTA, static stabilization, patella luxation, tibial fracture repair, etc.).

CONTRAINDICATIONS

- Skin infection or other lesions at the intended puncture site.

- Peripheral nerve disease affecting the pelvic limb.

- Any patient or procedure where prolonged motor blockade of the **mm. quadriceps femoris** and/or **adductor** is not desirable.

- Allergic reactions to local anesthetics.

POTENTIAL SIDE EFFECTS AND COMPLICATIONS

- Due to the proximity of the external iliac vessels, there is potential for vascular puncture and intravascular injection if the needle passes through the **m. iliopsoas**.

- Intra-abdominal injection and abdominal organ puncture/laceration are possible if overly long needles are used and/or US visualization of the needle tip is not maintained.

- Intraneural injection is possible if the operator does not monitor for resistance to injection and visualize the distribution of the local anesthetic in the proximity of the nerve.

GENERAL CONSIDERATIONS
CLINICAL ANATOMY

In dogs, the **femoral nerve** primarily arises from the L5 nerve root, with various contributions from the L4 and L6 spinal nerves (Evans and de Lahunta 2012). In cats, the **femoral nerve** mainly arises from the L5 and L6 nerve roots (Haro et al. 2012). The **obturator nerve** arises mainly from the L6 spinal nerve, with various contributions from the L5 and L4 spinal nerves, the latter sometimes being absent (Evans and de Lahunta 2012).

After leaving the vertebral canal, the spinal nerves run caudally in close proximity to the lumbar vertebral bodies. The **femoral** and **obturator nerves** are formed within the caudomedial portion of the **m. psoas major**, which is also variably referred to as the "psoas or lumbar compartment." Caudally, while the **femoral nerve** becomes embedded in the **m. iliopsoas**, the **obturator nerve** leaves this muscle dorsomedially and enters the pelvis at the ventromedial aspect of the shaft of the ilium.

(a)

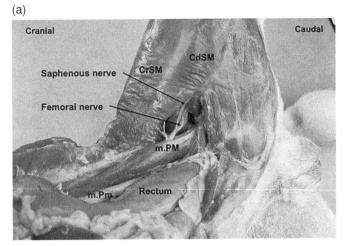

(b)

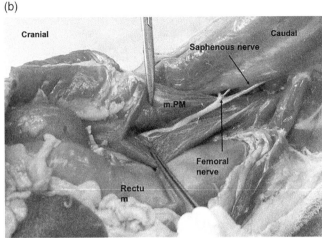

FIGURE 21.1   (a) Gross anatomy of the **femoral nerve** as it leaves the *m. iliopsoas* before and (b) after splitting the muscle. The *m. iliacus* component is not visible. m.PM, *m. psoas major*; m.Pm, *m. psoas minor*; Crm.S, cranial part of the *m. sartorius*; Cdm.S, caudal part of the *m. sartorius*. Source: E. Betti and C. Guintard.

The **femoral nerve** travels in a caudo–ventro–lateral direction within the *m. iliopsoas* (Figure 21.1). During its course, the **femoral nerve** branches to form the **saphenous nerve** and both nerves exit the *m. iliopsoas* caudally at the level of the muscular lacuna. The **saphenous nerve** continues distally along the medial aspect of the *m. quadriceps femoris*. The **saphenous** (or the **femoral**) **nerve** gives off muscular branches to the cranial and caudal parts of the *m. sartorius*, sensory branches to the hip joint capsule, and enters the *m. quadriceps femoris* between the *m. vastus medialis* and the *m. rectus femoris*.

EXPECTED DISTRIBUTION OF ANESTHESIA

Successful blockade of the **femoral nerve** within the *m. iliopsoas* will provide motor blockade of the *mm. quadriceps femoris* and *sartorius*. Depending on the distribution of local anesthetic within the *m. iliopsoas*, concurrent blockade of the **obturator nerve** may result in motor blockade of the *mm. external obturator, pectineus, gracilis,* and *adductor*.

The distribution of sensory blockade of the **femoral nerve** at this level will affect the nerve fibers that innervate the cranioventral portion of the hip joint and upper limb (e.g. femur). Distribution of local anesthetic around the **obturator nerve** will also block the sensory distribution of this nerve (i.e. the caudal portion of the hip joint and the medial and cranial portions of the stifle joint).

LOCAL ANESTHETIC: DOSE, VOLUME, AND CONCENTRATION

Any local anesthetic (e.g. bupivacaine, ropivacaine, and levobupivacaine) can be used to perform a **femoral nerve** block, with or without the coadministration of an adjuvant

(e.g. dexmedetomidine, dexamethasone, and buprenorphine). Shimada et al. (2017) documented successful **femoral nerve** blockade within the *m. iliopsoas* with 0.1 ml kg⁻¹. Tayari et al. (2017), O Cathasaigh et al. (2018), and Portela et al. (2018) recommended volumes of 0.15, 0.15, and 0.1 ml kg⁻¹, respectively. The author most commonly uses 0.1 ml kg⁻¹.

PATIENT PREPARATION AND POSITIONING

The patient can be positioned in dorsal recumbency (with the pelvic limb to be blocked extended caudally) (Figure 21.2) or in lateral recumbency (with the pelvic limb to be blocked in a neutral position). Although the latter technique has the advantage that the patient does not have to be repositioned between performing the **femoral nerve** block and a **sciatic nerve** block, in the author's experience, the *m. iliopsoas* is easier to identify using US when the patient is positioned in the dorsal recumbency with the limb extended caudally. This position also facilitates identification of the **femoral nerve** lying within the muscle itself.

The inguinal area and ventrolateral abdomen, up to the cranial aspect of the ilium, should be clipped free of hair and standard surgical preparation of the skin over the injection site should be performed.

STEP-BY-STEP PERFORMANCE

SURFACE ANATOMY AND LANDMARKS TO BE USED

In most patients, the *m. iliopsoas* is palpable along the ventral aspect of the caudal lumbar transverse processes; however, palpation of the muscle can be challenging in overweight patients. In skinny and/or small patients (less than ~2 kg), the *m. iliopsoas* may be very poorly developed and its

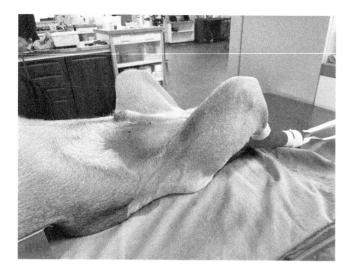

FIGURE 21.2   Patient positioned for right-sided US-guided **femoral nerve** block in the **m. iliopsoas**. The head of the dog is on the left. Source: Matt Read.

identification using manual palpation may be subtle. After the **m. iliopsoas** is identified, the US transducer should be positioned ventral and perpendicular to its long axis with the marker directed such that the needle, when introduced in the plane of the US beam, will approach the muscle in the same orientation on the US screen that it does in the patient (Figure 21.3). Using this approach, short axis views of the **m. iliopsoas** and the **femoral nerve** should be observed. If additional surface landmarks are desired, the transducer can be initially placed cranial to the ilium and the inguinal nipple,

(which is why this technique is often being referred to as the "*ventral supra-inguinal approach*" (Echeverry et al. 2012b; Shimada et al. 2017).

ULTRASOUND ANATOMY

Since it is used as the primary anatomical landmark, the **m. iliopsoas** should be identified and its image optimized and centered on the US screen by moving the transducer and adjusting the depth and gain settings. In large dogs (>30 kg), centering the **m. iliopsoas** on the screen may require firm pressure on the transducer. Next, the external iliac artery and vein should be identified medial to the **m. iliopsoas** (Figure 21.4). The use of color Doppler can be helpful to positively identify these important vascular structures and their locations. At no point during performance of the block should the needle tip be advanced as far as these vessels.

In its short axis, the **femoral nerve** will typically appear within the body of the **m. iliopsoas** as a round structure with a thin hyperechoic peripheral rim and hypoechoic center. Once it is identified, the **femoral nerve** can usually be followed along its entire intramuscular course by gliding the transducer cranially and caudally along the belly of the **m. iliopsoas**. Cranially, at the level of L5–L6, the **femoral nerve** will be located in the dorsomedial portion of the **m. iliopsoas** (i.e. in the far-field of the US screen). At that level, it is sometimes possible to also identify the **obturator nerve** adjacent to the **femoral nerve** as a similarly appearing structure. As the transducer is moved caudally, the **femoral nerve** will be seen to gradually reach a more superficial location in the ventrolateral portion of the **m. iliopsoas**. In the caudal third of the **m. iliopsoas**, the **femoral nerve** gives off the **sartorius**

(a)

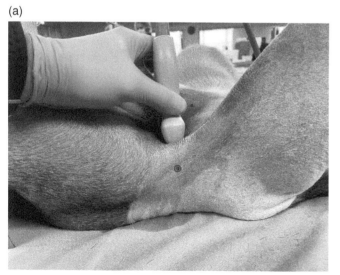

(b)

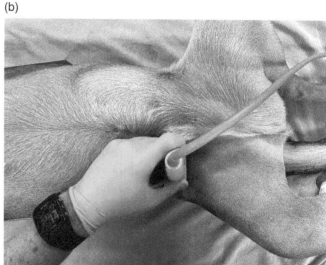

FIGURE 21.3   Positioning the ultrasound transducer to perform a right US-guided **femoral nerve** block in the **m. iliopsoas**. (a) Lateral and (b) overhead views. The head of the dog is on the left. The red dot indicates the approximate needle insertion site for an in-plane ultrasound approach to the **femoral nerve** within the **m. iliopsoas**. Source: Matt Read.

(a)
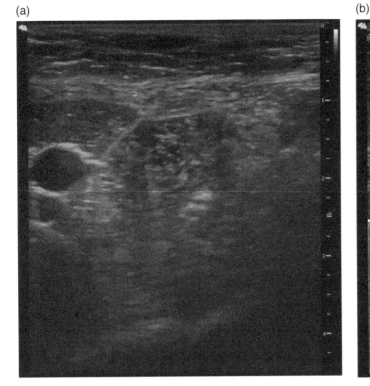

(b)
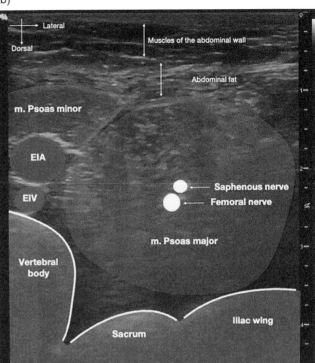

FIGURE 21.4   (a) Transverse ultrasound image of the **femoral nerve** within the *m. iliopsoas*, with annotations (b). Abdominal contents have been displaced medially so that no digestive structures are trapped between the abdominal wall and the *m. iliopsoas*. EIA, External iliac artery; EIV, External iliac vein.

nerve (motor) and both nerves remain close together within the muscle.

To perform a **femoral nerve** block using this approach, the desired image will show the **femoral nerve** in the approximate center of the *m. iliopsoas*. Mogicato et al. (2015) showed that the distance between the external iliac artery and the **femoral nerve** has a reproducible value in beagle dogs and cats and can help identify the **femoral nerve** within the *m. iliopsoas*.

In some patients, muscle fibers of the *m. iliopsoas* may also appear as round hypoechoic structures with a thin hyperechoic rim. To help differentiate the **femoral nerve** from surrounding muscle fibers, it is sometimes helpful to exploit the US principle of anisotropy as it relates to different tissues. Since muscle tissue and fasciae are slightly more anisotropic than nerves, by tilting the transducer back and forth a few degrees, the muscle fibers will become darker and/or disappear, making the nerve more obvious.

Haro et al. (2012) described the appearance of the **femoral nerve** in its long axis in cats. This image is obtained by starting from the previous view and rotating the US transducer 90°. In the obtained longitudinal views, the **femoral nerve** should appear as a hypoechoic tubular structure with hyperechoic margins.

NEEDLE INSERTION TECHNIQUE

The needle should be advanced in-plane, on a lateral-to-medial trajectory through the skin and the lateral aspect of the fascia that envelopes the *m. iliopsoas* (Figure 21.5). Ideally, the correct trajectory for the needle should be determined before the needle enters the *m. iliopsoas* fascia since attempts to modify the trajectory of the needle once it is in the muscle tend to bend the needle rather than alter its trajectory. If a "flat" needle trajectory (i.e. parallel to the transducer) is desired for better visualization, use the depth markers on the US screen to determine how deep the nerve is under the ventral skin surface prior to needle placement. The needle should be positioned on the lateral surface of the patient so that it penetrates the skin at this depth relative to the transducer.

Once through the skin, the needle should be slowly advanced into the muscle toward the **femoral nerve**. Once the tip of the needle is close to the **femoral nerve** (Figure 21.6), a test dose of the local anesthetic solution should be administered to observe the dispersion of the local anesthetic and confirm correct needle position.

In some patients, particularly overweight individuals, it may be difficult to identify the **femoral nerve** within the *m. iliopsoas*. In these cases (or simply when learning to perform the block), the use of nerve stimulation can be helpful

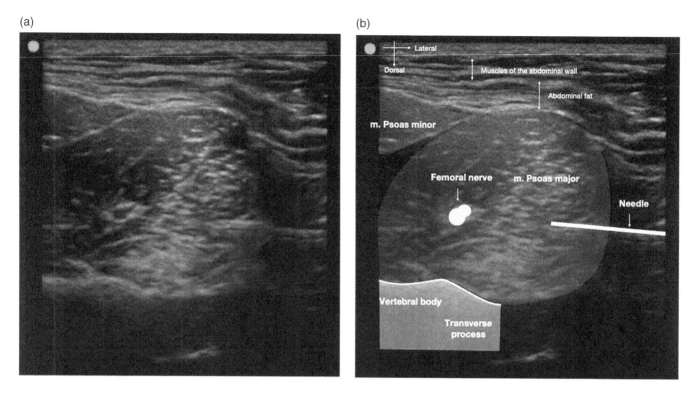

FIGURE 21.5 (a) In-plane introduction of a needle into the *m. iliopsoas* on a lateromedial trajectory prior to blockade of the **femoral nerve**. (b) Same image, with annotations.

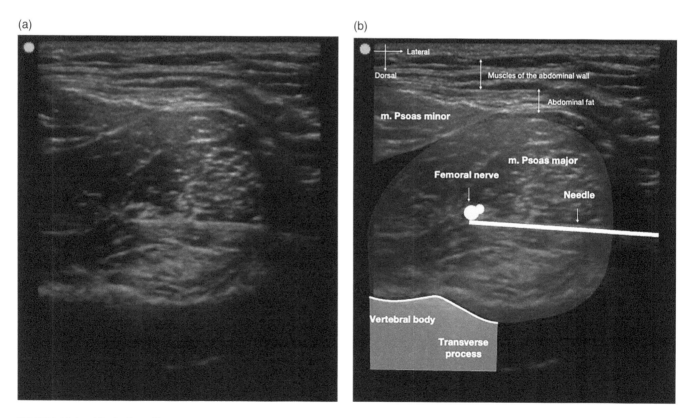

FIGURE 21.6 (a) Final needle position before injection of a local anesthetic for blockade of the **femoral nerve** within *m. iliopsoas*. (b) Same image, with annotations.

(a)

(b)

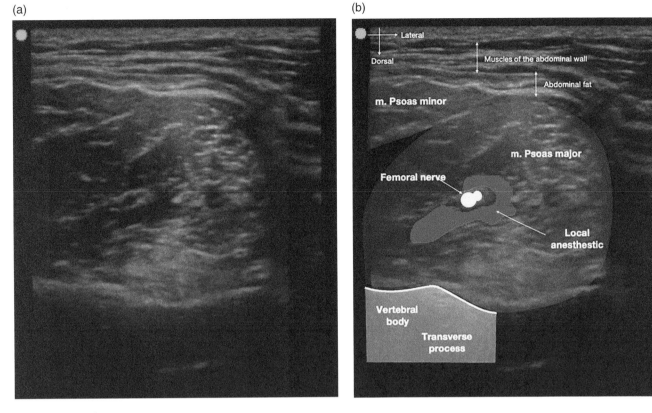

FIGURE 21.7   (a) Final distribution of local anesthetic around the **femoral nerve** following blockade of the **femoral nerve** within *m. iliopsoas*. (b) Same image, with annotations.

when trying to correctly identify the **femoral nerve** and confirm its location within the *m. iliopsoas* prior to drug administration (see below).

EXPECTED MOTOR RESPONSES FROM NERVE STIMULATION

If nerve stimulation is used, motor responses resulting from **femoral nerve** stimulation will result in contraction of the *m. quadriceps femoris* and extension of the stifle joint. Since stimulation of the **obturator nerve** elicits motor responses that result in abduction and inward rotation of the limb, they must be differentiated from those resulting from **femoral nerve** stimulation for the desired sensory block to be effective.

ADMINISTRATION OF LOCAL ANESTHETIC – WHAT TO LOOK FOR, WHAT TO FEEL FOR, DECISION POINTS

Local anesthetic injected into the *m. iliopsoas* spreads between the muscle fibers and may not necessarily pool close to, or even around, the **femoral nerve**. To obtain optimal distribution of the local anesthetic around the nerve, the needle tip may need to be repositioned slightly while the solution is

being injected. In this instance, the operator may not necessarily see the characteristic "*doughnut sign*" pattern that has been described for other nerve blocks (Figure 21.7).

It should be noted that in cats and small dogs, the total volume of local anesthetic solution is relatively small, which may limit its distribution around the target nerve unless the needle is repositioned.

In all cases, injections should be performed slowly and no resistance to injection should be encountered. If resistance to injection occurs, the injection should be stopped and the needle repositioned.

BLOCK EFFECTS (SENSORY, MOTOR, ETC.) AND PATIENT MANAGEMENT

The characteristic effects following **femoral nerve** blockade are complex, especially since it is usually combined with a **sciatic nerve** block in most clinical settings and there is potential to also block the **obturator nerve**. In dogs, following administration of 0.15–0.2 ml kg⁻¹ of bupivacaine 0.5%, the duration of sensory and motor blockade of the **femoral nerve** was 10.0 ± 1.4 hours and 10.2 ± 1.3 hours (Shimada et al. 2017), and 15 (10–18) hours and 11 (6–14) hours (O Cathasaigh et al. 2018), respectively. As such, post-block management of the patient should include adequate assessment of limb function and monitoring for skin abrasions for an extended period.

In an experimental study involving cats, **femoral nerve** blockade under sedation created an inability to bear weight on the blocked limb and cats were unable to flex the stifle joint, resulting in the limb being extended caudally (Haro et al. 2016). This observation is rarely seen in clinical patients as the discomfort caused by the disease, the surgical procedure, and/or the bandage discourages the use of the leg. The consequences of the paralysis of the adductor muscles and psoas major muscle have not been assessed.

COMPLICATIONS AND HOW TO AVOID THEM

Since the needle is manipulated away from major blood vessels (e.g. external iliac artery and vein), the approach described here for performing a **femoral nerve** block carries a low risk of intravascular injection or hemorrhage. Firm pressure on the transducer is sometimes required to bring the transducer close to the **m. iliopsoas**, and to displace the bowel and/or bladder away from the area of interest when attempting to identify the **m. iliopsoas**. As a result of this manipulation, the external iliac vein may collapse and may not always be visible. To correctly identify the vein (usually located dorso–medial to the artery) and confirm its position relative to the tip of the needle, pressure on the transducer should be adjusted and/or color Doppler used. The needle should always be advanced under visual guidance to prevent inadvertent vascular or abdominal cavity penetration.

COMMON MISTAKES AND HOW TO AVOID THEM

A common mistake is not advancing the needle at the right depth. Since it is difficult to change the trajectory of the needle once it has penetrated the **m. iliopsoas**, it can be challenging to successfully redirect the needle towards the nerve, which wastes time and potentially results in patient injury. In situations when the needle is not on an optimal trajectory, it is often easier to simply withdraw the needle from the patient and repeat the entire procedure again after determining the depth of the nerve within the muscle and determining a more ideal location on the skin for the needle to enter the patient.

HOW TO TALK TO CLIENTS/PROFESSIONAL COLLEAGUES

The average duration of effect following a **femoral nerve** motor block with bupivacaine is approximately 10 hours. If the patient is to be sent home the same day as surgery, the owner may notice a motor deficit. In practice, the discomfort caused by the primary disease, the surgical procedure, and/or the bandage will make any neurological deficit that the owner may notice barely visible. If the clinician or owner has any concerns, motor function and sensitivity should be assessed within 24–48 hours. If the animal is hospitalized, this assessment is made the day after the surgery.

It is always advisable to exclude neurological deficits from the **femoral nerve** block before considering long-term immobilization. A light bandage can be applied to prevent the animal from injuring itself as a result of dragging the affected limb.

REFERENCES

Echeverry DF, Laredo FG, Gil F et al. (2012a) Ventral ultrasound-guided suprainguinal approach to block the femoral nerve in the dog. Vet J 192, 333–337.

Echeverry DF, Laredo FG, Gil F et al. (2012b) Ultrasound-guided "two-in-one" femoral and obturator nerve block in the dog: an anatomical study. Vet Anaesth Analg 39, 611–617.

Evans HE, de Lahunta A (2012) Miller's Anatomy of the Dog, 4th Edition. Elsevier, St Louis (MO).

Graff SM, Wilson DV, Guiot LP et al. (2015) Comparison of three ultrasound guided approaches to the lumbar plexus in dogs: a cadaveric study. Vet Anaesth Analg 42, 394–404.

Haro P, Laredo F, Gil F et al. (2012) Ultrasound-guided dorsal approach for femoral nerve blockade in cats: an imaging study. J Fel Med Surg 15, 91–98.

Haro P, Laredo F, Gil F et al. (2016) Validation of the dorsal approach for the blockade of the femoral nerve using ultrasound and nerve electrolocation in cats. J Fel Med Surg 18, 620–625.

Huang CH, Hou SM, Yeh LS (2013) The innervation of canine hip joint capsule: an anatomic study. Anat. Histol. Embryol. 42, 425–431.

Mahler SP (2012) Ultrasound guidance to approach the femoral nerve in the iliopsoas muscle: a preliminary study in the dog. Vet Anaesth Analg 39, 550–554.

Marhofer P, Harrop-Griffiths W, Willschke H et al. (2010) Fifteen years of ultrasound guidance in regional anaesthesia: Part 2-recent developments in block techniques. Br J Anaesth 104, 673–683.

Mogicato G, Layssol-Lamour C, Mahler S et al. (2015) Anatomical and ultrasonographic study of the femoral nerve within the iliopsoas muscle in beagle dogs and cats. Vet Anaesth Analg 42, 425–432.

Monticelli P, Drozdzynska M, Stathopoulou T et al. (2016) A description of a technique for ultrasound-guided lumbar plexus catheter in dogs: cadaveric study. Vet Anaesth Analg 43, 453–456.

O'Connor BL, Woodbury P (1982) The primary articular nerves to the dog knee. J Anat 134, 563–572.

O Cathasaigh M, Read M, Atilla A et al. (2018) Blood concentration of bupivacaine and duration of sensory and motor block following ultrasound-guided femoral and sciatic nerve blocks in dogs. PLoS One 13(3): e0193400.

Papadopoulos G, Duckwitz V, Doherr MG (2022) Femoral and sciatic nerve blockade of the pelvic limb with and without obturator nerve block for tibial plateau levelling osteotomy surgery in dogs. Vet Anaesth Analg 49, 407–416.

Portela DA, Verdier N, Otero PE (2018) Regional anesthetic techniques for the pelvic limb and abdominal wall in small animals: a review of the literature and technique description. Vet J 238, 27–40.

Shimada S, Shimizu M, Kishimoto M (2017) Ultrasound-guided femoral nerve block using a ventral suprainguinal approach in healthy dogs. Vet Anaesth Analg 44, 1208–1215.

Tayari H, Tazioli G, Breghi G et al. (2017) Ultrasound-guided femoral and obturator nerves block in the psoas compartment in dog: anatomical and randomized clinical study. Vet Anaesth Analg 44, 1216–1226.

Warrit K, Griffenhagen G, Goh C et al. (2019) Comparison of ultrasound-guided lumbar plexus and sciatic nerve blocks with ropivacaine and sham blocks with saline on perianesthetic analgesia and recovery in dogs undergoing tibial plateau leveling osteotomy. Vet Anaesth Analg 46, 673–681.

Ultrasound-Guided Femoral Nerve Block (Inguinal Approach)

CHAPTER 22

Luis Campoy

BLOCK AT A GLANCE

What is it used for?

- To supplement anesthesia for surgeries involving the stifle and other anatomical structures distal to it such as tibial plateau leveling osteotomy (TPLO), tibial tuberosity advancement (TTA), and correction of patellar luxation (when used in combination with a **sciatic nerve** block).

Landmarks/transducer position:

- The ultrasound transducer should be placed at the junction of the proximal thigh and inguinal region (femoral triangle), perpendicular to the long axis of the femur.

- The needle puncture site is located on the cranial aspect of the thigh, in-plane with the US transducer, on the cranial belly of the *m. sartorius*.

What equipment and personnel are required?

- 21G 100 mm (or similar) blunt atraumatic needle
- Syringe of drug(s)
- Ultrasound machine
- High frequency (15–6 MHz) linear array transducer +/− protective sleeve
- Gloves
- Coupling agent (e.g. alcohol)
- Assistant to help position the leg and perform the injection

When do I perform the block?

- Prior to surgery, after the limb is clipped and skin preparation is complete. Final skin preparation will still be needed prior to surgery.

What volume of local anesthetic is used?

- 0.1 ml kg^{-1}

Goal:

- During injection, the local anesthetic should spread around the **femoral nerve**, deep to the femoral artery and fascia iliaca, cranial to *m. rectus femoris*.

Complexity level:

- Intermediate

Clinical Pearl:

- This block **will** produce motor paralysis of the quadriceps muscle group; therefore, the patient will not be able to bear any weight on the affected leg.

WHAT DO WE ALREADY KNOW?

Campoy et al. (2012a) first described an US-guided inguinal approach to the **femoral nerve** using a combination of methylene blue and lidocaine (0.1 ml kg^{-1}). Later, Campoy et al. (2012b) reported on the use of this approach (combined with a **sciatic nerve** block) in dogs undergoing stifle surgery using procedural sedation. Campoy et al. (2012b) and McCally et al. (2015) reported no differences in postoperative pain scores or opioid consumption when this technique was compared with epidural injection in dogs undergoing TPLO. McCally et al. (2015) also reported higher pain scores and higher incidence of rescue analgesia requirements when comparing the **femoral nerve** block alone with using combined **femoral** and **sciatic nerve** blocks in dogs undergoing unilateral TPLO procedures. Campoy et al. (2012a) also reported a higher incidence of urinary retention in dogs that received epidural analgesia compared to those that received nerve blocks.

Despite the analgesic efficacy of using this approach, Echeverry et al. (2010) discussed the difficulty with using US to identify the **femoral nerve** at its inguinal location, making it potentially challenging for novices to adopt into clinical practice. To this end, Garcia-Pereira et al. (2018) considered

Small Animal Regional Anesthesia and Analgesia, Second Edition. Edited by Matt Read, Luis Campoy, and Berit Fischer.
© 2024 John Wiley & Sons, Inc. Published 2024 by John Wiley & Sons, Inc.

the regional anatomy around the **femoral nerve** at its inguinal location and suggested using the circumflex iliac artery as an easily identifiable US landmark to assist with **femoral nerve** recognition prior to needle placement and local anesthetic injection.

Marolf et al. (2021) compared the use of epidural, **femoral nerve** block, **sciatic nerve** block, or a combined **femoral/sciatic nerve** block in dogs undergoing TPLO. The authors reported no observed differences in intra- and early postoperative opioid consumption when a combined **femoral/sciatic nerve** block was compared with epidural anesthesia. They did report, however, that higher opioid consumption was observed in the groups that received either standalone **femoral** or **sciatic nerve** blocks. It is worth noting that block failures were reported within each of the epidural, femoral-only and sciatic-only groups, which could have accounted for the observed differences.

Ferrero et al. (2021) retrospectively compared several different peripheral nerve blockade techniques (including US-guided and electrolocation-guided approaches) with epidural anesthesia for pelvic limb surgery in dogs. Those authors reported no differences between combined preiliac **femoral** and **sciatic nerve** blocks, **saphenous** and **sciatic nerve** blocks, and epidural anesthesia in terms of postoperative rescue analgesia requirement in dogs undergoing pelvic limb surgeries. Intraoperative hypotension and postoperative urinary retention were observed in a greater number of dogs in the epidural group.

Acquafredda et al. (2021) evaluated the effects of combining dexmedetomidine ($1\,\mu g\,ml^{-1}$) with lidocaine for combined **femoral** and **sciatic nerve** blocks in dogs undergoing stifle surgery. An increase in the duration of the sensory and proprioception blockade ($\times 2.5$) was observed when dexmedetomidine was added as a co-adjuvant. In this study, an increase in the duration of the sensory and proprioception blockade ($1.5\times$) was also observed when dexmedetomidine was administered intravenously (Acquafredda et al. 2021). In a two-center study, Marolf et al. (2022) evaluated the addition of dexmedetomidine ($0.5\,\mu g\,kg^{-1}$) per block to ropivacaine 0.5% as part of a combined **femoral** and **sciatic nerve** block on postoperative opioid requirements in 60 dogs undergoing TPLO in a 24-hour observational period. The addition of dexmedetomidine to ropivacaine yielded differences in opioid consumption in only one of the two centers. The authors attribute these differences to the lack of standardization between centers regarding surgical technique and assessors collecting postoperative data (Marolf et al. 2022).

PATIENT SELECTION

INDICATIONS FOR THE BLOCK

This block can be applied to a wide range of surgical procedures. Used in combination with a **sciatic nerve** block, complete anesthesia of the stifle can be achieved. Surgical procedures that may benefit from a **femoral nerve** block include TPLO, TTA, extracapsular lateral suture stabilization, meniscectomies, patellar tendon ruptures, correction of medial or lateral patellar luxations, distal femoral fracture repair, tibial fracture repair, and tarsal arthrodesis.

CONTRAINDICATIONS

- Skin infection or other lesions at the intended puncture site.

- Inability to identify the relevant anatomy during US scanning.

- Peripheral nerve disease affecting the pelvic limb.

- In patients presenting with instability of the contralateral limb. Inadvertent injury could occur since this block causes complete motor paralysis of the quadriceps muscle group. In these patients, a **saphenous nerve** blocks may be a better option.

POTENTIAL SIDE EFFECTS AND COMPLICATIONS

- Use of this block will result in motor paralysis of the quadriceps muscle group and the patient will, therefore, be unable to bear weight on the affected limb.

- The incidence of vascular puncture is very low as long as the needle tip is kept in the field of view as it is being advanced. This complication may be higher if the circumflex iliac artery is used as a landmark and is not maintained in constant view during needle manipulation.

- There is potential for nerve injury from inadvertent needle trauma, particularly if the operator has difficulty identifying the **femoral nerve**.

GENERAL CONSIDERATIONS
CLINICAL ANATOMY

The **femoral nerve** arises from the cranial portion of the lumbar plexus and is formed by the ventral branches of the L4, L5, and L6 spinal nerves. As it continues caudally, it follows a course through the center of the *m. iliopsoas*. At the caudal aspect of the *m. iliopsoas* (referred to as the *muscular lacuna*), the **femoral nerve** exits the muscle and courses across the femoral triangle (delineated by the *m. iliopsoas* proximally, the *m. pectineus* caudally, and the *m. sartorius* cranially) before continuing distally down the pelvic limb. Within the femoral triangle, the **femoral nerve** is located cranial to the femoral artery and vein and is covered by the caudal belly of the *m. sartorius* and the fascia iliaca. It then trifurcates into the **saphenous nerve** (sensory function) and into motor/muscular branches to the

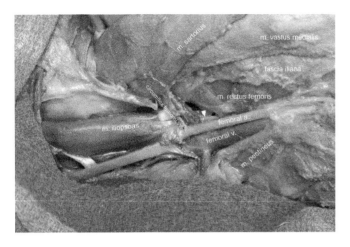

FIGURE 22.1   Dissection of the femoral triangle region of the left pelvic limb. The caudal belly of the sartorius muscle has been displaced cranially to allow for visualization of the **femoral nerve**. Observe the relationship of the femoral artery and vein as well as the circumflex femoral vessels, the **femoral nerve** (white arrowhead), *m. pectineus, m. vastus medialis,* and *m. rectus femoris*. The fascia iliaca (partially disrupted) is superficial to the *m. rectus femoris* and **femoral nerve**.

m. quadriceps and *m. sartorius*, entering the *m. quadriceps femoris* between the *m. vastus medialis* and *m. rectus femoris* (Figure 22.1).

EXPECTED DISTRIBUTION OF ANESTHESIA

A successful **femoral nerve** block will provide sensory anesthesia to the femur (mid- to distal diaphysis), medial and cranial aspects of the stifle joint capsule and intra-articular structures, the medial aspect of tibia, the skin of the dorsomedial tarsus, and the first digit.

LOCAL ANESTHETIC: DOSE, VOLUME, AND CONCENTRATION

Any local anesthetic (e.g. bupivacaine, ropivacaine, and levobupivacaine) can be used, with or without an adjuvant (e.g. dexmedetomidine, dexamethasone, and buprenorphine). The author most commonly uses bupivacaine 0.5% combined with dexmedetomidine ($1\,\mu g\,ml^{-1}$) at a volume of $0.1\,ml\,kg^{-1}$. This combination provides approximately 14 (6–24) hours [median (min–max)] of analgesic effect until rescue analgesia is needed following stifle surgery (Campoy et al. 2012a).

PATIENT PREPARATION AND POSITIONING

The patient should be positioned in lateral recumbency with the pelvic limb to be blocked positioned uppermost, abducted 90°, and extended caudally. The leg should be clipped free of hair and standard surgical preparation of the skin over the injection site should be performed.

STEP-BY-STEP PERFORMANCE

SURFACE ANATOMY AND LANDMARKS TO BE USED

The US transducer should be positioned over the femoral triangle, overlying the *m. pectineus* with the marker positioned caudally (i.e. toward the surface of the table). The transducer should be oriented perpendicular to the femoral artery so that a short-axis view of the artery can be obtained (Figure 22.2).

ULTRASOUND ANATOMY

Using the depth and gain controls, the image should be optimized so that the femoral artery appears jet black and is positioned in the upper left quadrant of the screen. This will put the structures of interest in the area of highest resolution so small details will be easier to see.

The femoral artery will be visualized in the near-field as a round, hypoechoic, and pulsatile structure (Figure 22.3). The femoral vein is rarely seen adjacent (caudal) to the artery, as it will usually be compressed from the pressure exerted by the US transducer. The **femoral nerve** will be located cranial and deep to the femoral artery and the fascia iliaca (seen as an intense hyperechoic line), caudal to the *m. rectus femoris*. It can be identified as a nodular, hyperechoic structure (often with a honeycomb appearance) directly beneath the thin caudal belly of the *m. sartorius*. The skin puncture site is located on the proximal and cranial aspect of the thigh (through the cranial belly of the *m. sartorius*), in-plane with the transducer.

NEEDLE INSERTION TECHNIQUE

The needle should be advanced through the *m. sartorius* and *m. rectus femoris* toward the **femoral nerve**, keeping the needle tip in the field of view at all times (Figure 22.4).

EXPECTED MOTOR RESPONSES FROM NERVE STIMULATION

If a combined US/electrolocation technique is used, stimulation of the **femoral nerve** will result in contractions of the *m. quadriceps femoris*, resulting in extension of the stifle.

ADMINISTRATION OF LOCAL ANESTHETIC – WHAT TO LOOK FOR, WHAT TO FEEL FOR, DECISION POINTS

After appropriate needle positioning has been achieved and a negative aspiration test has been verified, the local anesthetic can be slowly injected. During injection, the **femoral nerve** will be highlighted by the contrast produced by the hypoechoic fluid distributing around the nerve. No resistance to injection should be appreciated.

(a)

(b)

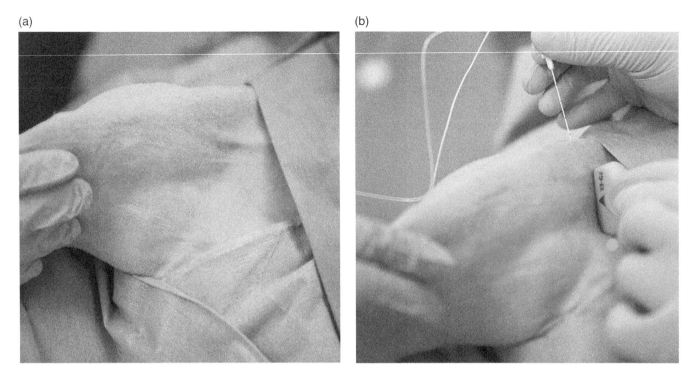

FIGURE 22.2 (a) Medial aspect view of the right pelvic limb of a dog positioned for a right **femoral nerve** block. The dog is in lateral recumbency with the leg to be blocked abducted and extended caudally. (b) Transducer and needle position for a right femoral nerve block at the level of the inguinal area. Note the transducer positioned in the medial aspect of the thigh, over the *m. pectineous* and perpendicular to the direction of the femur. The marker (green circle) is oriented caudally. Observe that the needle is parallel and in-plane relative to the transducer.

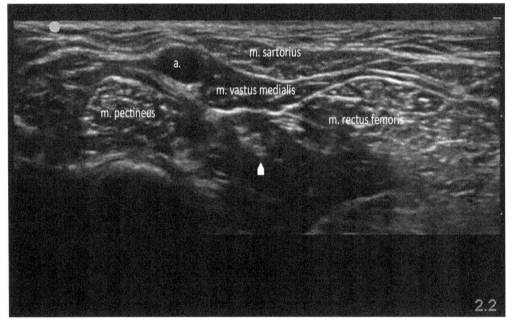

FIGURE 22.3 Ultrasound image of the **femoral nerve**. Cross-section view (short axis) at the level of the inguinal area in a dog. This image was obtained with the transducer positioned in the medial aspect at the level of the femoral triangle and perpendicular to the femur. The marker (green circle) is oriented caudally. Note the white arrowhead indicating the **femoral nerve**. a., femoral artery.

(a)

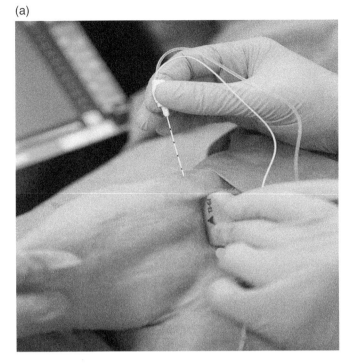

(b)

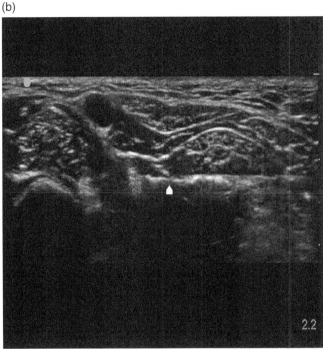

FIGURE 22.4   (a) Right **femoral nerve** block being performed in a dog positioned in lateral recumbency with the leg to be blocked abducted and extended caudally. The ultrasound transducer is positioned over the medial aspect of the thigh, over the inguinal region, with the marker (green circle) oriented caudally (towards the table). The needle is advanced in-plane and parallel to the transducer. (b) Corresponding cross-section (short-axis) ultrasound image. The needle (arrowhead) is advanced towards the **femoral nerve** through the *m. rectus femoris*.

BLOCK EFFECTS (SENSORY, MOTOR, ETC.) AND PATIENT MANAGEMENT

Blockade of the **femoral nerve** at this level will result in motor paralysis of the *m. quadriceps femoris* and the patient will be unable to fix the knee and support its own weight. A modified Robert Jones bandage may help to stabilize the pelvic limb in the absence of *m. quadriceps femoris* tone if desired.

COMPLICATIONS AND HOW TO AVOID THEM

The caudal fascia of the *m. rectus femoris* is very flexible and, as the needle is advanced, sudden perforation of this fascial plane may risk needle trauma to the femoral nerve. To minimize this risk, the needle should be advanced on a trajectory that places the tip just deep to the femoral nerve.

COMMON MISTAKES AND HOW TO AVOID THEM

If the needle does not perforate the *m. rectus femoris*, injection of the local anesthetic will be made into the belly of the muscle itself, resulting in block failure. Ensure that perforation of this fascia occurs and that the needle is correctly placed in close proximity to the **femoral nerve** prior to drug administration.

HOW TO TALK TO CLIENTS/PROFESSIONAL COLLEAGUES

- For an experienced clinician, a **femoral nerve** block should take less than four minutes to perform.

- Depending on the local anesthetic that is used, a **femoral nerve** block will provide analgesia to the affected area for up to 18–24 hours.

- Additional pain management in the postoperative period should include icing of the incision site (15 minutes, three to four times a day) and administration of oral analgesics (e.g. NSAIDs, pregabalin) for the following 5–7 days.

- Due to the motor blockade of the quadriceps muscle group, patients will be unable to bear weight on the affected leg following recovery from anesthesia.

- Patients can eat four to six hours post recovery and should be able to void.

REFERENCES

Acquafredda C, Stabile M, Lacitignola L et al. (2021) Clinical efficacy of dexmedetomidine combined with lidocaine for femoral and sciatic nerve blocks in dogs undergoing stifle surgery. Vet Anaesth Analg 48, 962–971.

Campoy L, Martin-Flores M, Ludders JW et al. (2012a) Comparison of bupivacaine femoral and sciatic nerve block versus bupivacaine and morphine epidural for stifle surgery in dogs. Vet Anaesth Analg 39, 91–98.

Campoy L, Martin-Flores M, Ludders JW et al. (2012b) Procedural sedation combined with locoregional anesthesia for orthopedic surgery of the pelvic limb in 10 dogs: case series. Vet Anaesth Analg 39, 436–440.

Echeverry DF, Gil F, Laredo F et al. (2010) Ultrasound-guided block of the sciatic and femoral nerves in dogs: a descriptive study. Vet J 186, 210–215.

Ferrero C, Borland K, Rioja E (2021) Retrospective comparison of three locoregional techniques for pelvic limb surgery in dogs. *Vet Anaesth Analg* 48, 554–562.

Garcia-Pereira FL, Boruta D, Tenenbaum S et al. (2018) Ultrasonographical identification of the superficial circumflex iliac artery as a landmark for location of the femoral nerve in dogs. Vet Anaesth Analg 45, 703–706.

Marolf V, Spadavecchia C, Müller N et al. (2021) Opioid requirements after locoregional anaesthesia in dogs undergoing tibial plateau levelling osteotomy: a pilot study. Vet Anaesth Analg 48, 398–406.

Marolf V, Selz J, Picavet P et al. (2022) Effects of perineural dexmedetomidine combined with ropivacaine on postoperative methadone requirements in dogs after tibial plateau levelling osteotomy: a two-centre study. Vet Anaesth Analg 49, 313–322.

McCally RE, Bukoski A, Branson KR, et al. (2015) Comparison of short-term postoperative analgesia by epidural, femoral nerve block, or combination femoral and sciatic nerve block in dogs undergoing tibial plateau leveling. Vet Surg 44, 983–987.

Ultrasound-Guided Saphenous Nerve Block

Luis Campoy

CHAPTER 23

BLOCK AT A GLANCE

What is it used for?

- A **saphenous nerve** block can be used to supplement anesthesia for surgeries involving the stifle joint and other anatomical structures distal to it, such as tibial plateau leveling osteotomy (TPLO), tibial tuberosity advancement (TTA), and correction of patellar luxation when used in combination with a **sciatic nerve** block.

- Can also be used to supplement anesthesia for fracture repair of bones distal to the stifle (when used in combination with a **sciatic nerve** block).

- To provide pain management for patients with severe stifle osteoarthritis.

Landmarks/transducer position:

- Position the dog in lateral recumbency, with the pelvic limb to be blocked positioned uppermost, abducted 90°, and extended caudally.

- The ultrasound transducer should be placed on the medial aspect of the midthigh, distal to the *m. pectineus,* and perpendicular to the long axis of the femur with the marker oriented caudally.

- The needle puncture site is located on the cranial aspect of the thigh, on the cranial belly of the *m. sartorius*.

What equipment and personnel are required?

- 21G 100 mm (or similar) blunt atraumatic needle
- Syringe of drug(s)
- Ultrasound machine
- High frequency (15–6 MHz) linear array transducer +/− protective sleeve
- Gloves
- Coupling agent (e.g. alcohol)
- Assistant to help position the leg and perform the injection

When do I perform the block?

- Prior to surgery, after the limb is clipped and skin preparation is complete. Final skin preparation will still be needed prior to surgery.

What volume of local anesthetic is used?

- 0.1 ml kg^{-1}

Goal:

- During injection, the local anesthetic should spread within the neurovascular bundle around the **saphenous nerve**, resulting in expansion of the neurovascular bundle and compression of the femoral artery that can be visualized using US.

Complexity level:

- Intermediate

Clinical pearl:

- This block **does not** cause motor paralysis of the quadriceps group.

WHAT DO WE ALREADY KNOW?

The use of a **saphenous nerve** block can be applied to a wide range of surgical procedures. Used in combination with a **sciatic nerve** block, anesthesia of almost the entire pelvic limb can be achieved without losing motor function of the quadriceps muscle group, allowing the patient to remain ambulatory.

Costa-Farré et al. (2011) first described the use of US-guidance to block the **saphenous nerve** in dogs using lidocaine 2% (0.1 ml kg^{-1}). Those authors reported successful sensory blockade (tested by pinching the skin with a hemostat) of the **saphenous nerve** dermatome after 15 minutes that was still present at 1 hour. After two hours, the sensory function had returned to baseline levels in each of the five dogs enrolled in their study. A similar approach to performing the block was reported by Otero et al. (2019) and is the one that is described here.

Using 0.3 ml kg^{-1} of methylene blue in 10 dog cadavers (20 injections total), Castro et al. (2018) investigated a different technique and reported a 55% success rate for staining the **saphenous nerve** following a bilateral US-guided approach to the adductor canal that is located between the *m. pectineus* and the *m. adductor magnus*. The same authors reported migration of the injectate into the popliteal fossa and subsequent staining of the tibial and peroneal branches of the **sciatic nerve** in 30% and 20% of the limbs, respectively.

Marolf et al. (2021) evaluated the effects of ropivacaine for US-guided combined **saphenous** and **sciatic nerve** blocks. Their results showed a significant nociceptive blockade prolongation when dexmedetomidine was added as co-adjuvant (250 minutes versus 445 minutes), but no prolongation of effect was observed if ropivacaine was used for the nerve blocks and the same amount of dexmedetomidine was administered intravenously (280 minutes).

Kalamaras et al. (2021) compared the effects of perioperative **saphenous** and **sciatic nerve** blocks using ropivacaine 0.5%, epidural anesthesia with ropivacaine 0.5% and morphine, or an intravenous infusion of morphine, lidocaine, and ketamine in dogs undergoing unilateral TPLO surgery. Although pain scores were lower in the blocked group, no dogs in any group required rescue analgesia based on the authors' criteria. The sedative effects of the intravenous constant infusion (that was discontinued at the end of surgery) were significant and there were still significant differences between groups at eight hours post recovery.

Ferrero et al. (2021) retrospectively compared the efficacy of electrostimulation-guided pre-iliac **femoral nerve** block combined with **sciatic nerve** blocks, US-guided **saphenous** and **sciatic nerve** blocks using bupivacaine 0.5% or ropivacaine 0.75%, and epidural anesthesia with morphine and either bupivacaine 0.5% or ropivacaine 0.75% for pelvic limb surgery. Those authors concluded that both US-guided **saphenous** and **sciatic nerve** blocks or electrostimulation-guided pre-iliac **femoral** and **sciatic nerve** blocks provided analgesia that was similar in quality and duration to epidural anesthesia. However, the incidence of intraoperative hypotension and postoperative urinary retention was significantly higher in the epidural group.

The histological, electrophysiological, and clinical effects of radiofrequency ablation of the **saphenous nerve** have been reported by Boesch et al. (2019–2020) for the treatment of severe stifle osteoarthritis.

PATIENT SELECTION

INDICATIONS FOR THE BLOCK

Surgical procedures that may benefit from the use of an US-guided **saphenous nerve** block include TPLO, tibial tuberosity advancement, extracapsular lateral suture stabilization, meniscectomies, patellar tendon ruptures, correction of medial or lateral patellar luxation, distal femoral fracture repair, tibial fracture repair, tarsal arthrodesis, etc. Additionally, this block has been successfully used to provide analgesia in cases of severe stifle osteoarthritis.

CONTRAINDICATIONS

- Skin infection or other lesions at the intended puncture site.

- Peripheral nerve disease affecting the pelvic limb.

- Small patient sizes (i.e. small breed dogs, cats, approx. <5 kg) can present technical challenges since the introduction of the needle tip within the neurovascular sheath itself may be difficult and the useable volume of local anesthetic is relatively small and may not result in complete blockade of the nerve.

- Allergic reactions to local anesthetics.

POTENTIAL SIDE EFFECTS AND COMPLICATIONS

- Due to the proximity of the femoral artery, there is potential for the needle to puncture the artery (or the femoral vein if the needle is out of position caudally). This could result in hemorrhage/hematoma formation.

- If the proximal caudal femoral artery (PCFA) is not identified prior to needle placement, there is also risk of inadvertently puncturing this vessel as the needle is advanced toward the **saphenous nerve**.

- The risk of vascular puncture is low if the needle tip is visualized continuously (sometimes difficult because of the oblique trajectory of the needle in regards to the transducer) while it is being advanced and the trajectory or position is corrected before the needle penetrates the lateral margin of the neurovascular bundle and encounters a vessel.

- If a vessel is punctured without the operator recognizing the issue and a local anesthetic is administered at an excessive dose, there is potential for local anesthetic systemic toxicity. At the local anesthetic doses recommended here, this complication is unlikely to manifest even if vascular puncture occurs (so long it is venous and not arterial) and an injection is made.

- As it is being injected, there is potential for the local anesthetic to flow backwards along the needle where it may accumulate outside the neurovascular bundle in the *m. vastus medialis*. This will be observed as fluid/cavitation outside the characteristic triangular shape of the neurovascular bundle. Depending on how much local anesthetic remains in contact with the **saphenous nerve**, the block may fail and/or the presence of local anesthetic in the muscle may cause transient muscle weakness and alter ambulation.

GENERAL CONSIDERATIONS

CLINICAL ANATOMY

The **saphenous nerve** is the terminal, strictly sensory branch of the **femoral nerve**. As soon as it leaves the *m. iliopsoas* (and oftentimes within the muscle), the **femoral nerve** gives off the **saphenous nerve** which then courses along the medial aspect of the *m. tensor fasciae latae*. The **saphenous nerve** continues distally along the medial aspect of the quadriceps muscle (*m. vastus medialis*) and sends sensory branches to the skin of the medial surface of the thigh and the cranial and lateral aspects of the crus. Additionally, the **saphenous nerve** gives off branches that accompany the descending genicular vessels, reaching the deep structures of the medial aspect of the stifle. The **saphenous nerve** then continues distally, supplying cutaneous branches to the medial aspect of limb, including the first digit (together with the **superficial peroneal nerve**) (Figure 23.1).

EXPECTED DISTRIBUTION OF ANESTHESIA

A successful **saphenous nerve** block will provide sensory anesthesia to the anteromedial aspect of the stifle, the medial aspect of tibia, and the first toe. The **medial articular nerve** arises from the **saphenous nerve** and supplies the medial and cranial aspects of the stifle. It may also send branches to the cranial attachment of the caudal cruciate ligament. Occasionally, the **medial articular nerve** receives additional sensory fibers from the **obturator** and/or **femoral nerves** (O'Connor and Woodbury 1982). In patients that have this innervation pattern (while recognizing that there is no way to appreciate this beforehand), performing a **saphenous nerve** block to facilitate certain surgical procedures of the stifle could result in incomplete blockade of all the desired anatomical struc-

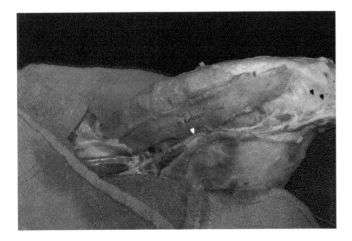

FIGURE 23.1   Dissection of the medial aspect of the left thigh. The **saphenous nerve** (white arrowhead) branches out of the **femoral nerve** as it enters the inguinal area. It then continuous distally to provide the sensory innervation to the stifle via the median articular branches (black arrowheads).

tures. This might manifest as lightening of the anesthetic plane and/or increases in heart rate and blood pressure because of surgical stimulation during capsular incision. It is the author's opinion that, postoperatively, the incomplete sensory block would not be noticeable or clinically relevant.

LOCAL ANESTHETIC: DOSE, VOLUME, AND CONCENTRATION

Any local anesthetic (e.g. bupivacaine, ropivacaine, and levobupivacaine) can be used to perform a **saphenous nerve** block, with or without the coadministration of an adjuvant (e.g. dexmedetomidine, dexamethasone, and buprenorphine).

Costa-Farré et al. (2011) reported the use of a volume of $0.1\,\mathrm{ml\,kg^{-1}}$ when performing **saphenous nerve** blocks. Otero and Portela (2019) recommended a volume of $0.05{-}0.1\,\mathrm{ml\,kg^{-1}}$. The author most commonly uses bupivacaine 0.5% combined with dexmedetomidine ($1\,\mathrm{\mu g\,ml^{-1}}$) at a volume of $0.1\,\mathrm{ml\,kg^{-1}}$.

PATIENT PREPARATION AND POSITIONING

The patient should be positioned in lateral recumbency, with the pelvic limb to be blocked positioned uppermost, abducted 90°, and extended caudally. The leg should be clipped free of hair and standard surgical preparation of the skin over the injection site should be performed.

STEP-BY-STEP PERFORMANCE

SURFACE ANATOMY AND LANDMARKS TO BE USED

The US transducer should be positioned on the medial aspect of the midthigh, over the distal aspect of the *m. pectineus*, with the marker positioned caudally (toward the surface of the table). The transducer should be oriented perpendicular to the femoral artery so that a short-axis view of the artery can be obtained (Figure 23.2).

ULTRASOUND ANATOMY

Using the depth and gain controls, the image should be optimized so that the femoral artery appears jet black and is positioned in the center (from top to bottom) of the screen. This will put the structures of interest in the area of highest resolution so small details will be easier to see. If desired, slide the transducer on the skin to position the artery left of center, giving more information about the anatomic structures that will be in the needle's planned path and allowing the needle to be observed as it is slowly advanced toward the target.

The femoral artery will be located between the *m. vastus medialis* and the *m. adductor*, deep to the *m. sartorius* and cranial to the *m. pectineus*. The **saphenous nerve** may not always be readily visible in all patients but can usually be appreciated within the neurovascular bundle as a small, round, and hypoechoic structure immediately cranial to the femoral artery (Figure 23.3).

(a)

(b)

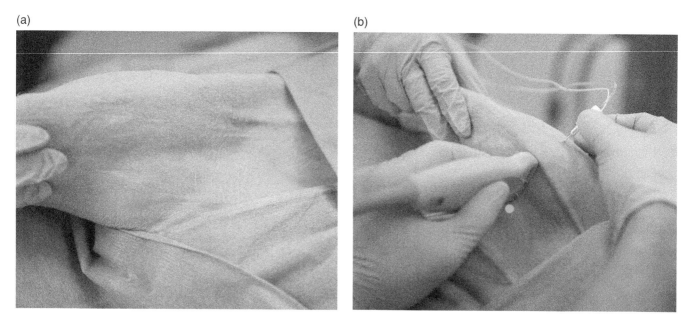

FIGURE 23.2 (a) Medial aspect view of the right pelvic limb in a dog positioned or a right **saphenous nerve** block. The dog is in lateral recumbency with the leg to be blocked abducted and extended caudally. (b) Transducer and needle position for a right **saphenous nerve** block at the level of midthigh. Note the transducer is positioned on the medial aspect of the thigh, distal to the *m. pectineous* and perpendicular to the direction of the femur. The marker (green circle) is oriented caudally. Observe that the needle is oblique to the ultrasound beam and it is in-plane relative to the transducer.

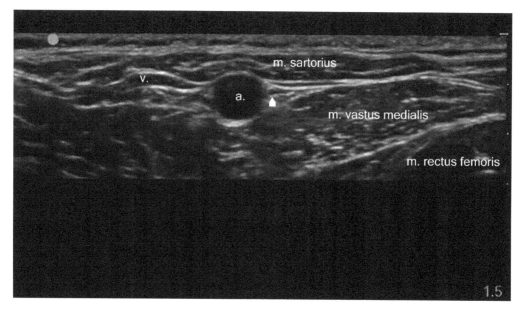

FIGURE 23.3 Ultrasonographic image of the **saphenous nerve** at the level of the midthigh. Cross-section view (short axis) in a dog. This image was obtained with the transducer positioned in the medial aspect at the level of the midthigh and perpendicular to the femur. The marker (blue circle) is oriented caudally. The **saphenous nerve** (arrowhead) is located within the neurovascular sheath, adjacent (cranial) to the femoral artery (a.) and vein (v.)

NEEDLE INSERTION TECHNIQUE

To successfully perform this block, it is very important to advance the needle on the correct trajectory. To do so, the needle should be advanced in-plane through the *m. rectus femoris* and *m. vastus medialis*, aiming toward the cranial aspect of the femoral artery. To achieve the ideal trajectory, the needle should enter the US screen from a 4:00 or 5:00 position and be advanced across the screen toward a 10:00–11:00 position. As visualized on the screen, the medial femoral fascia that surrounds the neurovascular bundle will be pierced by the needle on a deep-to-superficial trajectory. The fascia can be challenging to penetrate in some patients and the needle may require slight pressure to be applied (or to twist it along its long axis) to successfully puncture the fascia and enter the neurovascular space.

Depending on the size of the patient, after the fascia has been punctured, the needle may need to be withdrawn until the tip is located within the neurovascular sheath, cranial to the femoral artery. An image should be saved and stored to document the needle's final position prior to drug administration.

If the needle is advanced in-plane toward the femoral artery from a relatively cranial position (i.e. the needle appears to be parallel to the surface of the skin and the US transducer and is advanced from a 3:00–9:00 position on the US screen), it will be difficult to puncture the neurovascular sheath without risking puncturing the artery. By advancing the needle using the "deep-to-superficial" approach described above, an angle is produced that will be sufficient to clear the artery in the case of inadvertent, excessive, or uncontrolled needle advancement. It should be noted that using this approach can be risky in small patients or in those whose femoral artery/neurovascular bundles are very superficial. Since the needle is being advanced on a trajectory toward the US transducer (heading toward 10:00 or 11:00), it is very important to always visualize the needle tip and control the needle as it is pushed through the lateral fascia. If needle movement is not controlled, it is possible to advance the needle too far. If this happens, the needle may puncture the skin, damaging the US transducer with the needle tip (Figure 23.4).

EXPECTED MOTOR RESPONSES FROM NERVE STIMULATION

Since the **saphenous nerve** is strictly sensory, no motor responses ("twitches") will be elicited if nerve stimulation is

used. For this reason, the use of peripheral nerve stimulation is not necessary when performing **saphenous nerve** blocks.

ADMINISTRATION OF LOCAL ANESTHETIC – WHAT TO LOOK FOR, WHAT TO FEEL FOR, DECISION POINTS

After appropriate needle positioning has been achieved and a negative aspiration test has been verified, the local anesthetic can be slowly injected. During injection, the **femoral nerve** will be highlighted by the contrast produced by the hypoechoic fluid distributing around the nerve. No resistance to injection should be appreciated. Dispersion of the local anesthetic will be observed as distention of the sheath and, if needle positioning is correct, compression of the femoral artery will be observed as the local anesthetic is being injected. Following injection of the planned volume of local anesthetic, an image should be saved and stored to document the appearance of the relevant anatomical structures following drug administration. In most cases, the presence of the local anesthetic in the sheath will result in the **saphenous nerve** being visible on the screen, even if it was not able to be identified prior to drug administration.

BLOCK EFFECTS AND PATIENT MANAGEMENT

This block should not cause paralysis of the quadriceps muscle group, making it especially useful for day-surgery of the knee. However, since it is typically combined with a **sciatic nerve** block for full anesthesia of the operative limb, postoperative

(a)

(b)

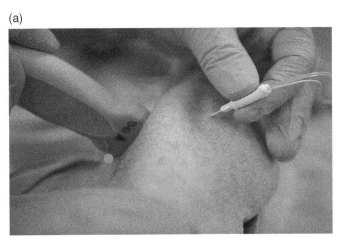
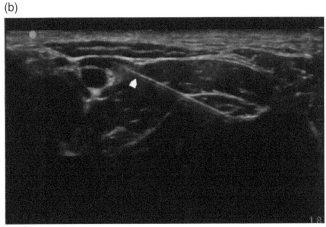

FIGURE 23.4   (a) Right **saphenous nerve** block being carried out in a dog positioned in lateral recumbency with the leg to be blocked abducted and extended caudally. The ultrasound transducer is positioned over the medial aspect of the midthigh with the marker (blue circle) oriented caudally (toward the table). The needle is advanced in-plane and is slightly oblique to the ultrasound beam. This will provide the correct angulation of the needle to achieve an ideal trajectory toward the cranial aspect of the femoral artery. (b) Corresponding cross-section (short-axis) ultrasound image. Note the needle (arrowhead) inside the neurovascular sheath. Observe the distension of the sheath and the compression of the arterial wall during the injection.

management of the patient should include monitoring for skin abrasions or ulcers on the dorsal aspect of the patient's foot that may result from knuckling following the **sciatic nerve** block.

COMPLICATIONS AND HOW TO AVOID THEM

Close monitoring of needle position using US is crucial to patient safety and success of this block. As described above, it is possible to inadvertently puncture the femoral artery as the needle is advanced through the medial femoral fascia toward the neurovascular bundle. Additionally, depending on the location along the limb, it is possible to inadvertently puncture the PCFA with the needle when it is advanced into the neurovascular bundle. This vessel typically branches off the femoral artery near the distal aspect of the *m. pectineus* so it is recommended that the target area be scanned to identify the PCFA (consider using color Doppler to verify its position) before inserting the needle. Once the PCFA is identified, the US transducer should be moved to a more proximal or distal location (i.e. away from the PCFA) where the needle can be safely advanced toward the target area.

Negative blood aspiration should be verified prior to drug administration to prevent an intravascular injection.

COMMON MISTAKES AND HOW TO AVOID THEM

A common mistake is to incorrectly position the tip of the needle in the *m. vastus medialis* (i.e. outside the neurovascular sheath), resulting in administration of the local anesthetic outside the neurovascular sheath and failure of the nerve block (Figure 23.5). A test injection should be performed using US visualization to ensure correct needle positioning before the full volume of local anesthetic is administered.

HOW TO TALK TO CLIENTS/PROFESSIONAL COLLEAGUES

- For an experienced clinician, a **saphenous nerve** block should take less than four minutes to perform.

- Depending on the local anesthetic that is used, a **saphenous nerve** block will provide analgesia to the affected area for up to 18–24 hours.

- Additional pain management in the postoperative period should include icing of the incision site (15 minutes, 3–4 times a day) and administration of oral analgesics (e.g. NSAIDs, pregabalin) for the following 5–7 days.

- Patients are usually able to walk immediately following recovery from anesthesia and can eat four to six hours post recovery and should be able to void.

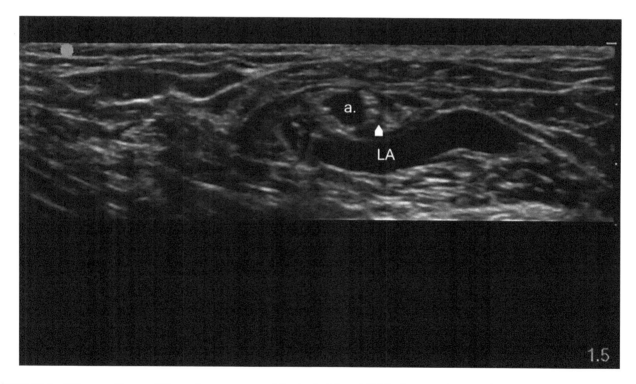

FIGURE 23.5   Ultrasound image of the **saphenous nerve** at the level of the midthigh. Cross-section view (short axis) in a dog. This image was obtained post injection with the transducer positioned in the medial aspect at the level of the midthigh and perpendicular to the femur. The marker (blue circle) is oriented caudally. Note the local anesthetic (LA) outside the neurovascular sheath pooling within the *m. vastus medialis*. The **saphenous nerve** (arrowhead) is located within the neurovascular sheath, adjacent (cranial) to the femoral artery. a. femoral artery.

Boesch JM, Campoy L, Martin-Flores M et al. (2020) Thermal radiofrequency ablation of the saphenous nerve in dogs with pain from naturally-occurring stifle osteoarthritis. Vet Anaesth Analg 47, 417–418.

Boesch JM, Campoy L, Southard T et al. (2019) Histological, electrophysiological and clinical effects of thermal radiofrequency therapy of the saphenous nerve and pulsed radiofrequency therapy of the sciatic nerve in dogs. Vet Anaesth Analg 46, 689–698.

Castro DS, Garcia-Pereira F, Giglio RF (2018) Evaluation of the potential efficacy of an ultrasound-guided adductor canal block technique in dog cadavers. Vet Anaesth Analg 45, 566–574.

Costa-Farré C, Blanch XS, Cruz JI et al. (2011) Ultrasound guidance for the performance of sciatic and saphenous nerve blocks in dogs. Vet J 187, 221–224.

Ferrero C, Borland K, Rioja E (2021) Retrospective comparison of three locoregional techniques for pelvic limb surgery in dogs. Vet Anaesth Analg 48, 554–562.

Kalamaras AB, Aarnes TK, Moore SA et al. (2021) Effects of perioperative saphenous and sciatic nerve blocks, lumbosacral epidural or morphine-lidocaine-ketamine infusion on postoperative pain and sedation in dogs undergoing tibial plateau leveling osteotomy. Vet Anaesth Analg 48, 415–421.

Marolf V, Ida KK, Siluk D et al. (2021) Effects of perineural administration of ropivacaine combined with perineural or intravenous administration of dexmedetomidine for sciatic and saphenous nerve blocks in dogs. Am J Vet Res 82, 449–458.

O'Connor BL, Woodbury P (1982) The primary articular nerves to the dog knee. J Anat 134, 563–572.

Otero PE, Portela DA (2019) Manual of small animal regional anesthesia. In: Block of the Saphenous and Medial Articular Nerves: Proximal and Distal Medial Approach, 2nd edition). Otero PE, Portela DA (eds.) Inter-Medica, Buenos Aires. pp. 168–177.

Ultrasound-Guided Parasacral Lumbosacral Trunk Block

CHAPTER 24

Diego A. Portela

BLOCK AT A GLANCE

What is it used for?

- To provide anesthesia and analgesia for surgical procedures involving the proximal pelvic limb such as hip surgery, femoral fracture repair, or pelvic limb amputation, when combined with a lumbar plexus block (e.g. psoas compartment block).

Landmarks/transducer position:

- The ultrasound transducer should be placed over the area between the sacrum and the iliac wing, perpendicular to the course of the lumbosacral trunk (i.e. oriented approximately at a 45° angle to a line connecting the cranial dorsal iliac spine and the medial angle of the ischiatic tuberosity) with the marker directed laterally. An in-plane or out-of-plane technique can be used.

What equipment and personnel are required?

- 22G 50 mm for dogs <5 kg; 21G 75 or 100 mm for dogs >5 kg, short-bevel needle
- Syringe of drug(s)
- Ultrasound machine
- High frequency (15–6 MHz) linear array transducer +/− protective sleeve
- Gloves
- Coupling agent (e.g. alcohol)
- Assistant to help perform the injection

When do I perform the block?

- The lumbosacral trunk block is ideally performed prior to surgery, after the limb is clipped and skin preparation is complete. Final skin preparation will still be needed prior to surgery. It is essential to respect the onset time of the local anesthetic used to guarantee an adequate sensory block when the surgical procedure starts (e.g. approximately 10–20 minutes depending on the long-acting local anesthetic used).

- In animals with traumatic lesions of the pelvic limb that require stabilization before surgery, the block can be performed under sedation to alleviate the pain associated with the injury and facilitate the initial stabilization.

What volume of local anesthetic is used?

- 0.15–0.2 ml kg^{-1}

Goal:

- During injection, the local anesthetic should be observed spreading within the pelvic fascia in close proximity to the lumbosacral trunk.

Complexity level:

- Intermediate to advanced

Clinical pearl:

- In small patients, a 25 mm linear (or hockey stick) transducer may be necessary.

WHAT DO WE ALREADY KNOW?

The parasacral lumbosacral trunk block is used to anesthetize the **sciatic nerve** close to its origin before it runs over the greater ischiatic foramen (ischiatic notch) (Figures 24.1 and 24.2). When a local anesthetic solution is injected at this location, it promotes blockade of the lumbosacral trunk at the origin of the **sciatic nerve**, the **cranial** and **caudal gluteal nerves**, and possibly the **caudal cutaneous femoral nerve**.

Small Animal Regional Anesthesia and Analgesia, Second Edition. Edited by Matt Read, Luis Campoy, and Berit Fischer.
© 2024 John Wiley & Sons, Inc. Published 2024 by John Wiley & Sons, Inc.

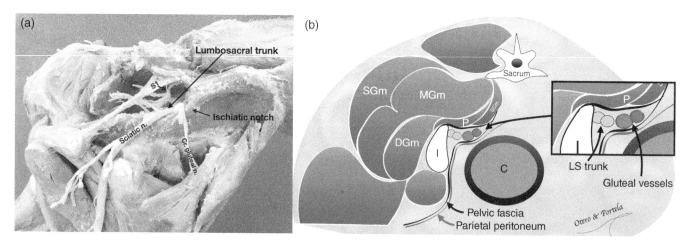

FIGURE 24.1 Anatomical preparation of the lumbosacral trunk and cross-sectional schematic of the parasacral area. C, Colon; DGm, *m. gluteus profundus*; I, ilium; LS trunk, lumbosacral trunk; MGm, *m. gluteus medius*; P, *m. piriformis*; SCm, *m. sacrocaudalis*; SGm, *m. gluteus superficialis*.

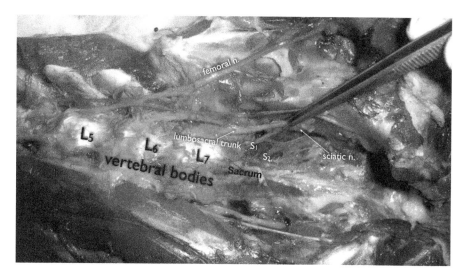

FIGURE 24.2 Anatomical dissection of the lumbosacral trunk. Ventral view of the lumbar plexus and the lumbosacral trunk after removing the abdominal and pelvic contents and the *mm. psoas*. The forceps are holding the lumbosacral trunk and the origin of the **sciatic nerve**.

A US-guided parasacral approach to the lumbosacral trunk was first described in an experimental study by Shilo et al. (2010). In that study, the lumbosacral trunk was initially visualized using a short-axis view in the parasacral region. The transducer was subsequently rotated 90° to obtain a long-axis view of the nerve. Using an in-plane needle technique, bupivacaine 0.5% at 0.03, 0.06, or 0.13 ml kg⁻¹ was injected perineurally, resulting in a 67% success rate of sensory blockade following each of the different doses. The low success rate may be explained by the use of a low-frequency US transducer, inadequate distribution of the local anesthetic around the neural structures, and the relatively insensitive method of assessing block efficacy via response to toe pinch.

Recently, Marolf et al. (2019) described the parasacral approach to the lumbosacral trunk using a short-axis view of the target nerve and an in-plane needle technique. The first phase of their study was performed in canine cadavers and showed that injection of 0.2 ml of new methylene blue resulted in lumbosacral trunk staining in 93% of the injections. In the second phase of the study, the authors showed that administration of 0.2 ml kg⁻¹ of levobupivacaine 0.5% achieved an 86% success rate for sensory blockade in live dogs. The motor deficit that resulted from the block lasted for a median (interquartile range) of 60 (30–210) minutes. However, the ability to reposition the limb (proprioception test) was not different between dogs injected with levobupivacaine or saline (Marolf et al. 2019).

PATIENT SELECTION
INDICATIONS FOR THE BLOCK

This block is typically combined with a lumbar plexus block (psoas compartment block) for procedures involving the proximal third of the pelvic limb, including procedures of the hip, femoral head, and proximal femur. As well, combining these blocks can serve as an effective alternative to neuraxial anesthesia for patients undergoing pelvic limb amputation. This block can also be used to alleviate pain in animals with osteosarcomas of the pelvic limb, for which surgical treatment is not an option. In this case, using a low concentration of local anesthetic with adjuvants can improve the quality of the animal's life for several days.

CONTRAINDICATIONS

- Skin infection or other lesions at the intended needle puncture site.

- Inability to identify the relevant anatomy. For example, dogs with traumatic fractures of the proximal femur, including the femoral head, can have a substantial hematoma present in the gluteal region, compromising clear visualization of the target structures.

- Peripheral nerve disease affecting the pelvic limb.

- Small patient sizes (i.e. small dogs, cats, approx. <5 kg) can present technical challenges since the footprint of the US transducer may be too large (even a 25 mm transducer). In these cases, the use of an out-of-plane needle technique can facilitate the procedure.

POTENTIAL SIDE EFFECTS AND COMPLICATIONS

- Inadvertent puncture of intrapelvic structures (e.g. colon).

- Potential puncture of the caudal gluteal vessels resulting in hematoma formation.

- Iatrogenic nerve injury. Avoid injection of the local anesthetic if resistance is perceived during injection and spread of the local anesthetic around the nerve is not observed.

- A local anesthetic solution injected in the parasacral area can potentially spread further than intended and block the sacral nerves that become the **pudendal** and **perineal nerves**. The clinical effects of inadvertently blocking these nerves, especially in animals with preexisting fecal incontinence, are unknown.

- Local anesthetic systemic toxicity.

GENERAL CONSIDERATIONS
CLINICAL ANATOMY

The lumbosacral trunk is formed by the ventral branches of L6, L7, and S1 **spinal nerves**. Occasionally, the S2 spinal nerve may also contribute. After leaving the ***m. psoas major***, the lumbosacral trunk is covered by the pelvic fascia and, during its intrapelvic course, crosses the shaft of the ilium on its dorsal aspect. The **cranial** and **caudal gluteal nerves** arise from the intrapelvic portion of the lumbosacral trunk and lie above the pelvic fascia on the medial aspect of the ilium in close proximity to the gluteal vessels. The lumbosacral trunk courses through the intrapelvic and parasacral spaces surrounded by the ***mm. sacrocaudalis ventralis lateralis*** (medially), ***levator ani*** (laterally), and ***mm. gluteus medius***, ***gluteus superficialis***, and ***piriformis*** (dorsally) (Evans and de Lahunta 2013). Caudally, the trunk exits the pelvis and crosses over the ischiatic notch, where it continues distally down the limb as the **sciatic nerve** (Figure 24.1).

EXPECTED DISTRIBUTION OF ANESTHESIA

This technique desensitizes the craniolateral and caudolateral portions of the hip joint as a result of blockade of the **articular branches** that originate from the **cranial gluteal** and **sciatic nerves**, respectively (Huang et al. 2013). Since the lumbosacral trunk is blocked proximal to the origin of the **gluteal nerves**, the ***mm. gluteus medius***, ***gluteus superficialis***, ***internal obturator***, ***gemelli***, ***quadratus femoris***, ***biceps femoris***, ***semimembranosus,*** and ***semitendinosus*** will also be blocked (Campoy 2019).

Combining a lumbar plexus block (e.g. psoas compartment block) with a parasacral lumbosacral trunk block would be expected to result in complete desensitization of the pelvic limb.

LOCAL ANESTHETIC: DOSE, VOLUME, AND CONCENTRATION

Any local anesthetic (e.g. bupivacaine, ropivacaine, and levobupivacaine) can be used to perform a lumbosacral trunk block, with or without the coadministration of an adjuvant (e.g. dexmedetomidine, dexamethasone, and buprenorphine). High concentrations ($\geq$0.5%) promote more consistent levels of sensory and motor blockade, whereas lower concentrations ($\leq$0.2%) tend to induce blockade of the sensory fibers with potentially limited (i.e. shorter duration) motor blockade (Ford et al. 1984; Yao et al. 2012; Kii et al. 2014).

Volumes ranging from 0.05 to 0.13 ml kg^{-1} resulted in variable effects in early research studies (Portela et al. 2010; Shilo et al. 2010). Levobupivacaine 0.5% (0.2 ml kg^{-1}) was associated with a high success rate in an experimental study (Marolf et al. 2019). Clinical reports that used 0.15 ml kg^{-1} of bupivacaine 0.5% or 0.1 ml kg^{-1} of bupivacaine 0.75% were associated with high rates of success (Romano et al. 2016; Congdon et al. 2017). Volumes of 0.15–0.2 ml kg^{-1} are currently recommended for this technique (Portela et al. 2018; Campoy 2019).

PATIENT PREPARATION AND POSITIONING

The patient should be deeply sedated or anesthetized and positioned in lateral recumbency, with the limb to be blocked positioned uppermost, and resting in a natural position. Alternatively, sternal recumbency can be used, particularly if the patient is small. The area over the dorsolateral gluteal area should be clipped free of hair and standard surgical preparation of the skin over the injection site should be performed.

STEP-BY-STEP PERFORMANCE
SURFACE ANATOMY AND LANDMARKS TO BE USED

The transducer should be positioned over the dorsal gluteal area between the wing of the ilium and the sacrum just caudal to the sacroiliac joint (Figure 24.3). Orientation of the probe will be slightly oblique (~35°–45° angle) to the long axis of the

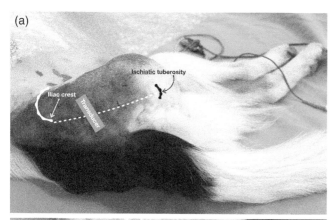

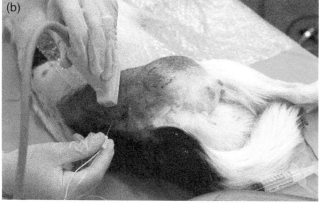

FIGURE 24.3   (a) Surface anatomy and initial ultrasound transducer position (blue rectangle) to perform a parasacral lumbosacral trunk block on a dog. The transducer should be positioned caudal to the sacroiliac joint at the junction of the cranial and middle thirds of an imaginary line connecting the cranial dorsal iliac spine of the sacral tuberosity and the medial angle of ischiatic tuberosity.
(b) After image optimization, the ultrasound transducer has been rotated laterally to facilitate in-plane needle introduction.

ilium with the marker directed laterally. To help with correct transducer positioning, an imaginary line can be drawn connecting the cranial dorsal iliac spine at the level of the sacral tuberosity with the medial angle of the ischiatic tuberosity. The transducer should be positioned perpendicular to this line, approximately at the junction of its cranial and middle thirds. After obtaining a clear image of the target structures, the transducer should be slightly rotated to a 35°–45° angle to the line connecting the iliac crest with the medial angle of ischiatic tuberosity to prevent the needle from contacting the sacrum or the coccygeal vertebrae.

ULTRASOUND ANATOMY

The ilium is the main sonographic landmark to be identified (Figure 24.4). It will appear as a hyperechoic line casting an acoustic shadow. The lumbosacral trunk is located medial to the ilium, ventral to the **m. piriformis** (which in turn is deep to the **m. gluteus medius**) and is surrounded by the pelvic fascia. Ultrasonographically, the lumbosacral trunk is identifiable as a round, hypoechoic structure surrounded by a hyperechoic rim. In some animals, the lumbosacral trunk can be seen as a double-rounded structure (similar to the **sciatic nerve**). Following the lumbosacral trunk cranially (proximally), it will disappear under the acoustic shadow of the ilium. Followed caudally, it will be observed crossing the ilium dorsally at the ischiatic notch and then continuing distally along the proximal thigh as the **sciatic nerve**.

The caudal gluteal artery can be identified as an anechoic, round, and pulsatile structure located medial to the lumbosacral trunk. Color Doppler can be used to verify its identity and position. Both the lumbosacral trunk and the caudal gluteal vessels share the same interfascial plane within two layers of the pelvic fascia (Figures 24.1 and 24.4). Ventromedial to the neurovascular bundle, the colon can be seen deep to the parietal peritoneum (Benigni et al. 2007).

At this location, the **mm. gluteus superficialis**, **gluteus medialis**, and **piriformis** are located dorsal to the lumbosacral trunk. The gluteal fascia lies between the skin and the **m. gluteus superficialis.** The dorsal branches of the **lumbar** and **sacral cutaneous nerves** run between the gluteal fascia and the skin but are rarely visible on US.

CLINICAL PEARL

In dogs with large gluteal muscles, the lumbosacral trunk will be located deeper than 4 cm. In these situations, it is recommended that the "penetration" setting be used on the US machine to improve nerve visualization, appreciating that using this setting may reduce the overall resolution/quality of the image. A low-frequency convex or micro-convex transducer may also be used in some cases when the lumbosacral trunk is located deeper than 4–5 cm. In small dogs, a 25 mm footprint linear array transducer may be needed to fit between the ilium and the sacrum.

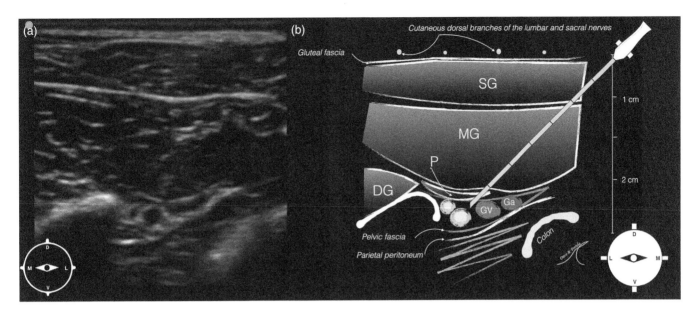

FIGURE 24.4   (a) Ultrasound image and (b) schematic representation of the parasacral lumbosacral trunk block. The ultrasound image was obtained using a linear high-frequency (15 MHz) transducer. D, dorsal; DG, ***m. gluteus profundus***; Ga, gluteal artery; Gv, gluteal vein; L, lateral; M, medial; MG, ***m. gluteus***; SG, ***m. gluteus superficialis***; V, ventral. Lumbosacral trunk is indicated in yellow. Source: With permission from Pablo Otero and Diego Portela.

NEEDLE INSERTION TECHNIQUE

Once the anatomical features of the lumbosacral trunk are identified, the transducer can be rotated, 35°–45° to an imaginary line connecting the iliac crest and the medial angle of ischiatic tuberosity (Figure 24.3). This oblique orientation of the transducer facilitates the introduction of the needle in-plane. The needle is then advanced on a ventrolateral trajectory through ***mm. gluteus superficialis***, ***gluteus medialis***, and ***piriformis*** (Figures 24.3 and 24.4). The needle's angle should be adjusted to approach the target nerve on its dorsomedial aspect so as to avoid puncture of the caudal gluteal vessels. Alternatively, the needle can be advanced out-of-plane. The tip of the needle, the vessels, and the target nerves should motor responses from nerve stimulation always be visualized as the needle is being advanced.

EXPECTED MOTOR RESPONSES FROM NERVE STIMULATION

A combined US-guided/electrostimulation technique may be used to aid in confirming correct positioning of the needle and to reduce the chances of administering an intraneural injection. The nerve stimulator should initially be set to deliver a current at 0.5 mA, 0.1 ms, and 1 Hz to elicit appropriate motor responses (i.e. of the ***mm. gluteus superficialis***, ***gluteus medialis***, ***semimembranosus***, and ***semitendinosus***). Occasionally, only a gluteal muscle response may be observed, indicating that the needle tip is located too far laterally. If this motor response is observed, the needle should be repositioned prior to injection. If muscular responses are elicited with current <0.3 mA, the needle

should be slightly withdrawn because the tip of the needle may be in contact with the nerve trunk itself.

ADMINISTRATION OF LOCAL ANESTHETIC – WHAT TO LOOK FOR, WHAT TO FEEL FOR, DECISION POINTS

Once the tip of the needle is thought to be correctly located, inject a small amount of local anesthetic to confirm its distribution around the nerve trunk. The total volume of local anesthetic recommended for this block is 0.15–0.2 ml kg^{-1}. As it is being injected, the local anesthetic should be seen spreading within the layers of the pelvic fascia. If necessary, move the needle carefully while injecting the local anesthetic to ensure an even distribution of the drug around the target nerve. If resistance to injection is perceived, it might indicate that the local anesthetic is being injected intraneurally. In this situation, administration of the local anesthetic should immediately be discontinued and the needle repositioned.

BLOCK EFFECTS AND PATIENT MANAGEMENT

This technique produces motor blockade of the muscle groups that stabilize the hip. As a result, weakness of the gluteal and hamstring muscles may be present, affecting the patient's ability to flex the hip during ambulation. Moreover, blockade of the **common peroneal nerve** as part of the **sciatic nerve** affects proprioceptive responses of the foot. Patients should be monitored for prolonged/unexpected duration of blockade and their distal limbs protected if trauma is observed.

COMPLICATIONS AND HOW TO AVOID THEM

- If the needle tip is advanced too deep, there is potential for piercing the parietal peritoneum and entering the colon. Visualization of the needle tip during needle movements reduces the risk of potential intrapelvic puncture.

- Inadvertent puncture of the caudal gluteal vessels may occur resulting in hematoma formation. Color flow Doppler can help differentiate neural structures from vascular structures. To avoid accidental intravascular injection, always ensure a negative aspiration test.

- Nerve trauma can result from an intraneural injection. Avoiding injection when increased resistance is encountered or when the animal shows a nociceptive response during injection is imperative to avoid this complication.

COMMON MISTAKES AND HOW TO AVOID THEM

During an in-plane needle advancement, the needle tip may contact the ilium or the sacrum. In this situation, the direction of the needle should be adjusted to a more medial or lateral orientation, respectively. If the transducer is not positioned in an oblique orientation, the needle generally enters at a very steep angle and it may encounter the sacrum or the coccygeal vertebrae on its path. Inserting the needle at a steep angle impairs needle visualization when linear transducers are used, making the technique more challenging.

In some instances, muscular responses will not be obtained even if the tip of the needle is touching the nerve (Portela et al. 2013). Therefore, it is advised to proceed with the injection of local anesthetic if the needle tip appears to be in the correct position and there is adequate visualization of the lumbosacral trunk and the caudal gluteal vessels even if muscular twitches are not obtained at 0.5 mA. This could help avoid potential nerve trauma that may occur with additional needle movements.

In dogs with large muscle mass over the target area, the lumbosacral trunk can be deeper than 4 cm. In these cases, a low-frequency transducer (i.e. convex or microconvex) can facilitate the performance of this block.

HOW TO TALK TO CLIENTS/PROFESSIONAL COLLEAGUES

When planning a parasacral block of the lumbosacral trunk, it is important to advise the surgeon about the pros and cons of this technique. The lumbosacral trunk block is less invasive than neuraxial techniques and selectively blocks only the target limb. Therefore, the animal can use the contralateral limb immediately after surgery. It is also important to highlight that this technique, combined with a lumbar plexus block, is an excellent alternative to epidural blocks in patients that require pelvic limb amputations.

The surgeon(s) and personnel who will be evaluating the patient in the postoperative period should be advised that motor deficits will be produced by this block, as well as the expected duration of the motor block based on the drugs that were used. This allows mitigation strategies, such as sling walking and bandaging, to be implemented in the postoperative period.

REFERENCES

Benigni L, Corr SA, Lamb CR (2007) Ultrasonographic assessment of the canine sciatic nerve. Vet Radiol Ultrasound 48, 428–433.

Campoy L (2019) Locoregional anesthesia for hind limbs. Vet Clin North Am Small Anim Pract 49, 1085–1094.

Congdon JM, Boscan P, Goh CSS et al. (2017) Psoas compartment and sacral plexus block via electro-stimulation for pelvic limb amputation in dogs. Vet Anaesth Analg 44, 915–924.

Evans HE, de Lahunta A (2013) Chapter 17 – The spinal nerves. In: Miller's Anatomy of the Dog, 4th edition. Evans HE, de Lahunta A (eds.) Elsevier Saunders, St Louis, MI. pp. 611–657.

Ford DJ, Raj PP, Singh P et al. (1984) Differential peripheral nerve block by local anesthetics in the cat. Anesthesiology 60, 28–33.

Huang CH, Hou SM, Yeh LS (2013) The innervation of canine hip joint capsule: an anatomic study. Anat Histol Embryol 42, 425–431.

Kii N, Yamauchi M, Takahashi K et al. (2014) Differential axillary nerve block for hand or forearm soft-tissue surgery. J Anesth 28, 549–553.

Marolf V, Rohrbach H, Bolen G et al. (2019) Sciatic nerve block in dogs: description and evaluation of a modified ultrasound-guided parasacral approach. Vet Anaesth Analg 46, 106–115.

Portela DA, Otero PE, Tarragona L et al. (2010) Combined paravertebral plexus block and parasacral sciatic block in healthy dogs. Vet Anaesth Analg 37, 531–541.

Portela DA, Otero PE, Biondi M et al. (2013) Peripheral nerve stimulation under ultrasonographic control to determine the needle-to-nerve relationship. Vet Anaesth Analg 40, e91–99.

Portela DA, Verdier N, Otero PE (2018) Regional anesthetic techniques for the pelvic limb and abdominal wall in small animals: a review of the literature and technique description. Vet J 238, 27–40.

Romano M, Portela DA, Breghi G et al. (2016) Stress-related biomarkers in dogs administered regional anaesthesia or fentanyl for analgesia during stifle surgery. Vet Anaesth Analg 43, 44–54.

Shilo Y, Pascoe PJ, Cissell D et al. (2010) Ultrasound-guided nerve blocks of the pelvic limb in dogs. Vet Anaesth Analg 37, 460–470.

Yao J, Zeng Z, Jiao Z-H et al. (2012) Optimal effective concentration of ropivacaine for postoperative analgesia by single-shot femoral–sciatic nerve block in outpatient knee arthroscopy. J Int Med Res 41, 395–403.

Ultrasound-Guided Sciatic Nerve Block (Caudal Approach)

CHAPTER 25

Luis Campoy

What is it used for?

- A **sciatic nerve** block can be used to supplement anesthesia for surgeries involving the stifle and other anatomical structures distal to it, such as tibial plateau leveling osteotomy (TPLO), tibial tuberosity advancement (TTA), and correction of patellar luxation when used in combination with a **femoral** or **saphenous nerve** block.

- It can also be used to supplement anesthesia for fracture repair of bones distal to the stifle (when used in combination with a **femoral** or **saphenous nerve** block).

- It can also be used to supplement anesthesia for surgical procedures involving the tibia and foot, usually in combination with either a **femoral** or a **saphenous nerve** block (though not always, depending on the location of the procedure).

Landmarks/transducer position:

- The ultrasound (US) transducer should be placed on the lateral aspect of the midthigh, over the ***m. biceps femoris***, perpendicular to the direction of the femur with the marker oriented cranially.

- The needle puncture site will be located on the caudal aspect of the thigh.

What equipment and personnel are required?

- 21Ga 100mm (4in.) (or similar) blunt atraumatic needle

- Syringe of drug(s)

- Ultrasound machine

- High frequency (15–6MHz) linear array transducer +/− protective sleeve

- Gloves

- Coupling agent (e.g. alcohol)

- Assistant to perform the injection

When do I perform the block?

- Prior to surgery, after the limb is clipped and skin preparation is complete. Final skin preparation will still be needed prior to surgery.

What volume of local anesthetic is used?

- 0.05–0.1 ml kg^{-1}

Goal:

- During injection, the local anesthetic should be seen spreading around the sciatic nerve. Detachment from the fascia of the ***m. biceps femoris*** muscle does not appear to provide any additional clinical benefit.

Complexity level:

- Basic

WHAT DO WE ALREADY KNOW?

A caudal approach to performing US-guided **sciatic nerve** blocks was originally described by Campoy et al. (2010) and Echeverry et al. (2010). Since those original reports, there have been no major changes or refinements to the technique. Other authors have further documented the clinical use of US-guided **sciatic nerve** blocks: Vettorato et al. (2012), Gurney and Leece (2014), and Portela et al. (2018). Haro et al. (2012) described the use of a similar approach for use in cats.

Marolf et al. (2021) observed no differences in intra- and early postoperative opioid consumption in dogs undergoing TPLO procedures that received either combined **femoral** and **sciatic nerve** blocks or epidural anesthesia. Higher opioid consumption was observed, however, in the dogs that received either standalone **femoral** or **sciatic nerve** blocks.

In a retrospective study, Ferrero et al. (2021) reported results comparing the effects and benefits of using several different locoregional anesthetic techniques (including US-guided and electrolocation-guided nerve blocks) with epidural anesthesia to facilitate pelvic limb surgery in dogs. Those authors reported no differences observed between using combined preiliac-**femoral** (psoas compartment) and **sciatic nerve** blocks, combined **saphenous** and **sciatic nerve** blocks, or epidural anesthesia on postoperative rescue analgesia requirement in dogs. Complications such as intraoperative hypotension and postoperative urinary retention were observed in a greater number of dogs in the epidural group. Acquafredda et al. (2021) evaluated the effects of adding dexmedetomidine (1 μg ml⁻¹) to lidocaine for combined **femoral** and **sciatic nerve** blocks in dogs undergoing stifle surgery. An increase in the duration of sensory and proprioceptive blockade (~2.5-fold) was observed when dexmedetomidine was added as a co-adjuvant, while an increase in the duration of these same two effects (~1.5-fold) was observed when dexmedetomidine was administered intravenously. Marolf et al. (2022), in a two-center study, evaluated the effects of adding dexmedetomidine to ropivacaine for **sciatic nerve** blocks on the opioid requirements of dogs undergoing TPLO procedures. Less opioid consumption was observed in only one of their two centers when dexmedetomidine was used as a co-adjuvant. A different, more proximal approach for performing **sciatic nerve** blocks (similar to the parasacral approach described elsewhere in this book) was reported by Shilo et al. (2010). In that study, the **sciatic nerve** was imaged along its long axis and an overall 67% success rate with variable duration of effect was reported.

PATIENT SELECTION

INDICATIONS FOR THE BLOCK

A **sciatic nerve** block, when used in combination with either a **femoral** or **saphenous nerve** block, is indicated for surgical procedures involving the stifle and structures distal to it (e.g. TPLO, TTA, extracapsular lateral suture stabilization, meniscectomies, patellar tendon ruptures, correction of medial or lateral patellar luxation, distal femoral fracture repair, tibial fracture repair, tarsal arthrodesis, etc.).

CONTRAINDICATIONS

- Skin infection or other lesions at the intended puncture site.
- Peripheral nerve disease affecting the pelvic limb.
- Allergic reactions to local anesthetics.

POTENTIAL SIDE EFFECTS AND COMPLICATIONS

Blockade of the **sciatic nerve** at this location will result in motor paralysis of the flexors and extensors of the paw, leading to an inability to flex the tarsus and loss of proprioception. These, in turn, will lead to knuckling and an abnormal gait (pseudohypermetric gait).

GENERAL CONSIDERATIONS

CLINICAL ANATOMY

The *muscular branches* of the **sciatic nerve** branch off proximal to where the US-guided approach is typically performed and run in a caudo–distal direction to provide motor innervation to the ischiotibial muscles (***mm. semimembranosus, semitendinosus,*** and ***biceps femoris***). These muscular branches can be found branching out of the **sciatic nerve** at the level of the greater trochanter and run distally and caudal to the **sciatic nerve** along the cranial edge of the ***m. semimembranosus*** (Figure 25.1).

At the level of the midthigh where the block is usually performed, the **sciatic nerve** is located between the ***m. biceps femoris*** (lateral), the ***m. semimembranosus*** (caudal and medial), and the ***m. adductor*** (medial). It then divides into its two primary branches, the **tibial nerve** (medially) and the **common peroneal nerve** (laterally), lateral to the ***m. gastrocnemius***. In most cases, if the US transducer is placed over the ***m. biceps femoris***, the **sciatic nerve** can be observed directly underneath the muscle at its deepest point.

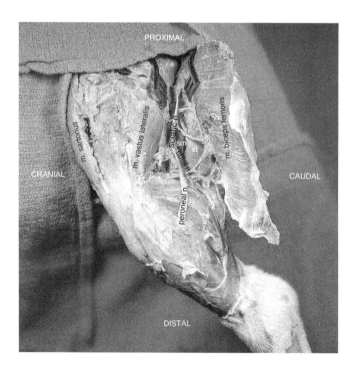

FIGURE 25.1 Dissection of the lateral aspect of the left thigh of a canine cadaver in lateral recumbency showing the **sciatic nerve**. The ***m. biceps femoris*** has been transected and reflected caudally to allow for easier visualization of the **sciatic nerve** and its surrounding structures. sm, semimembranosus; st, semitendinosus.

EXPECTED DISTRIBUTION OF ANESTHESIA

An US-guided caudal approach to the **sciatic nerve** block will result in anesthesia of the caudolateral aspect of the stifle (including part of the joint capsule and intra-articular structures), the tibia, the tarsus, the metatarsus (dorsal – **common peroneal nerve**; plantar – **tibial nerve**), and the second through fifth digits (i.e. the first digit and medial aspect of second digit are innervated by branches of the **saphenous nerve**). Using this US-guided caudal approach to the **sciatic nerve** block may spare the sensory and motor blockade of the ischiotrochanteric and ischiotibial muscles (***mm. semitendinosus*** and ***semimembranosus***) and the ***m. biceps femoris***, for at least the proximal two-thirds of the muscle belly.

LOCAL ANESTHETIC: DOSE, VOLUME, AND CONCENTRATION

Any local anesthetic (bupivacaine, ropivacaine, and levobupivacaine) can be used, with or without an adjuvant (e.g. dexmedetomidine, dexamethasone, and buprenorphine), at a volume of 0.05–0.1 ml kg^{-1}.

PATIENT PREPARATION AND POSITIONING

The patient should be positioned in lateral recumbency with the limb to be blocked positioned uppermost and extended in a natural position. In dogs, with extensive muscle atrophy, a roll of towels in between both pelvic limbs may facilitate

needle approach. The leg should be clipped free of hair and standard surgical preparation of the skin over the injection site should be performed.

STEP-BY-STEP PERFORMANCE

SURFACE ANATOMY AND LANDMARKS TO BE USED

Once the limb is clipped free of hair, the ***m. biceps femoris*** should be able to be identified and palpated on the lateral aspect of the thigh. The US transducer should be positioned over the ***m. biceps femoris*** distal to the ischiatic tuberosity, in a cranio–caudal direction (i.e. perpendicular to the long axis of the femur) with the marker oriented cranially (Figure 25.2). This should result in a short axis view of the ***m. biceps femoris*** and **sciatic nerve**.

ULTRASOUND ANATOMY

The ***m. biceps femoris*** should be observed beneath the US transducer (near field) (Figure 25.3). The **sciatic nerve** will be in direct contact with the medial fascia of the ***m. biceps femoris*** at its thickest part and will appear as two small circles (sometimes described as looking like a pair of eyeglasses) with hypoechoic centers and hyperechoic halos (known as paraneurium (Choquet et al. 2012). Its **tibial nerve** component will usually appear larger than its **common peroneal nerve** component and will be located caudally. The ***m. semimembranosus*** will be located caudal and deep to the ***m. biceps***

(a)

(b)

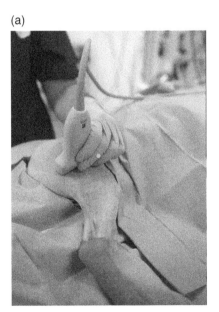
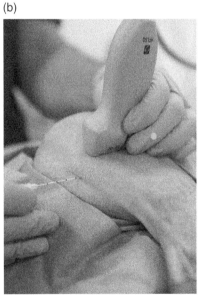

FIGURE 25.2   (a) Dog positioned in left lateral recumbency for a right **sciatic nerve** block (caudal approach). The ultrasound transducer is positioned over the midthigh, perpendicular to the femoral axis with the marker (green circle) oriented cranially. (b) Transducer and needle position for a right **sciatic nerve** block (caudal approach). The transducer is positioned over the ***m. biceps femoris*** perpendicular to the femur. The marker (green circle) is oriented cranially and the needle is advanced in-plane relative to the transducer.

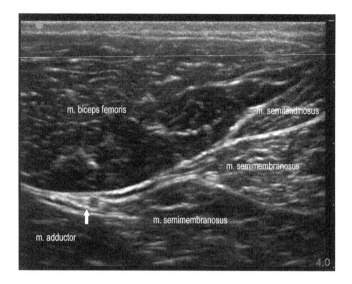

FIGURE 25.3 Ultrasonographic image of the **sciatic nerve** in short-axis view. The marker (green circle) is oriented cranially.

femoris and the *m. semitendinosus* will be seen in a more caudal location. Deep to the *m. biceps femoris* and **sciatic nerve**, the *m. adductor* will be seen.

NEEDLE INSERTION TECHNIQUE

The needle puncture site will be located somewhere on the caudal aspect of the thigh (Figure 25.4). Use the depth markers on the US screen to determine how deep the nerve is relative to the *m. biceps femoris* and the US transducer on the skin. The needle should puncture the skin on the caudal aspect of the limb at this approximate depth before slowly being advanced in-plane toward the nerve. This will allow the needle

to be perpendicular to the US beam, making it more visible and easier to track as it approaches the nerve. Keep the needle tip in the field of view at all times. Stop advancing the needle when the tip gets close to the **tibial** (i.e. caudal, closest to the needle) component of the **sciatic nerve**.

The muscular branches of the **sciatic nerve** are located in the intersection of the two bellies of the *m. semimembranosus* and the *m. biceps femoris*. If the needle path is near this location, involuntary contractions of the hamstrings may be observed as a result of direct physical or electrical stimulation of these branches (if nerve stimulation is being used).

EXPECTED MOTOR RESPONSES FROM NERVE STIMULATION

A positive response to **sciatic nerve** stimulation can be observed as either dorsiflexion or plantar extension of the tarsus (foot). Plantar extension of the tarsus will result from stimulation of the caudal aspect of the nerve (**tibial nerve** component) and will usually be observed first since the needle comes in close proximity to this aspect of the nerve first when approaching from a caudal direction. Dorsiflexion of the tarsus results from stimulation of the cranial aspect of the nerve (**common peroneal nerve** component). Both patterns of motor response are considered to be acceptable endpoints.

ADMINISTRATION OF LOCAL ANESTHETIC – WHAT TO LOOK FOR, WHAT TO FEEL FOR, DECISION POINTS

After appropriate needle positioning has been achieved and a negative aspiration test has been verified, the local anesthetic can be slowly injected. During injection, the **sciatic nerve** will

(a)

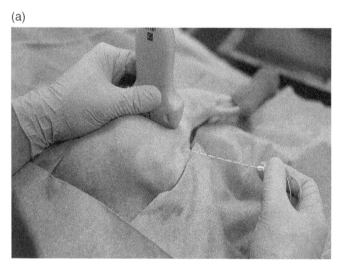

(b)

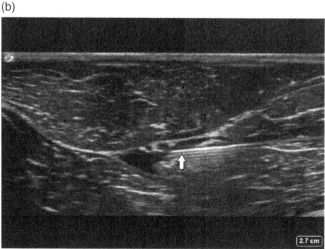

FIGURE 25.4 (a) Right **sciatic nerve** block in a dog. The ultrasound transducer is positioned on the lateral aspect of the midthigh over the *m. biceps femoris*. The marker (blue circle) is oriented cranially. (b) Corresponding ultrasonographic image. The blue logo is oriented cranially. Observe the needle tip (white arrow) located in the vicinity of the **sciatic nerve**. Local anesthetic (hypoechoic pocket) is being injected deep to the **sciatic nerve**.

be highlighted by the contrast produced by the hypoechoic fluid distributing around the nerve. No resistance to injection should be appreciated. As it is being administered, the local anesthetic should be seen dispersing under and around the nerve. It can be helpful to have an assistant perform the injection so the anesthetist can manipulate the needle in real-time under US guidance to ensure ideal dispersion of the administered solution. If certain fascial planes were not completely penetrated as the needle was advanced toward its final location, the local anesthetic will be observed dispersing away from the nerve, within the muscles themselves. In this case, breaking/piercing the cranial aspect of the fascia of the *m. semimembranosus* with the needle may help facilitate cranial diffusion of the local anesthetic solution around the **sciatic nerve**.

Although it is commonly observed during local anesthetic administration, complete detachment of the **sciatic nerve** away from the fascia of the *m. biceps femoris* is not considered essential or necessary to obtain a good block. Clinically, no differences in the intensity or duration of the resulting nerve block can be appreciated if the **sciatic nerve** is not completely surrounded in local anesthetic solution.

BLOCK EFFECTS AND PATIENT MANAGEMENT

Blockade of the **sciatic nerve** at this midthigh location will result in motor paralysis of the flexors and extensors of the paw. This will lead to an abnormal pseudohypermetric gait in which the stifle is raised excessively to overcome the inability to flex the tarsus. Additionally, proprioception will also be impeded, causing knuckling. Abrasions of the nails, toes, and dorsal aspect of the paw can be observed if this effect of the block is not addressed appropriately. Walking on rough or abrasive surfaces should be avoided, if possible (or a light bandage should be applied to the paw until the block has worn off).

COMPLICATIONS AND HOW TO AVOID THEM

It is good practice to scan the entire area involved in the nerve block prior to performing the procedure. Although muscles are the only tissues that would be expected to be present in the caudal aspect of the thigh where the block is performed (which is why it is such a good location to perform the block), in some patients, aberrant blood vessels in the vicinity of the planned needle track may be able to be detected using US. For this reason, it is useful to scan through the entire area where the needle may track toward the nerve prior to needle placement to make sure that the anatomy looks normal before the block is performed. If abnormal structures are found to be present, a different needle puncture site or trajectory can be planned.

In large dogs, the entire needle track (i.e. from the puncture site on the skin to the **sciatic nerve**) may not be able to fit on the US screen. In these situations, the transducer will initially need to be positioned caudally in order to locate the needle and glide it cranially as the needle is being advanced toward the nerve while keeping the needle tip in the field of view at all times.

COMMON MISTAKES AND HOW TO AVOID THEM

The muscular branches of the **sciatic nerve** are located at the intersection of the bellies of the *m. semimembranosus* and the *m. biceps femoris*. If the needle path is in close proximity to this location, involuntary contractions of the hamstrings may be observed as a result of direct physical or electrical stimulation of these branches. Avoidance of this area as the needle is being advanced is important to avoid causing unnecessary trauma of these nerves.

HOW TO TALK TO CLIENTS/PROFESSIONAL COLLEAGUES

- For an experienced clinician, the block should take less than three minutes to perform.

- Depending on the local anesthetic that is used, a **sciatic nerve** block will provide analgesia to the affected area for up to 18–24 hours, with nerve deficits being expected to last up to 24 hours.

- Additional pain management in the postoperative period should include icing of the incision site (e.g. for 15 minutes, 3–4 times a day) and administration of oral analgesics (e.g. NSAIDs, pregabalin) for the following 5–7 days.

REFERENCES

Acquafredda C, Stabile M, Lacitignola L et al. (2021) Clinical efficacy of dexmedetomidine combined with lidocaine for femoral and sciatic nerve blocks in dogs undergoing stifle surgery. Vet Anaesth Analg 48, 962–971.

Campoy L, Bezuidenhout AJ, Gleed RD et al. (2010) Ultrasound-guided approach for axillary brachial plexus, femoral nerve, and sciatic nerve blocks in dogs. Vet Anaesth Analg 37, 144–153.

Choquet O, Morau D, Biboulet P et al. (2012) Where should the tip of the needle be located in ultrasound-guided peripheral nerve blocks? Curr Opin Anaesthesiol 25, 596–602.

Echeverry DF, Gil F, Laredo F et al. (2010) Ultrasound-guided block of the sciatic and femoral nerves in dogs: a descriptive study. Vet J 186, 210–215.

Ferrero C, Borland K, Rioja E (2021) Retrospective comparison of three locoregional techniques for pelvic limb surgery in dogs. Vet Anaesth Analg 48, 554–562.

Gurney MA, Leece EA (2014) Analgesia for pelvic limb surgery. A review of peripheral nerve blocks and the extradural technique. Vet Anaesth Analg 41, 445–458.

Haro P, Laredo F, Gil F et al. (2012) Ultrasound-guided block of the feline sciatic nerve. J Feline Med Surg 14, 545–552.

Marolf V, Selz J, Picavet P et al. (2022) Effects of perineural dexmedetomidine combined with ropivacaine on postoperative methadone requirements in dogs after tibial plateau levelling osteotomy: a two-centre study. Vet Anaesth Analg 49, 313–322.

Marolf V, Spadavecchia C, Müller N et al. (2021) Opioid requirements after locoregional anaesthesia in dogs undergoing tibial plateau levelling osteotomy: a pilot study. Vet Anaesth Analg 48, 398–406.

Portela DA, Verdier N, Otero PE (2018) Regional anesthetic techniques for the pelvic limb and abdominal wall in small animals: a review of the literature and technique description. Vet J 238, 27–40.

Shilo Y, Pascoe PJ, Cissell D et al. (2010) Ultrasound-guided nerve blocks of the pelvic limb in dogs. In: Vet Anaesth Analg 37,. 460–470.

Vettorato E, Bradbrook C, Gurney M et al. (2012) Peripheral nerve blocks of the pelvic limb in dogs: a retrospective clinical study. In: Vet Comp Orthop Traumatol 25, 314–320.

Ultrasound-Guided Pudendal Nerve Block in Male Cats

CHAPTER 26

Chiara Adami

What is it used for?

- To improve perioperative analgesia in male cats undergoing perineal urethrostomy or potentially any other surgery involving the urethra and/or penis.

- To facilitate urethral stone retropulsion.

Landmarks/transducer position

- *Adami's approach* – The linear ultrasound (US) transducer should be positioned parasagittal to dorsal midline at the level of the pelvis, between the ischiatic tuberosity and the transverse processes of the caudal sacrum and first two coccygeal vertebrae. This should allow visualization of the pubic bone and the long axis of the urethra that are used as ultrasonographic landmarks.

- *Briley's approach (cadaveric study)* – With the cat in a frog-legged position, a micro-convex transducer is positioned over the dorsolateral aspect of the gluteal region to visualize the area of interest delimited by the sacral transverse process craniomedially, the ischiatic spine and the pelvic fascia caudolaterally, and the rectum ventrally. The needle may be inserted in this area, using an in-plane technique, from a position either cranial or caudal to the transducer.

What equipment and personnel are required?

- Urinary catheter
- 24–22G 50 mm blunt atraumatic needle
- Syringe of drug(s)
- Ultrasound machine
- High frequency (10–16 MHz) linear or micro-convex array transducer +/− protective sleeve
- +/− Disposable external needle guide
- Sterile gloves
- Coupling agent (e.g. alcohol)
- Ideally, an assistant to help position the patient and perform the injection

When do I perform the block?

- Prior to surgery, after the area is clipped and skin preparation is complete. Final skin preparation will still be needed prior to surgery.

What volume of local anesthetic is used?

- $0.3\,ml\,kg^{-1}$ to be divided equally and injected at two sites (i.e. left and right sides).

Goal:

- During injection, the local anesthetic should spread dorsal and lateral to the urethra.

Complexity level:

- Advanced

Clinical pearl:

- Empty the rectum prior to performing the block to improve visibility of the ultrasonographic landmarks.

- Use echogenic needles equipped with blunt tips to decrease the risk of iatrogenic puncture of the pelvic anatomical structures.

WHAT DO WE ALREADY KNOW?

The **pudendal nerve** block is an US-guided peripheral nerve block that can be used to provide analgesia to the penis and urethra of male cats. In a prospective, blinded, and controlled clinical study carried out on 18 cats undergoing perineal urethrostomy, when this block was performed using bupivacaine 0.5%, it provided effective pain relief during surgery and for up to four hours post-surgery (Adami et al. 2014).

Small Animal Regional Anesthesia and Analgesia, Second Edition. Edited by Matt Read, Luis Campoy, and Berit Fischer.
© 2024 John Wiley & Sons, Inc. Published 2024 by John Wiley & Sons, Inc.

Recently, an US-guided transgluteal technique for blocking the **pudendal nerve** near its sacral origin was described in cat cadavers (Briley et al. 2022). Although the analgesic efficacy of the technique was not tested in living cats, the **pudendal nerve** was successfully stained with dye in 75% of the cadavers with injection volumes of 0.1 and 0.2 ml kg⁻¹, which suggests that a US-guided transgluteal **pudendal nerve** block may be useful in cats. Further research in live animals is necessary before clinical use of this technique can be recommended.

PATIENT SELECTION

INDICATIONS FOR THE BLOCK

This block can be used to provide perioperative analgesia to male cats undergoing perineal urethrostomy surgery. It may also be used to facilitate urethral stone retropulsion as well as potentially provide analgesia to patients undergoing other surgical procedures involving the penis or urethra.

CONTRAINDICATIONS

- Any pathological condition affecting the pelvis that may alter the gross anatomy and/or the ultrasonographic appearance of the major landmarks.

- Obstipation, which can compromise the visualization and identification of relevant sonographic landmarks.

- Skin infections or lesions affecting the site(s) of needle insertion.

POTENTIAL SIDE EFFECTS AND COMPLICATIONS

- Urinary retention/dysfunction may result from detrusor muscle hypomotility.

- Loss of anal tone may result from concurrent blockade of the **rectal perineal nerve**.

- Penile protrusion may occur in patients in which amputation of the penis is not performed. This can result from blockade of sacral spinal nerves when there is cranio–dorsal spread of the injectate (Boggs et al. 2006; Tai et al. 2007; Yoo et al. 2008a).

- Other potential complications may include inadvertent or accidental puncture or laceration of the rectum, urethra, pelvic vessels, or sacral spinal nerves.

GENERAL CONSIDERATIONS

CLINICAL ANATOMY

The feline **pudendal nerve** is a multi-fasciculated trunk that arises at a mid-sacral level from the convergence of the S2 and S3 sacral spinal nerves. Before merging to form the main trunk of the **pudendal nerve** with the S2 spinal nerve,

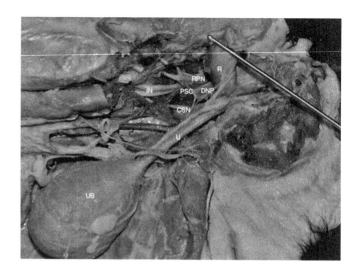

FIGURE 26.1   Dissection of the feline pelvic region showing the right **pudendal nerve** and related anatomy. The left hemipelvis and associated structures have been removed. CSN, **Cranial sensory nerve**; DNP, **dorsal nerve of the penis**; IN, **ischiatic (sciatic) nerve**; PSC, **pudendal nerve** (sensory component); RPN, **rectal perineal nerve**; U, urethra; UB, urinary bladder; R, rectum.

the S3 spinal nerve also supplies a branch to the **rectal perineal nerve**.

The sensory component of the **pudendal nerve** runs ventro–caudal from its sacral emergence until it reaches the dorsal aspect of the urethra, approximately midway between the penis and the neck of the urinary bladder. Some fibers derived from the sensory branch provide differential innervation of the proximal and distal urethra and will evoke pudendal reflexes, such as external urethral sphincter relaxation and contraction, if electrically stimulated. Dorsal to the urethra, the sensory trunk of the **pudendal nerve** branches into the **cranial sensory nerve**, which supplies the prostate, and the dorsal nerve of the penis, which provides sensory innervation to both the distal urethra and the penis (Mariano et al. 2008; Yoo et al. 2008b) (Figure 26.1).

EXPECTED DISTRIBUTION OF ANESTHESIA

The local anesthetic should be deposited bilaterally at the level of the dorsal aspect of the urethral flexure in order to reach both sensory branches of the **pudendal nerve** (**cranial sensory nerve** and **dorsal nerve of the penis**). When performed as described, the **pudendal nerve** block would be expected to produce sensory blockade of the penis, as well as to the portion of the urethra caudal to the urethral flexure.

LOCAL ANESTHETIC: DOSE, VOLUME, AND CONCENTRATION

Any local anesthetic (e.g. bupivacaine, ropivacaine, and levobupivacaine) can be used.

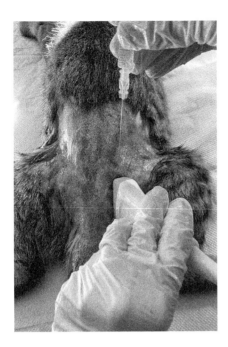

FIGURE 26.2 Performance of a **pudendal nerve** block in a cat. Note the positioning of the ultrasound transducer on a parasagittal plane, cranio–medial to the ischiatic tuberosity, and lateral to the vertebral column at the level of the base of the tail (first intercoccygeal junction). The needle is being advanced on an in-plane trajectory.

A total injection volume of 0.3 ml kg^{-1} should be used, with the volume being divided equally between the left and right sides.

PATIENT PREPARATION AND POSITIONING

The **pudendal nerve** block is performed with the patient under general anesthesia and positioned in sternal recumbency. A urinary catheter may be placed prior to performing the block to enhance urethral visualization. The pelvic limbs should be extended with the feet directed caudally ("frog-legged"). An area of skin over the dorsal pelvis, extending from mid-sacrum to the perineum, should be clipped and surgically prepared. The area to be clipped and prepared is considerably more extensive than for a standard urethrostomy, a drawback that may prevent some cat owners from giving their consent for the block (Figure 26.2).

STEP-BY-STEP PERFORMANCE

SURFACE ANATOMY AND LANDMARKS TO BE USED

Using the caudal sacrum and first two coccygeal vertebrae as palpable anatomic landmarks, the US transducer should be positioned on a parasagittal plane, cranio–medial to the ischiatic tuberosity, lateral to the caudal sacrum and the first coccygeal vertebra (i.e. the transducer should be positioned longitudinal to the long axis of the patient at the level of the base of the tail). A properly positioned transducer should be abaxial and parallel to the vertebral column with the midpoint marker on the transducer at the level of the first intercoccygeal junction (Adami et al. 2013). Positioned this way, the US beam will be aligned with the long axis of the urethra.

ULTRASOUND ANATOMY

The bulbourethral glands and pubic bone should be used as the primary ultrasonographic landmarks (Figure 26.3). The urinary catheter will appear as a hyperechoic double-line within the lumen of the urethra. After identifying these structures, the transducer can be tilted (so the beam aims medially) up to 45°with respect to the parasagittal plane to visualize the rectum and look for abnormalities. The transducer should then be tilted back into its original parasagittal plane prior to needle insertion (Adami et al. 2013).

A slightly different transgluteal approach, using a micro-convex transducer in an oblique, parasacral orientation, has recently been described in cat cadavers with the purpose of blocking the **pudendal nerve** trunk at the level of the ischiorectal fossa, prior to the point of bifurcation into the **sensory branch** and the **rectal perineal branch** (Briley et al. 2022). This approach allowed visualization of the sacral transverse process craniomedially, the ischiatic spine and the pelvic fascia caudolaterally, and the rectum ventrally within the same acoustic window.

NEEDLE INSERTION TECHNIQUE

The use of a disposable external needle-guide mounted onto the US transducer has been described as a way of facilitating accurate needle insertion when performing this block (Adami et al. 2013). The decision of whether a needle-guide will be used is influenced by the absolute need to maintain the needle in-plane with the US beam while it is being advanced. This is particularly important considering that the needle is being inserted into the pelvic cavity and puncture of important pelvic organs, and blood vessels must be avoided. An experienced anesthetist with advanced expertise in US-guided nerve blocks may be able to perform the block without the use of a needle guide.

The needle should be inserted using an in-plane technique from the cranial aspect of the US transducer, allowing the tip of the needle to be visualized throughout its course. The needle should be advanced towards the urethra until the needle tip reaches its final position on the dorsal aspect of the urethra.

EXPECTED MOTOR RESPONSES FROM NERVE STIMULATION

This block does not routinely involve the use of nerve stimulation.

(a)

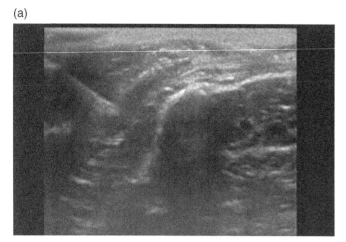

(b)

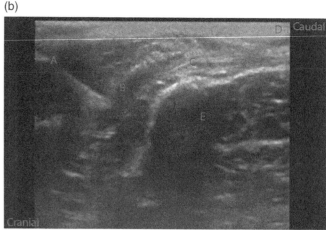

FIGURE 26.3   (a) Ultrasonographic landmarks for the para-coccygeal **pudendal nerve** block. (b) Same image, with labels. A, Needle; B, long axis of the urethra; C, urinary catheter; D, bulbourethral glands; E, pubic bone (shadow).

ADMINISTRATION OF LOCAL ANESTHETIC – WHAT TO LOOK FOR, WHAT TO FEEL FOR, DECISION POINTS

Aspiration to verify extravascular location of the needle tip should be performed prior to drug administration. As the local anesthetic is injected, it should distribute evenly and be visualized as a pocket of fluid dorsal and lateral to the urethra. Following injection, the needle should be withdrawn, and the procedure repeated on the contralateral side.

In patients where it is not possible to identify the required ultrasonographic landmarks or visualize the distribution of the local anesthetic during the injection, the block attempt should be aborted, and the needle withdrawn.

BLOCK EFFECTS (SENSORY, MOTOR, ETC.) AND PATIENT MANAGEMENT

The block provides effective pain relief intraoperatively and in the early postoperative period (for ~four hours) following perineal urethrostomy (Adami et al. 2014).

COMPLICATIONS AND HOW TO AVOID THEM

Complications can be potentially severe and, for this reason, the patient should be assessed frequently within the first 12 hours following the block.

- In case of urinary retention, the urethra should be catheterized to empty the urinary bladder.

- Loss of anal tone following surgery may result in contamination of the surgical site with feces, a complication that requires prompt intervention to avoid incisional infection and delayed healing.

- Overdilation of the urethra may predispose to urethral puncture when the needle approaches the dorsal urethral wall.

- Inadvertent puncture of the rectum during the block could result from poor technique and failure to visualize and locate the rectum within the acoustic window.

- Puncture of vessels, such as the pudendal vein and artery, with consequent hematoma formation, is another potential sequel of the block.

COMMON MISTAKES AND HOW TO AVOID THEM

When the US transducer is positioned too close to the sacrum, it may result in decreased visibility of the ultrasonographic landmarks owing to acoustic shadowing caused by the bony prominences. In small cats, this may be avoided by using a smaller US transducer. Attempting the block in the presence of feces or gas within the rectum may result in the identification of the ultrasonographic landmarks being more difficult. Moreover, the presence of an enlarged rectum will greatly increase the risk of rectal puncture during needle insertion. For these reasons, it is recommended to empty the rectum before attempting the nerve block.

HOW TO TALK TO CLIENTS/PROFESSIONAL COLLEAGUES

Extensive clipping should be discussed in advanced with the cat's owner to avoid misunderstandings and potential complaints when the cat is discharged. Performing the block should not take more than 10 minutes, although this may vary depending on the level of expertise of the anesthetist. If longer times are anticipated, it may be advisable to discuss this with the surgery team.

Adami C, Angeli G, Haenssgen K et al. (2013) Development of an ultrasound-guided technique for pudendal nerve block in cat cadavers. J Feline Med Surg 10, 901–907.

Adami C, Dayer T, Spadavecchia C et al. (2014) Ultrasound-guided pudendal nerve block in cats undergoing perineal urethrostomy: a prospective, randomised, investigator-blind, placebo-controlled clinical trial. J Feline Med Surg 16, 340–345.

Boggs JW, Wenzel BJ, Gustafson KJ et al. (2006) Frequency-dependent selection of reflexes by pudendal afferents in the cat. J Physiol 577, 115–126.

Briley JD, Keenihan EK, Mathews KG et al. (2022) Development of an ultrasound-guided transgluteal injection of the pudendal nerve in cats: a cadaveric study. Vet Anaesth Analg 49, 189–196.

Mariano TY, Boger AS, Gustafson KJ. (2008) The feline dorsal nerve of the penis arises from the deep perineal nerve and not the sensory afferent branch. Anat Histol Embryol 37, 166–168.

Tai C, Wang J, Wang X et al. (2007) Bladder inhibition or voiding induced by pudendal nerve stimulation in chronic spinal cord injured cats. Neurourol Urodyn 26, 570–577.

Yoo PB, Woock JP, Grill WM. (2008a) Somatic innervation of the feline lower urinary tract. Brain Res 1246, 80–87.

Yoo PB, Woock JP, Grill WM. (2008b) Bladder activation by selective stimulation of pudendal nerve afferents in the cat. Exp Neurol 212, 218–225.

Ultrasound-Assisted Epidural Anesthesia

Matt Read, Berit L. Fischer, and Luis Campoy

CHAPTER 27

BLOCK AT A GLANCE

What is it used for?

- Ultrasound can be used to assist with performance of epidural injections in patients where traditional methods of identifying the correct intervertebral space and/or confirmation that the drugs are being administered in the correct location are challenging.

Landmarks/transducer position

- Depending on the species and the technique to be used, the transducer should be placed over the regions of the lumbosacral and/or sacrococcygeal intervertebral spaces.

What equipment and personnel are required?

- 22G 1.5 in. or 20G 2.5 in. Tuohy needle (appropriate to the patient)

- Syringe of drug(s)

- Ultrasound machine

- High frequency (15–6 MHz) linear array transducer +/− protective sleeve

- +/− Mid-frequency curvilinear transducer +/− protective sleeve

- Sterile gloves

- Aseptic skin preparation solutions (e.g. chlorhexidine and alcohol)

- Coupling agent (e.g. alcohol)

- Skin marker pen

When do I perform the block?

- Prior to surgery, after the skin over the lumbosacral and/or sacrococcygeal intervertebral spaces has been clipped and skin preparation is complete.

What volume of local anesthetic is used?

- Like other epidural injections, drug choices (i.e. opioids, local anesthetic, etc.) and doses are based on patient and procedural considerations, with the goal of achieving the desired effects while minimizing side effects.

Goals:

- To use US imaging to identify the anatomical structures that can be used to localize the site for performing an epidural injection, to measure the distance from the skin to epidural space, to visualize needle placement in real time, and/or to visualize the injection being made at the correct location (i.e. in epidural space).

Complexity level:

- Basic to intermediate

WHAT DO WE ALREADY KNOW?

Epidural anesthesia has been used since the beginning of the twentieth century as a means of providing locoregional anesthesia for a variety of procedures in both human and veterinary medicine (Franco and Diz 2000; Otero and Campoy 2013). Traditional means of identifying the epidural space have included "*loss of resistance*" (low specificity) and/or "*hanging drop*" (high specificity, low sensitivity). However, both techniques demonstrate unreliability when used alone and can result in failure rates of up to 30% (Adami and Gendron 2017; Liotta et al. 2015). Other confirmatory methods, including the use of electrical stimulation and the detection of epidural pressure waves, either require specialized equipment, lack consensus on the methodology to be used, or lack sensitivity, preventing these techniques from being adopted more widely in clinical practice (Adami and Gendron 2017).

The use of US to assist and/or provide direct guidance for performing epidurals, either for single injections or for epidural catheter placement, has been described in humans, dogs, and cats (Cork et al. 1980; Liotta et al. 2015; Otero et al. 2016). Cork et al. (1980) performed one of the first blinded, randomized controlled trials in people that incorporated the use of US assistance to identify the desired intervertebral space and measure the distance from skin to the ligamentum flavum prior to performing epidural injections. In that study, successful epidural injections were achieved in 32/36 attempts and the predicted distances demonstrated excellent correlation to actual measured needle insertion depths. At that time, the clinical use of US for anesthesia purposes was still in its infancy and subsequent studies that utilized US imaging for epidural administration did not materialize for another 20 years.

In 2001, Grau and colleagues published the results of six different studies that described the ultrasonographic anatomy of the human spine and associated vasculature, compared various different transducer orientations for best visualization and access, and compared conventional methods of epidural space detection with the use of US in people (Grau et al. 2001a, b, c, d, e, f). These studies concluded that using US to assist with epidural injections was clinically feasible and likely provided benefits over conventional methods.

Since then, several meta-analyses and systematic reviews have examined the accuracy of needle placement and the efficacy, efficiency, and safety of using US assistance when performing neuraxial techniques compared to using palpation alone (Neal et al. 2016; Perlas et al. 2016; Sidiropoulou et al. 2021; Jain et al. 2022). Those reports concluded that: (1) the use of preprocedural US to determine the intervertebral level is more accurate than using palpation alone (71% versus 29%, respectively) (Perlas et al. 2016); (2) the depth to the epidural space that is measured with US is highly correlated with actual needle insertion depth ($r = 0.91$), often differing by less than 3 mm (Neal et al. 2016); (3) the use of US increases "first attempt" success rates and decreases the number of needle redirections that are needed before the needle enters the epidural space (Perlas et al. 2016; Sidiropoulou et al. 2021; Jain et al. 2022) – benefiting patients whose epidural injections might already be challenging (including elderly or pediatric patients, those with spinal abnormalities, and/or those with higher body mass index) (Chin 2018; Jain et al. 2022); and (4) the use of US resulted in a 31% decrease in overall epidural failure rates compared to conventional methods (a figure that increases to 47% in patients with spinal abnormalities or who are obese) (Sidiropoulou et al. 2021).

Although the overall incidence of complications following epidural injections is too low to be included in these meta-analyses, individual studies have shown that using US to assist with epidural injections decreases the risk of trauma, dural puncture, and procedural bleeding when compared to conventional methods (Perlas et al. 2016; Chin 2018; Jain et al. 2022).

The veterinary literature investigating the use of US assistance for epidural anesthesia is small in comparison. The first description of ultrasonographic anatomy of the canine lumbar and caudal spine was by Etienne et al. (2010) who were able to identify the L5–L6 interspace and successfully obtain cerebrospinal fluid samples from 8/10 live dogs. In 2014, Gregori et al. similarly described the ultrasonographic anatomy of the sacrococcygeal space in cadavers and clinical patients, followed by the use of an out-of-plane technique to perform epidurals at that location. That same year, Liotta et al. (2015) used US to perform both lumbosacral epidural injections and/or place epidural catheters in 20 dog cadavers and five live dogs, with the transducer positioned using a parasagittal orientation that allowed for in-plane advancement of a spinal or Touhy needle into the epidural space. Computed tomography (CT) scans following injections demonstrated successful epidural injections in all dogs; however, variable amounts of subarachnoid contamination were present in 85% of cadavers and 100% of live dogs.

Viscasillas et al. (2016) investigated four different approaches for accessing the epidural space in dog cadavers using US, followed by CT confirmation of needle placement. Those authors determined that the use of an in-plane technique was more successful for assisting epidural placement in the lumbar spine than an out-of-plane technique (95% versus 45%), with success being further dependent on the operator's level of experience with US-guided procedures, especially when performing out-of-plane techniques.

A study by Otero et al. (2016) was the first to describe the sonographic lumbar anatomy of cats, to predict needle depth insertion via preprocedural US measurements, and to successfully utilize color flow Doppler to verify epidural injection in real time. A similar, real-time method was utilized by Credie and Luna (2018) for confirming sacrococcygeal epidural injections in cats. Those authors, who recognized the difficulty in obtaining US images and performing injections at the same time in the sacrococcygeal location, obtained transverse views of the lumbosacral junction and observed the injections in the epidural space, visualized as the ventral displacement of the dura and enlargement of the epidural space.

More recently, attention has focused on the benefits of using US to assist with performing epidural injections in obese patients (da Silva et al. 2020; Credie and Luna 2022). Similar to the situation in obese people, performing epidural injections in this subpopulation of veterinary patients can be technically challenging due to the usual landmarks not being as readily palpable and the increased depth from the skin to the target. A study of seven obese dogs undergoing elective orthopedic surgery used US to measure the distance from skin to the epidural space and identify the optimal point of needle insertion on the skin (da Silva et al. 2020). Those authors were able to identify the lumbosacral junction, successfully access the epidural space in all dogs on the first attempt, and demonstrate a high correlation between the depth to the target site as measured by US and the actual needle insertion depth ($r = 0.996$).

Credie and Luna (2022) published the results of a study that compared the use of US assistance to palpation/loss of resistance techniques for performing epidural injections in both obese and nonobese dogs. Similar to what has been previously reported in people, those authors identified that, regardless of body condition, palpation techniques resulted in more needle-bone contact events (i.e. increased number of needle redirections) and a higher incidence of blood aspiration (11.1% and 22.2% in nonobese and obese dogs, respectively, versus 5.5% and 0% in the US groups).

The use of US for assisting epidural injections has not been adopted on a large scale in veterinary medicine to date since it is still considered by many people to be an advanced technique that is associated with a steep learning curve. This is also true in human patients, with some studies indicating that trainees need to perform a minimum of 10–20 supervised procedures before achieving competence (Chin 2018). Other reasons for its use not being widely incorporated into clinical practice may include the need for specialized equipment (e.g. an US machine with a high-frequency transducer) and the fact that its additional value may not be recognized, especially for patients with easily palpable landmarks or for experienced anesthetists who are adept at performing epidural injections in most of their patients.

PATIENT SELECTION

INDICATIONS FOR USING ULTRASOUND TO ASSIST WITH AN EPIDURAL INJECTION

When used to assist with performance of an epidural injection, US can help identify the puncture site and provide information regarding the ideal insertion angle for the needle, the expected depth to the target location, and to confirm that the injection is being made at the correct location.

CONTRAINDICATIONS

The use of epidural anesthesia and analgesia has several relative and absolute contraindications that have previously been described (Otero and Campoy 2013). The use of US to assist with performance of an epidural injection does not, in itself, have any contraindications and may, as described above, actually make the procedure safer for patients (Credie and Luna 2022).

In general, epidural anesthesia should not be performed, with or without the use of US-assistance, if any of the following are present:

- Skin infection or other lesions at the intended needle puncture site;

- Inability to identify the relevant anatomy during palpation or US scanning;

- Preexisting neurological deficits relating to the anatomical area to be blocked;

- Preexisting, uncorrected coagulopathy or thrombocytopenia;

- Spinal trauma or abnormal anatomy involving the lumbosacral area;

- Preexisting hemodynamic disturbances such as uncorrected hypovolemia or hypotension (if local anesthetics are being used).

GENERAL CONSIDERATIONS
CLINICAL ANATOMY

The target site for the majority of epidural injections in dogs and cats is the lumbosacral intervertebral space (L7–S1), although the sacrococcygeal intervertebral space has recently gained popularity. At the lumbosacral level, the transverse processes of the seventh lumbar vertebra are directed cranially and slightly ventrally and the cranial articular processes bear the mamillary processes. The caudal articular processes of the seventh lumbar vertebra articulate with the cranial articular processes of the sacrum. Caudally, the bodies and processes of the three sacral vertebrae are fused to form the sacrum. The median sacral crest represents the fusion of the three sacral spinous processes (Figure 27.1).

The supraspinous ligament attaches to the apices of the vertebral spinous processes while the interspinous ligament, formed by the fibrous tissue in between the two left and right epaxial muscles coming together, connects the spinous processes from top to bottom. The roof of the vertebral canal is formed by the *interarcuate ligament* (also called the "*ligamentum flavum*" or "*yellow ligament*"). At the lumbosacral level, the vertebral canal in dogs is elliptical in cross section and contains the epidural (extradural) space, the dural sac, and the *cauda equina*.

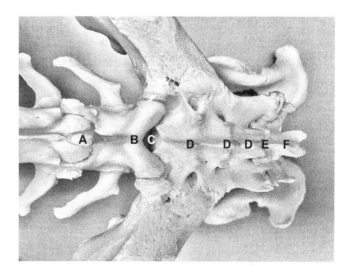

FIGURE 27.1   Dorsal view of a dog pelvis and caudal lumbar vertebrae. A, Spinous process of the seventh lumbar vertebra; B, caudal lamina of the seventh lumbar vertebra; C, lumbosacral intervertebral space; D, median sacral crest; E, sacrococcygeal intervertebral space; and F, first coccygeal vertebra.

Caudally, the spinal cord tapers into a conical structure called the *conus medullaris*. In large breed dogs, the spinal cord typically extends caudally as far as the sixth or seventh lumbar vertebrae, while in small breed dogs, it may continue to the level of the lumbosacral space (Fletcher and Kitchell 1966). From birth until four to six months of age, the spinal cord in dogs may extend caudally as far as the sacrum (Aarnes and Muir 2011). In adult cats, the spinal cord ends at the level of the sacrum (Maierl and Liebich 1998). Within the vertebral canal, the dural sac continues past the termination of the spinal cord to form the lumbar cistern, ending at the level of L6–L7 (Evans and de Lahunta 2013) (Figure 27.2).

The epidural space is located between the *dura mater* and the boundaries of the vertebral canal. In dogs, the epidural space is typically largest at the lumbosacral level where the dural sac tapers off. In cats, the average size of the epidural space at the lumbosacral level is 0.4 mm (Otero et al. 2016). The dorsal aspect of the epidural space is occupied exclusively by adipose tissue, while the wider ventrolateral compartments contain vascular, lymphatic, and neural structures (Figure 27.3).

The *cauda equina* comprises a bundle of nerve fibers formed by the roots of the caudal segments within and caudal to the dural sac, the sacrum, and around the *filum terminale*. In the dog, most of the *cauda equina* involves spinal roots with individual meningeal sheaths located within the epidural space at the level of the sacrum and the tail (Fletcher and Kitchell 1966). Caudal to the dural sac, the *dura mater* narrows, forming a thin tubular ligament (*filum durae matris spinalis*), which ensheaths the *filum terminale* and continues to the second or third coccygeal vertebrae (Figure 27.4).

PATIENT PREPARATION AND POSITIONING

In most cases, neuraxial techniques such as epidural injections are performed in dogs and cats while they are under general anesthesia, however, heavy sedation may be preferred

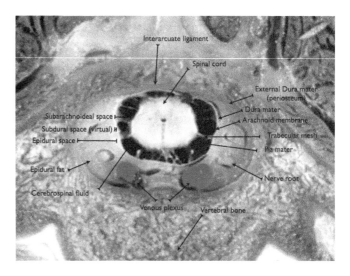

FIGURE 27.3   Transverse view (axial section) of a dog spine at the level of the fifth lumbar vertebra.

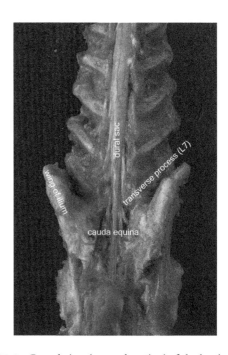

FIGURE 27.4   Dorsal view (coronal section) of the lumbar spine of a dog.

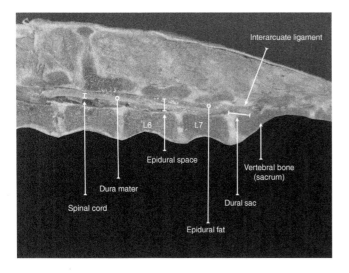

FIGURE 27.2   Lateral view (sagittal section) of the lumbar spine of a dog.

in some instances. In those situations, infiltration of the puncture site (i.e. skin and interspinous ligament) with 1% buffered lidocaine (e.g. commercially available – pH corrected) may increase patient tolerance to the procedure.

To perform an epidural injection, the animal may be placed in either sternal or lateral recumbency, depending on the patient's medical condition and clinician preference. In a study carried out on canine cadavers, no differences in the number of stained nerve roots were observed following epidural injection of new methylene blue solution when the dogs were positioned in lateral recumbency when compared with sternal recumbency (Gorgi et al. 2006).

The spine and other important landmarks are often easier to palpate when the patient is positioned in sternal recumbency, especially in obese animals. Puggioni et al. (2006)

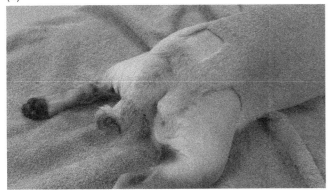

(a)

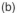

(b)

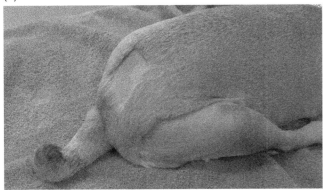

FIGURE 27.5   Positioning a Pug for a lumbosacral injection. (a) When the pelvic limbs are extended backward (i.e. frog-legged), the lumbosacral space will be narrowed, making needle placement more challenging. (a) When the pelvic limbs are extended forward, the lumbosacral space will be opened up, making needle placement easier.

showed that the greatest interarcuate space resulted when animals were in sternal recumbency with the spine flexed in a kyphotic position and the pelvic limbs were extended forward along either side of the dog's body (Figure 27.5a, b).

In lateral recumbency, the spine can be either in a neutral position or flexed. In some cases, lateral recumbency is preferred over sternal recumbency since it is easier to position a patient with pelvic or femoral fractures; however, it can be more difficult to appreciate dorsal midline in overweight patients. Regardless of the patient's position, appropriate clipping, skin preparation, and the following of aseptic technique are of paramount importance. Infections, even though rare, can be challenging to treat (Remedios et al. 1996).

ULTRASOUND-ASSISTED LUMBOSACRAL EPIDURAL INJECTION TECHNIQUE
SURFACE ANATOMY AND LANDMARKS TO BE USED

In most cases, the patient should be positioned in sternal recumbency with the legs pulled forward. The skin over the lumbosacral area should be clipped and prepared for an injection. Depending on the anesthetist's preference, the transducer can initially be positioned in either a transverse or a sagittal orientation, with the second step involving rotating the transducer 90° to verify the sonographic anatomy in a different plane. Alcohol can be used to improve skin coupling (Figure 27.6).

ULTRASOUND ANATOMY

All bony structures will appear as hyperechoic surfaces associated with distal acoustic shadowing (Liotta et al. 2015). The transducer should be positioned in a transverse orientation over the approximate level of the lumbosacral intervertebral space, with its marker oriented on the left side of the patient so the corresponding marker appears on the left side of the US

(a)

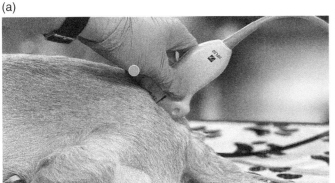

(b)

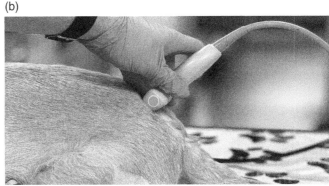

FIGURE 27.6   Orientations of an ultrasound transducer over the lumbosacral intervertebral space in a dog. (a) Sagittal orientation with marker (blue dot) oriented cranially; (b) Transverse orientation with marker (blue dot) on left side of patient, to correspond to images in Figures 27.8 and 27.7, respectively. Note the angle of the transducer is approximately 90° to the skin, similar to the trajectory that the needle will need to be advanced on.

(a)   (b)

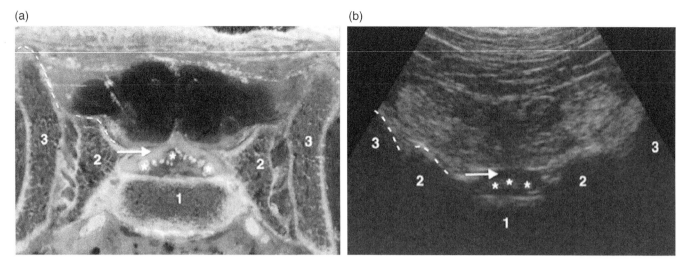

FIGURE 27.7   Comparison between the anatomic transverse slice (a) and the transverse ultrasonographic image (b) of the lumbosacral region of a dog. The sigmoid-shaped hyperechoic interface (dotted line) associated with distal acoustic shadow corresponds to the left wing of the sacrum (2) and to the left wing of the ilium (3). Within the vertebral canal, the epidural space appears hypoechoic (arrow) and surrounds the echoic internal nervous structures (*). The vertebral canal is ventrally bordered by the cranial epiphysis of the first sacral vertebra (1). Source: Liotta et al. (2015)/with permission from John Wiley & Sons, Inc.

screen. The transducer should be glided cranial and caudal and left and right until the spinous process of L7 becomes visible as a hyperechoic spot. The acoustic shadow of the spinous process of L7 should be identified (indicating midline) and the depth and gain adjusted to optimize the image (Figure 27.7).

Next, the transducer should be glided left or right to position midline in the center of the screen and tilted cranially and caudally until the optimal image of the relevant anatomy is obtained with the transducer perpendicular to the skin surface, representing the trajectory that the needle will need to be advanced along. Using the middle of the transducer as a guide, a mark(s) may be made on the skin with a pen (away from the transducer) to indicate midline.

To determine the correct level to make the injection (i.e. L7–S1), the transducer should be rotated 90° so the marker is located cranially and a sagittal view of the spinous process of L7 and the sacral crest are identified. This intervertebral space is easy to identify due to the relatively wide gap between the lamina of the last lumbar vertebra and the sacral crest (Viscasillas et al. 2016). The sacrum will appear as a continuous hyperechoic surface with three notches with distal acoustic shadowing (Liotta et al. 2015). Between the acoustic shadows of the last lumbar vertebra and the sacrum, the vertebral canal can be visualized as two straight hyperechoic lines separated by a hypoechoic space (Figure 27.8).

The transducer should then be glided cranially and caudally until the middle of the transducer is centered over the lumbosacral intervertebral space. Using the middle of the transducer as a guide, a mark(s) may be made on the skin with a pen (away from the transducer) to indicate the level of the L7–S1 space (Figure 27.9). Once the second mark is made, the

transducer can be removed and the skin should be aseptically prepared in preparation for needle placement. Alternatively, US guidance can be used to visualize a needle being advanced in-plane in a caudocranial direction under the caudal edge of the transducer until the tip of the needle is visualized in the vertebral canal (Viscasillas et al. 2016).

Visualized using a transverse transducer orientation, the vertebral canal will be hypoechoic and circular in profile and be bordered by the hyperechoic ligamentum flavum dorsally and the hyperechoic dorsal longitudinal ligament ventrally (Liotta et al. 2015). Using a sagittal transducer orientation, the vertebral canal will be visualized as a hypoechoic space between the hyperechoic ligamentum flavum dorsally and the hyperechoic dorsal longitudinal ligament ventrally (Viscasillas et al. 2016). Some authors refer to these (and their closely associated) structures as the *dorsal* and *ventral complexes* (Otero et al. 2016). Depending on the patient and the resolution of the US machine being used, the "dorsal complex" can sometimes be visualized as two discrete thin, hyperechoic lines that represent the ligamentum flavum and the dorsal dura mater, with the epidural space appearing as a thin hypoechoic line (representing fat) between them. The "ventral complex" usually appears as a second, thick hyperechoic structure on the ventral aspect of the vertebral canal. The individual components that comprise the ventral complex, the ventral dura mater, epidural space, and dorsal longitudinal ligament, may not always be distinguishable from each other as discrete structures and, more often than not, the ventral complex will simply appear as a single hyperechoic line (Figure 27.10).

Visualization of the nervous structures in the vertebral canal is variable and depends on patient size, body condition, and skin quality. Using canine cadavers, Liotta et al. (2015)

(a)

(b)

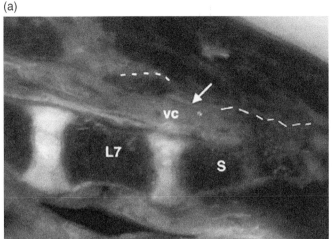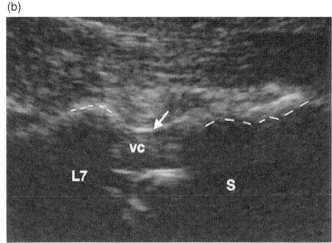

FIGURE 27.8   Comparison between the anatomic parasagittal slice (a) and the parasagittal ultrasonographic image (b) of the lumbosacral region. The caudal aspect of the lamina of the seventh lumbar vertebra (L7) appears as a curved hyperechoic line associated with distal acoustic shadow (curved dotted line). The lamina of the sacrum (S) appears as a notched hyperechoic line (notched dotted line) associated with distal acoustic shadow. The vertebral canal (VC) is bordered dorsally by a thin hyperechoic line (arrow) which corresponds to the interarcuate ligament (ligamentum flavum). Source: Liotta et al. (2015)/with permission from John Wiley & Sons, Inc.

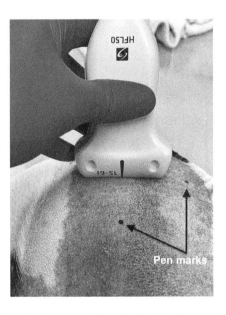

FIGURE 27.9   Looking caudally a dog that has been positioned in sternal recumbency for an epidural injection. Ultrasound has been used to identify midline and the level of the lumbosacral intervertebral space, which have been marked on the skin away from the planned injection site (that is immediately under the middle of the transducer). Once the transducer is removed, the skin can be prepared for needle placement.

were not able to differentiate the *conus medullaris* from the dural sac or nerve roots that form the *cauda equina*. In their study, transverse images showed the nervous structures as multiple, small, round hyperechoic spots, sometimes containing a hypoechoic center, while sagittal images showed the nervous structures as thin, tapering hyperechoic structures, sometimes with hypoechoic center lines.

NEEDLE INSERTION TECHNIQUE

Various approaches to using US to assist with needle placement in the epidural space of dogs and cats have been described (Gregori et al. 2014; Liotta et al. 2015; Otero et al. 2016; Viscasillas et al. 2016; Credie and Luna 2018; da Silva et al. 2020; Credie and Luna 2022). Depending on the patient, desired effects, available equipment, and skill of the anesthetist, the use of US can assist with pre-planning the injection, visualizing the needle as it is being advanced (using either an in-plane or out-of-plane technique), or monitoring the spread of the injectate in the epidural space.

After identifying the ideal location for the needle to puncture the skin and the trajectory for it to be advanced on, unless there is a desire to use US to visualize real-time needle placement, there is no need to continue to use US and routine techniques to place the needle in the epidural space may be used. In this situation, the skin over the injection site should be prepared aseptically prior to needle puncture. If real-time US guidance is to be used to further assist with the injection, the skin should be prepared for injection, and a sterile covering optionally placed over the transducer to maintain aseptic technique.

The transducer can be positioned using either a sagittal or oblique parasagittal orientation (when using an in-plane needle technique) or a transverse orientation (when using an out-of-plane needle technique) over the lumbosacral intervertebral space. Different approaches will variably allow the anesthetist to visualize the needle as it penetrates the ligamentum flavum and enters the epidural space. Alternatively, the needle can be placed into the sacrococcygeal epidural space (see below), and the US transducer placed over the lumbosacral intervertebral space to monitor the spread of injectate as it is

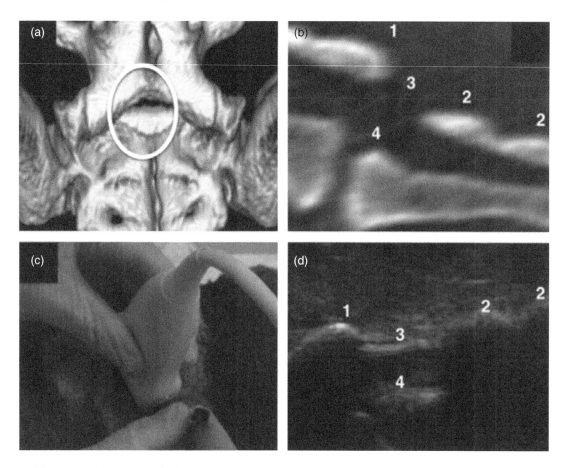

FIGURE 27.10   (a) Computed tomography (CT) image showing the dorsal view of the lumbosacral region of a dog. (b, d) Comparison between a sagittal CT image (b) and an ultrasound image (d) of the lumbosacral intervertebral space. (c) Position of a linear ultrasound probe and a needle for an in-plane approach. 1, Caudal lamina of the seventh lumbar vertebra; 2, sacrum; 3, ligamentum flavum; 4, floor of vertebral canal. Source: Viscasillas et al. (2016)/with permission from Elsevier.

being administered. Using this technique, US is used to visualize distention of the epidural space and compression of the dural sac as fluid is injected into the epidural space, resulting in separation of the dura mater from the ligamentum flavum and generation of turbulent flow that can be detected with color flow Doppler (Otero et al. 2016; Castro et al. 2020) (Figure 27.11 and 27.12).

Once the needle is in the epidural space, routine methods for checking for negative blood aspiration and assessing loss of resistance can be used prior to drug administration to optimize efficacy and safety and minimize the chances of encountering complications.

ULTRASOUND-ASSISTED SACROCOCCYGEAL EPIDURAL INJECTION TECHNIQUE

SURFACE ANATOMY AND LANDMARKS TO BE USED

In most cases, the patient should be positioned in sternal recumbency. The skin over the sacrococcygeal area from the lumbosacral area down to the proximal third of the tail should

be clipped and prepared for an injection. The transducer should be positioned in a transverse orientation over the sacrum, with its marker oriented on the left side of the patient so the corresponding marker appears on the left side of the US screen (Figure 27.13).

ULTRASOUND ANATOMY

The median sacral crest is a useful initial landmark to use and should be identified as a thin hyperechoic vertical structure that casts an anechoic shadow (Gregori et al. 2014). The sacral crest indicates midline and it should be centered on the US screen as the depth and gain are adjusted to optimize the image. Once the median sacral crest has been identified, while maintaining the shadow of the median sacral crest in the center of the US screen, the transducer should be glided caudally until the caudal sacral processes are identified as paired perpendicular hyperechoic lines. Depending on the patient and its positioning, the transducer may need to be tilted between 80° and 100° relative to the vertebral column in order to visualize the sacrococcygeal space and the floor of the

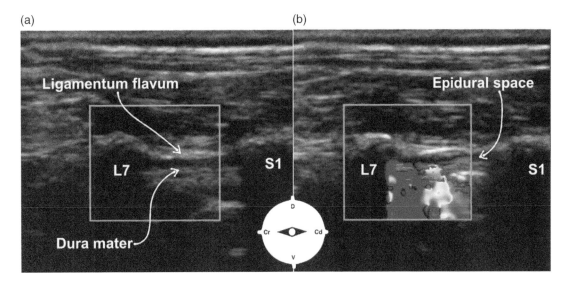

FIGURE 27.11   (a) Sonoanatomy of the lumbosacral epidural space in a dog showing the ligamentum flavum and the dura mater. (b) Positive color flow Doppler test at the lumbosacral space after a sacrococcygeal epidural injection. The red color depicts the injectate flowing in the epidural space and around the dural sac. Cd, Caudal; Cr, cranial; D, dorsal; L7, lamina of the seventh lumbar vertebra; S1, first sacral vertebra; V, ventral. Source: Castro et al. (2020)/with permission from Elsevier.

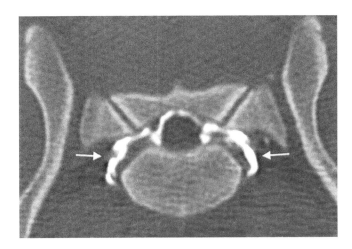

FIGURE 27.12   Transverse CT image (bone window) of the lumbosacral region of a dog showing the presence of contrast medium in the epidural space and at the exit of the intervertebral foramina (arrows). Source: Liotta et al. (2015)/with permission from John Wiley & Sons, Inc.

vertebral canal immediately caudal to the median sacral crest and caudal sacral processes (Gregori et al. 2014). The sacrococcygeal space will be visualized as a hypoechoic circular structure caudal to the sacrum, characterized by thin hyperechoic horizontal lines that represent the dorsal lamina and body of the first caudal vertebra (Figure 27.14).

NEEDLE INSERTION TECHNIQUE

A pen can be used to mark the location on the skin over the sacrococcygeal space and the angle of the transducer will represent the trajectory that the needle will likely need to be

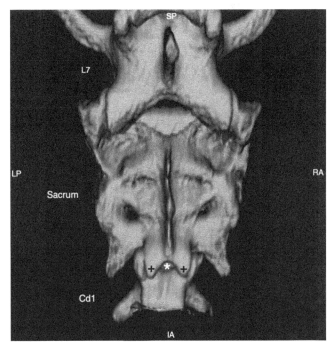

FIGURE 27.13   CT three-dimensional volume rendering of the sacrococcygeal area of a dog cadaver. The sacrococcygeal space (*) is located between the caudal aspect of the sacrum and the first caudal vertebra (Cd1). Caudal sacral processes (+), seventh lumbar vertebra (L7). Source: Gregori et al. (2014)/with permission from John Wiley & Sons, Inc.

advanced in order to enter the space. Alternatively, an out-of-plane needle technique can be used, whereby the needle is advanced along the cranial aspect of the transducer into the epidural space, with the tip of the needle being visualized in

(a)

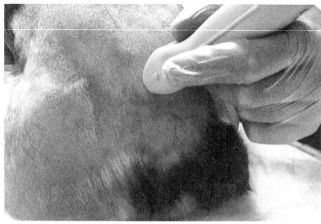

(b)

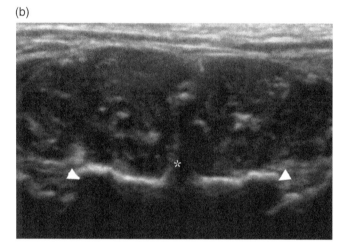

FIGURE 27.14   (a) Cadaver of a dog in sternal recumbency with hindlimbs pulled cranially. The ultrasound probe is positioned transverse to the vertebral column and the initial anatomical landmarks used to find the sacrococcygeal space were the median sacral crest (*) and the caudal sacral processes (arrowheads) (b). Source: Gregori et al. (2014)/with permission from John Wiley & Sons, Inc.

real-time entering the sacrococcygeal space and being advanced until it contacts the floor of the vertebral canal.

Once the needle is in the epidural space, routine methods for checking for negative blood aspiration and assessing loss of resistance can be used prior to drug administration

(a)

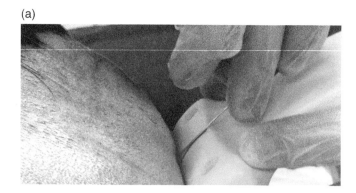

(b)

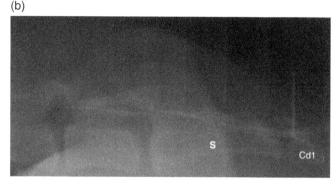

FIGURE 27.15   (a) Ultrasound-guided insertion of a needle using a 45°–60° angle in a canine cadaver. (b) Lateral horizontal beam view of the sacral area after epidural sacrococcygeal injection of 0.15 ml of iodinated contrast in the same canine cadaver showed in (a). The contrast spread to the cranial aspect of the seventh lumbar vertebra. Cd1, First caudal vertebra; S, sacrum. Source: Gregori et al. (2014)/ with permission from John Wiley & Sons, Inc.

to optimize efficacy and safety and minimize the chances of encountering complications (Figure 27.15).

CONCLUSIONS

Although the use of US to assist with epidural and intrathecal injections is still a relatively new development in dogs and cats, it holds obvious promise from both teaching and clinical standpoints. Additional prospective studies, case reports, and case series are needed to further document the potential benefits and risks of using US assistance for epidural injections and catheter placement, especially in terms of efficacy and patient safety.

REFERENCES

Aarnes T, Muir W (2011) Pain assessment and management. In: Small Animal Pediatrics: The First 12 Months of Life, 1st edition. Peterson ME, Kutzler MA (eds.) Saunders, Elsevier, USA. pp 220–232.

Adami C, Gendron K (2017) What is the evidence? The issue of verifying correct needle position during epidural anaesthesia in dogs. Vet Anaesth Analg 44, 212–218.

Castro D, Portela DA, Otero PE (2020) Positive color flow Doppler test used to confirm sacrococcygeal epidural injection in a dog. Vet Anaesth Analg 47, 280–281.

Chin KJ (2018) Recent developments in ultrasound imaging for neuraxial blockade. Curr Opin Anesthesiol 31, 608–613.

Cork RC, Kryc JJ, Vaughan RW et al. (1980) Ultrasonic localization of the lumbar epidural space. Anesthesiology 52, 513–516.

Credie L, Luna S (2018) The use of ultrasound to evaluate sacrococcygeal epidural injections in cats. Can Vet J 59, 143–146.

Credie LFGA, Luna SPI (2022) Real-time ultrasound-guided lumbosacral epidural anaesthesia in obese or appropriate body condition score dogs: a randomized clinical trial. Vet J 280, 105791.

da Silva LCBA, Pacheco PF, Sellera FP et al. (2020) The use of ultrasound to assist epidural injection in obese dogs. Vet Anaesth Analg 47, 137–140.

Etienne AL, Peeters D, Busoni V (2010) Ultrasonographic percutaneous anatomy of the caudal lumbar region and ultrasound-guided lumbar puncture in the dog. Vet Radiol Ultrasound 51, 527–532.

Evans EH, de Lahunta A (2013) Spinal nerves. Miller's Anatomy of the Dog, 4th edition. Elsevier, Missouri. pp. 611–657.

Fletcher TF, Kitchell RL (1966) Anatomical studies on the spinal cord segments of the dog. Am J Vet Res 27, 1759–1767.

Franco A, Diz JC (2000) The history of the epidural block. Curr Anesth Crit Care 11, 274–276.

Gorgi AA, Hofmeister EH, Higginbotham MJ et al. (2006) Effect of body position on cranial migration of epidurally injected methylene blue in recumbent dogs. Am J Vet Res 67, 219–221.

Grau T, Leipold RW, Conradi R et al. (2001a) Ultrasound imaging facilitates localization of the epidural space during combined spinal and epidural anesthesia. Reg Anesth Pain Med 26, 64–67.

Grau T, Leipold RW, Conradi R et al. (2001b) Ultrasound control for presumed difficult epidural puncture. Acta Anaesthesiol Scand 45, 766–771.

Grau T, Leipold R, Conradi R et al. (2001c) Ultrasonography and peridural anesthesia. Technical possibilities and limitations of ultrasonic examination of the epidural space. Anaesthesist 50, 94–101.

Grau T, Leipold RW, Horter J et al. (2001d) Paramedian access to the epidural space: the optimum window for ultrasound imaging. J Clin Anesth 13, 213–217.

Grau T, Leipold RW, Horter J et al. (2001e) The lumbar epidural space in pregnancy: visualization by ultrasonography. Brit J Anaesth 86, 798–804.

Grau T, Leipold RW, Horter J et al. (2001f) Colour doppler imaging of the interspinous and epidural space. Eur J Anaesthesiol 18, 706–712.

Gregori T, Viscasillas J, Benigni L (2014) Ultrasonographic anatomy of the sacrococcygeal region and ultrasound-guided epidural injection at the sacrococcygeal space in dogs. Vet Rec 175, 68.

Jain D, Hussain SY, Ayub A (2022) Comparative evaluation of landmark technique and ultrasound-guided caudal epidural injection in pediatric population: a systematic review and meta-analysis. Pediatr Anesth 32, 35–42.

Liotta A, Busani V, Carrozzo MV et al. (2015) Feasibility of ultrasound-guided epidural access at the lumbo-sacral space in dogs. Vet Radiol Ultrasound 56, 220–228.

Maierl J, Liebich HG (1998) Investigations on the postnatal development of the macroscopic proportions and the topographic anatomy of the feline spinal cord. Anat Histol Embryol 27, 375–379

Neal JM, Brull R, Horn JL, et al. (2016) The second american society of regional anesthesia and pain medicine evidence-based medicine assessment of ultrasound-guided regional anesthesia: executive summary. Reg Anesth Pain Med 41, 181–194.

Otero PE, Campoy L (2013) Epidural and spinal anaesthesia. In: Small Animal Regional Anesthesia and Analgesia. Campoy L, Read MR (eds.) Wiley, USA. pp. 227–259.

Otero PE, Verdier N, Zaccagnini AS et al. (2016) Sonographic evaluation of epidural and intrathecal injections in cats. Vet Anaesth Analg 43, 652–661.

Perlas A, Chaparro LE, Chin KJ (2016) Lumbar neuraxial ultrasound for spinal and epidural anesthesia: A systematic review and meta-analysis. Reg Anesth Pain Med 41, 251–260.

Puggioni A, Arnett R, Clegg T et al. (2006) Influence of patient positioning on the L5–L6 mid-laminar distance. Vet Radiol Ultrasound 47, 449–452.

Remedios AM, Wagner R, Caulkett NA et al. (1996) Epidural abscess and discospondylitis in a dog after administration of a lumbosacral epidural analgesic. Can Vet J 37, 106–107.

Sidiropoulou T, Christodoulaki K, Siristatidis C (2021) Pre-procedural lumbar neuraxial ultrasound – a systematic review of randomized controlled trials and meta-analysis. Healthcare 9, 479.

Viscasillas J, Gregori T, Castiñeiras D et al. (2016) Description and evaluation of four ultrasound-guided approaches to aid spinal canal puncture in dogs. Vet Anaesth Analg 43, 444–452.

Complications Associated with Locoregional Anesthesia

CHAPTER 28

Berit L. Fischer and Manuel Martin-Flores

> The first step in the risk management process is to acknowledge the reality of risk.
>
> —Charles Tremper

Similar to other facets of medicine, the execution of locoregional techniques is not without risk. Those performing them must, therefore, have knowledge of the pertinent anatomy, use of the equipment, and be well-versed in the pharmacology of the individual local anesthetic drugs and adjuvants used. Likewise, a solid understanding of the inherent risk associated with implementing these techniques into practice and the causative factors, such as direct nerve trauma, that can result in patient morbidity and mortality is imperative.

WHAT DO WE KNOW ALREADY?

INCIDENCE

The incidence and severity of complications associated with locoregional blockade differ depending on the type of block (i.e. anatomical location, peripheral nerve block versus neuraxial), technique (blind, electrolocation, ultrasound-guided), and drug(s) used. The suspected overall incidence of severe complications arising from either neuraxial or peripheral nerve blocks is very low. The paucity of veterinary literature on the subject, lack of reporting, and inability to detect subtle or subclinical lesions in nonverbal species, however, prevents a true, objective determination.

The American Society of Regional Anesthesia and Pain Medicine (ASRA) published a practice advisory on neurologic complications associated with regional anesthesia in 2015, reporting that the rate of long-term injury following peripheral nerve blockade in humans is 2–4 per 10,000 blocks. Neuraxial techniques carry an overall higher incidence of complications that is dependent on health of the patient and reason for performing the block, however, of those that occur, only 0.01–0.05% of them are categorized as serious (Neal et al. 2015). Studies of similar breadth do not exist in the veterinary literature. Still, a retrospective clinical study in 2012 examined the prevalence of complications following femoral and

sciatic nerve blockade in 265 dogs using peripheral nerve stimulation. No dogs demonstrated evidence of prolonged neurologic complications both after recovery and when evaluated six weeks later (Vettorato et al. 2012). In 2016, this same author performed a similar study on 69 cats with an identical result (Vettorato and Corletto 2016). While this does provide some basis, it is likely these studies are underpowered, indicating that large-scale, prospective, multicenter studies are needed in veterinary medicine to answer this question.

TYPES OF COMPLICATIONS

Complications associated with peripheral nerve blockade can generally be divided into those caused by nerve injury, inadvertent puncture of nearby anatomical structures, migration of injectate away from the desired location eliciting unintended effects, and local anesthetic systemic toxicity (LAST).

NERVE INJURY

Damage to a nerve can occur directly as a result of needle trauma or indirectly from other physical or cytotoxic mechanisms during performance of a local anesthetic technique. The anatomy of nerves provides that they are fairly resilient structures making severe, irreversible damage an uncommon complication. However, when a patient does suffer nerve damage from a block, there is potential for it to be catastrophic. Manifestations of peripheral nerve injury may present as sensorimotor deficits that extend beyond what would be expected from the individual block and local anesthetic used. When sensorimotor deficits persist, it remains prudent to investigate all possible sources of injury, including patient positioning, underlying patient risk factors, use of tourniquets, etc., in addition to peripheral nerve blockade.

Relevant Anatomy

The anatomy of peripheral nerves is designed to shield the individual nerve fibers from physical and metabolic harm by the provision of three different connective tissue layers. Grossly, individual axons are surrounded by loosely organized collagen fibers (referred to as the "*endoneurium*") and are

Small Animal Regional Anesthesia and Analgesia, Second Edition. Edited by Matt Read, Luis Campoy, and Berit Fischer.
© 2024 John Wiley & Sons, Inc. Published 2024 by John Wiley & Sons, Inc.

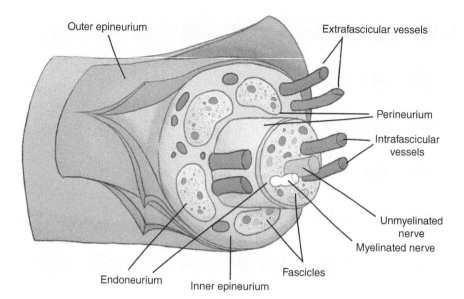

FIGURE 28.1   Diagram depicting anatomy of a peripheral nerve. Source: Image created by Abigail L. Fischer. Used with permission.

grouped together into one or more "*fascicles*" (Figure 28.1). Each fascicle is surrounded by a "*perineurium*," an organized, multilayered, mixed cellular, and collagen fiber layer that limits diffusion of substances across it through the presence of tight junctions (Mizisin and Weerasuriya 2011). Multiple fascicles are encapsulated within a final, external layer of connective tissue known as the "*epineurium*" that serves as a protective barrier but is penetrable and allows the diffusion of numerous substances, including local anesthetics, along their concentration gradients (Franco and Sala-Blanch 2019).

Direct

Needle Trauma When performing peripheral nerve blocks, the goal is to deposit local anesthetic "perineurally" within the tissue space in close apposition to, but outside of, the epineurium to maximize the chances of successful blockade while minimizing the risk of nerve trauma (Franco and Sala-Blanch 2019). Direct needle trauma can occur when the needle tip breaches the epineurium and becomes intraneural. The risk of inadvertent intraneural needle puncture and nerve fiber damage is dependent on several factors, including anatomy of the nerve itself, needle size, bevel type, insertion angle, needle tip location within the nerve, the opening injection pressure, and the rate and volume of the injection (Selander et al. 1977; Rice and McMahon 1992; Hadzic et al. 2004; Kapur et al. 2007; Steinfeldt et al. 2010a, b; Laredo et al. 2020).

The incidence of intraneural injections is likely higher than suspected; however, the development of post-block neurologic complications is rare. Over the past two decades, research has determined that intraneural–extrafascicular blocks seldom result in clinically relevant sensorimotor deficits, whereas puncture of the perineurium and injection within the fascicle itself carries significant risk of harm (Hadzic et al. 2004; Mornjaković et al. 2005; Kapur et al. 2007).

Intraneural injections under both direct visualization and ultrasound (US) guidance have been performed in a variety of species and a relationship between opening injection pressure, intrafascicular needle tip location, and post-block neurologic dysfunction has been determined.

Hadzic et al. (2004) and Kapur et al. (2007) both examined injection pressures following perineural and intraneural lidocaine injections of the sciatic nerves of dogs. In cases of perineural and intraneural injections where injection pressures did not exceed 12 psi, return of normal sensory and motor function occurred within 24 hours and no evidence of nerve injury was documented on histology seven days later. Contrary to this, it was determined that injection pressures that exceeded 25 or 20 psi, respectively, resulted in sensorimotor deficits of the affected limbs that did not resolve prior to the end of each study (Figure 28.2). Additionally, the affected nerves had severe histologic damage characterized by axonal degeneration and infiltration with inflammatory cells. The distinction between extra- and intrafascicular injection pressures and resulting nerve fiber damage was further investigated by Mornjaković et al. (2005) who demonstrated that mean injection pressures during intrafascicular injections were almost four times higher (28.7 psi versus 7.7 psi) and were associated with significant axonal damage extending proximal and distal from the injection site when compared to extrafascicular injections.

Recovery from neurologic injury following peripheral nerve blockade is promising, with the people who have persistent deficits declining 100-fold over the course of a year to 0.2% (Neal et al. 2015). Studies in veterinary patients that document long-term neurologic recovery following locoregional techniques are lacking.

Peripheral nerves vary considerably in the number of fascicles they contain, the neural-to-nonneural tissue ratio, and even the organization of the fascicles within the nerve.

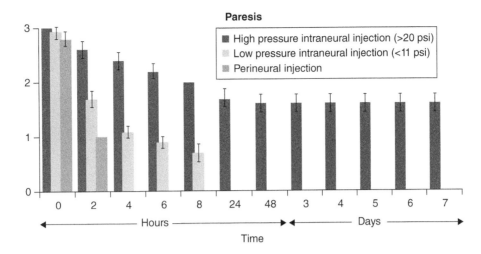

FIGURE 28.2   Duration of limb paresis following high-pressure intraneural (>20 psi), low-pressure intraneural (<11 psi), or perineural sciatic nerve injection in dogs with lidocaine 20 mg ml⁻¹. 0, no paresis: 1, slight paresis; 2, moderate paresis; 4, flaccid extremity. Data represent mean ± standard deviation. Source: Kapur et al. (2007). Used with permission of John Wiley & Sons.

It is suspected that as the number of fascicles decreases and the neural-to-nonneural tissue ratio increases, the risk of intrafascicular injection with resultant nerve injury is greater (Choquet et al. 2012; Rambhia and Gadsden 2019). Fascicle orientation within the epineurium may also determine an individual nerve's susceptibility to damage. A recent study examining 3-D reconstructions of pig lingual and median nerves theorized that the median nerve's wavy fascicles may allow them to be more flexible in the face of intraneural injection and thereby be more resistant to injury, as opposed to the straight fascicular orientation of the lingual nerve (Prats-Galino et al. 2018).

Needle size and bevel type can affect not only the incidence but also the severity of nerve injury during peripheral nerve blocks. Experiments have demonstrated that short-bevel needles (45°) are less likely to pierce the perineurium and enter the fascicle than long-bevel needles (14°). The damage they evoke, however, can be considerably worse, particularly if oriented perpendicular to the nerve or when a larger gauge is used (Selander et al. 1977; Rice and McMahon 1992; Steinfeldt et al. 2010a, b). Most commercially available needles for performing peripheral nerve blocks have a 30° bevel which could offer certain advantages over those utilized in experiments (Figure 28.3).

(a) (b)

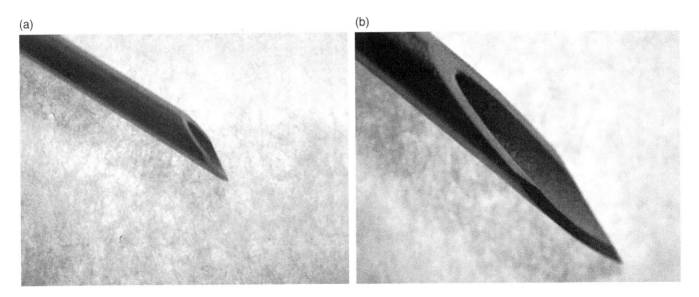

FIGURE 28.3   (a) Short (30°) and (b) long (15°) bevel needles shown here at 25×. The blunt end of a short-bevel needle may help to prevent intraneural placement when performing regional anesthetic blocks. If pierced, however, short-bevel needles are noted to impart greater damage to nerves than long-bevel needles.

Prevention of Intraneural Injection

Despite the rarity of neurologic sequelae following locoregional anesthesia, methods to prevent intraneural injection should always be employed. Studies evaluating the use of electrical nerve stimulation, US guidance, and opening injection pressure for determining intraneural needle location have been performed, however, limitations exist for each.

Electrical Nerve Stimulation When electrical nerve stimulators were first incorporated into locoregional blockade, they were originally thought to minimize the risk of intraneural injection as users were advised against injecting when motor movement was present at currents less than 0.3 mA. This recommendation was based on Coulomb's law, which defined the inverse relationship between needle–nerve distance and minimum current needed to depolarize the target nerve and the assumption that currents <0.3 mA were highly specific for intraneural needle tip location (Raw et al. 2013). The sensitivity of this method in humans was evaluated by Perlas et al. (2006) who determined that with current set at 0.5 mA, 25% of patients where needle–nerve contact was present did not demonstrate a motor response. These findings were confirmed in dogs by Portela et al. (2013) when evaluating needle–nerve relationships using both electrical stimulation and US guidance. The investigators showed that the minimum electrical current required to produce a motor response decreased as the needle was advanced toward the nerve (as expected), but once the needle contacted the epineurium, a current of less than 0.3 mA only resulted in a motor response in 17% to 40% of dogs with a stimulus duration of 0.1 ms or 0.3 ms, respectively.

Various mechanisms for lack of motor response despite needle–nerve contact when using low currents have been proposed. These include changes in electrical conductance and resistance of the nerve itself versus other tissues, decreased electrical resistance of neighboring tissues driving current away from the nerve, and possible overstimulation of the nerve resulting in hyperpolarization and conduction block (Gadsden 2021). Regardless, these findings indicate electrical stimulation, when used alone, may be unreliable for preventing intraneural injection.

Ultrasound US guidance allows direct visualization of the needle tip as it is advanced towards the target nerve. Real-time ultrasonographic imaging was expected to result in a decrease in needle–nerve contact and a subsequent decrease in the incidence of intraneural injections, however, the current literature has not been able to document this (Neal 2016). Operator experience, available equipment, and individual patient characteristics such as obesity can significantly impact image quality. Likewise, image artifacts, anatomical obstructions, or need for steep needle angles can further contribute to difficult needle visualization, thereby increasing the risk of making an intraneural injection.

Once injection has been initiated, the use of US can provide evidence of needle tip location. Perineural spread of hypoechoic local anesthetic often highlights the nerve against other tissues demonstrating appropriate deposition. In cases of intraneural injection, however, operators may observe swelling of the nerve itself or fascicular separation (Choquet et al. 2012). Considering this visual feedback occurs during injection, its use as a method to prevent intraneural injection is limited.

Opening Injection Pressure An opening injection pressure greater than 15 psi may be indicative of making an intrafascicular injection. Multiple factors can influence injection pressures, including rate of injection, needle length and manufacturer, syringe size, and needle contact with high-resistance tissues, including the epineurium and fascia (Claudio et al. 2004). The subjective ability of an operator to detect when this threshold has been passed, regardless of experience, is poor (Claudio et al. 2004; Smith et al. 2021). A simulation using 30 anesthesiologists determined that when estimating pressure by "syringe feel," 70% of injections had pressures greater than 20 psi at some point during an injection of 40 ml of saline (Claudio et al. 2004). Objective methods of measuring injection pressure have since been developed; however, some have failed to be incorporated into veterinary clinical practice due to steep learning curves, time, and cost.

The compressed air injection technique ("CAIT") is a simple method that uses Boyle's law to indirectly indicate injection pressure. Boyle's law states that when temperature is constant, the product of pressure and volume is constant (i.e. if volume is decreased by 50%, pressure must double). To use CAIT for monitoring injection pressure, a small air bubble (~1–3 ml) should be drawn into the syringe containing local anesthetic prior to injection. Assuming a normal barometric pressure of ~14.7 psi at sea level, if the volume of air decreases by half as the injection is being made, it suggests that the pressure in the syringe has doubled, reflecting resistance to injection that could be the result of an intrafascicular injection with an injection pressure greater than the threshold that induces histologic injury (Figure 28.4). Therefore, as long as the air bubble does not compress more than 50% during injection, pressure cannot have increased above this threshold without the anesthetist noticing. An *in vitro* study examining this method found excellent correlation ($r = 0.99$) between different reductions in air bubble volume and increases in injection pressure as measured via an inline pressure transducer, indicating this method may be beneficial for helping to avoid making intraneural injections (Tsui et al. 2006).

B. Braun Medical Inc. has advanced this theory to develop a disposable inline manometer (BSmart™) that detects opening injection pressures. As injection pressure rises, a piston is lifted within the device to display a pressure indicator. The anesthetist is then able to visualize either a white (<15 psi), yellow (15–20 psi), or red (>20 psi) line that correlates with the pressure they are exerting during injection

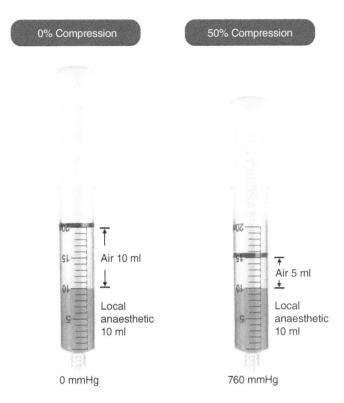

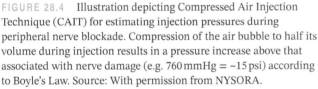

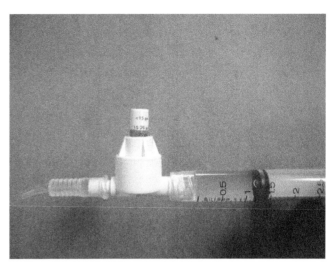

FIGURE 28.5   BSmart™ manometer (B. Braun Medical Inc., Germany) used for monitoring injection pressure during performance of peripheral nerve blocks. The color-coded pressure indicator provides real-time feedback to inform the operator if injection pressure exceeds those associated with neurologic damage.

FIGURE 28.4   Illustration depicting Compressed Air Injection Technique (CAIT) for estimating injection pressures during peripheral nerve blockade. Compression of the air bubble to half its volume during injection results in a pressure increase above that associated with nerve damage (e.g. 760 mmHg = ~15 psi) according to Boyle's Law. Source: With permission from NYSORA.

(Figure 28.5). Smith et al. (2021) evaluated the effectiveness of the BSmart™ versus "syringe feel" for reducing the incidence of high-pressure injections during a simulated nerve block. While the use of the BSmart™ did reduce the number of high-pressure injections (>15 psi) from 62% to 21%, it did not eliminate these injections from occurring entirely.

A combination of electrical nerve stimulation, US, and an in-line pressure monitor, referred to as "triple monitoring," was evaluated by Pascarella et al. (2021) in 60 patients undergoing interscalene brachial plexus blocks. When using US in combination with nerve stimulation, needle–nerve contact was determined in 30% more patients than when using US guidance alone. This number increased an additional 25% when injection pressure monitoring was employed. Based on this, the increased sensitivity of incorporating all three systems to prevent needle–nerve contact should be considered in veterinary patients as well.

Indirect

Vascular Injury/Neuronal Ischemia Nerve damage following locoregional anesthesia may occur not as the result of direct needle trauma, but from other mechanisms as well. "Indirect" injury can result from external mechanical injury, vascular injury that results in nerve ischemia, or cytotoxic injury from nerve exposure to high concentrations of the local anesthetic solution, adjuvants, and/or preservatives used.

The blood supply to peripheral nerves is two-fold; it is initially supplied by blood vessels in the epineurium that penetrate the perineurium and anastomose with small endoneurial capillaries. Local anesthetics can cause vasoconstriction of the larger epineurial vessels, depending on the agent that is used, its concentration, and the duration of exposure. The use of vasoconstrictive adjuvants, such as epinephrine, may exacerbate this effect (Myers and Heckman 1989). Vascular puncture of these capillaries or surrounding blood vessels during needle advancement may also increase the risk of nerve ischemia and injury as hemorrhage and/or hematoma formation could potentially increase intraneural pressure in excess of capillary pressure in the area affected.

Certain patient populations may be more at risk of ischemic nerve injury following peripheral nerve blockade than others, specifically, patients with preexisting neurologic dysfunction. Diabetes mellitus is described as a causative factor of peripheral neuropathy in humans, dogs, cats, and rodents and is associated with loss of nerve fiber and endoneurial capillary density histologically (Estrella et al. 2008; Lirk et al. 2015; Morgan et al. 2008). The duration of sensory and motor blockade following locoregional anesthesia in diabetics is, therefore, expected to be prolonged (Lirk et al. 2015). Currently, locoregional blockade is not an absolute contraindication in this population of human patients, however, it is recommended that clinicians utilize caution by using lower doses and concentrations of local anesthetics (Baeriswyl et al. 2018).

Migration of Local Anesthetic Excessive migration of the local anesthetic solution following injection can lead to unexpected consequences. Specific blocks may lend themselves to this complication more than others due to their location and associated anatomical structures. For example, migration of local anesthetic into the epidural space has been observed following erector spinae plane (ESP) and interscalene brachial plexus blocks in people, resulting in transient bilateral symptoms (Stundner et al. 2016; Pratheep et al. 2022). Unilateral **phrenic nerve** blockade following brachial plexus block has also been reported and can be a source of respiratory morbidity in patients (Stundner et al. 2016).

These are considered rare complications and have decreased in incidence with the use of US guidance and lower local anesthetic volume requirements (Neal 2016).

Cadaver studies examining the distribution of injectate following US-guided quadratus lumborum and paravertebral brachial plexus blocks have been performed in dogs and epidural migration and phrenic nerve staining have both been identified (Monticelli et al. 2018; Alaman et al. 2022). The relevance of these findings to clinical patients is currently unknown, but considering the relatively small number of cadaver subjects used in the studies and the fact that these complications were observed at all, it would seem that the possibility is real and more research is indicated.

Horner's Syndrome Transient Horner's syndrome has been documented in dogs following lumbar epidural and spinal anesthesia, as well as following regional blocks of the thoracic limb and caudal cervical spine (Bosmans et al. 2009; Son et al. 2015; Chouette et al. 2017). It most often occurs when there is disruption of sympathetic transmission between preganglionic sympathetic fibers originating from spinal nerves T1–T3 and their postganglionic terminations within the eyes, vessels, and sweat glands of the face. This disruption results in miosis, ptosis, and enophthalmos with elevation of the third eyelid due to loss of sympathetic tone to the iris dilator muscle and smooth muscles within the orbit (Figure 28.6) (Zwueste and Grahn 2019). In humans, Horner's syndrome is often associated with neuraxial anesthesia following obstetric procedures, with the incidence reportedly ranging between 0.13% and 4.0% (Chambers and Bhatia 2018). A combination of cephalad spread and sensitivity of preganglionic sympathetic nerves to local anesthetics is the most probable cause in this situation.

In dogs, the literature contains a single case report that documented the occurrence of Horner's syndrome following L7–S1 epidural administration of 0.75% ropivacaine with saline (total volume $0.23\,ml\,kg^{-1}$) (Bosmans et al. 2009). In an experimental study, Son et al. (2015) examined the administration of four different volumes of lidocaine via epidural catheter in five dogs. With the catheter tip located at T7, 40% of all trials within the crossover design and 100% of trials with the highest volume resulted in blockade of spinal nerves T1–T3 with subsequent unilateral or bilateral Horner's syndrome. Sympathetic blockade in some cases extended

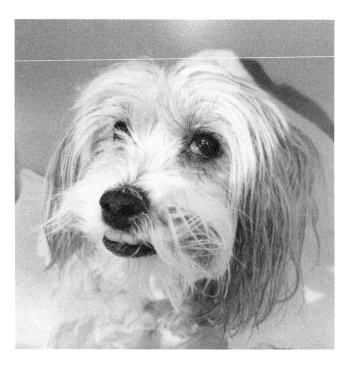

FIGURE 28.6   Horner's syndrome following subscalene brachial plexus block in a dog. Note elevated third eyelid, mild ptosis. Dog also had miosis of the left pupil when compared to the right.

further cranial than somatosensory blockade as determined by nociceptive responses to stimuli at associated dermatomes (Son et al. 2015).

Regional anesthetic blocks of the thoracic limb or caudal cervical spine can also lead to the development of Horner's syndrome. The brachial plexus nerve roots ([C5]C6–T1[T2]) run within the deep fascia of the neck, lateral to *m. longus colli,* just cranial to the first rib. The middle cervical and cervicothoracic ganglia containing preganglionic sympathetic fibers lie in close apposition to the first rib, deep to *m. longus colli* (Fitzmaurice 2020). Local anesthetic migration away from the intended injection site could therefore result in sympathetic blockade and subsequent Horner's syndrome. Scattered case reports in veterinary medicine have documented Horner's syndrome following both subscalenic and paravertebral approaches to the brachial plexus block, including an experimental study in eight dogs where 25% of study subjects developed Horner's syndrome following paravertebral brachial plexus block (Choquette et al. 2017). Fortunately, when this complication is observed, the effects are transient and no reports of sustained deficits exist.

COMPLICATIONS ASSOCIATED WITH NEURAXIAL ANESTHESIA

Hemodynamic

Hypotension is the most common complication reported following neuraxial local anesthetic administration in humans and veterinary species and is associated with sympathetic nervous system blockade from cranial migration of local anesthetic. Sympatholysis leads to vasodilation of the splanchnic circulation and lower extremities, causing a reduction in venous return with subsequent arterial hypotension (Holte et al. 2004; Iff and Moens 2008; Bosmans et al. 2009).

Bradycardia, sometimes culminating in asystole, can also occur following cranial spread via several proposed mechanisms. These have historically included extension of block to the T1–T4 cardioaccelerator fibers, alterations in vasomotor tone through increased subarachnoid pressure, and cardiotoxicity following accidental intravascular injection (Iff and Moens 2008). Currently, it is believed that the most likely cause of sudden and severe bradycardia is via idiosyncratic activation of parasympathetic pathways in the face of decreased venous return (Kinsella and Tuckey 2001). Reflex pathways thought to contribute to this complication are described by Lacey et al. (2022) and include the "Bezold-Jarisch," "reverse Bainbridge," and "pacemaker stretch" reflexes.

Despite the high incidence of hypotension and bradycardia, the overall incidence of cardiac arrest following neuraxial anesthesia is low. In humans, cardiac arrest following epidural administration is approximately 0.01% but increases three to six-fold when the deposition of local anesthetic is subarachnoid (Limongi and Lins 2011). Isolated case reports in veterinary literature describe rapid onset of asystole with successful resuscitation following epidural administration of local anesthetics in dogs (Mosing et al. 2008; Savvas et al. 2006). These reports document careful measures to ensure proper needle location, absence of CSF or blood, and appropriate doses of drugs prior to injection, thereby suggesting a vagally mediated mechanism of action in each instance.

The above reports indicate that the incidence of hypotension and bradycardia can most likely be mitigated by ensuring patients are euvolemic prior to drug administration and avoiding excessive cranial spread of a local anesthetic-containing solution. Several factors have been shown to result in excessive cranial spread, including increased age, obesity, pregnancy, subarachnoid versus epidural administration, increasing volume of injectate, patient positioning, and anatomical variations of the epidural space (Lee et al. 2004; Gorgi et al. 2006; Veering 2006; Iff and Moens 2008; Moll et al. 2014). Surprisingly, a study in dogs examining the relationship between injection speed and epidural pressure on cranial migration of injectate determined that, despite significant increases in epidural pressure, faster injection did not notably affect local anesthetic spread (Son et al. 2014).

Treatment of hypotension and bradycardia following neuraxial anesthesia often includes the administration of anticholinergic and sympathomimetic drugs. Using crystalloids or colloids to restore venous return has been shown to often be ineffective due to persistent sympatholysis (Holte et al. 2004; Bosmans et al. 2009). In humans, combinations of atropine, selective α-1 adrenoreceptor agonists, and the mixed α- and β-agonist, ephedrine, have been used to restore heart rate and blood pressure (Kinsella and Tuckey 2001). The use of selective

α-1 adrenoreceptor agonists alone in the face of bradycardia is cautioned against since additional baroreceptor-mediated decreases in heart rate can occur (Kinsella and Tuckey 2001). Iff and Moens (2008) reported bradycardia and hypotension in two dogs following administration of epidural anesthesia for cranial cruciate ligament repair. One dog responded to the administration of atropine, however, the other dog's heart rate returned to acceptable levels over time without intervention. While a specific treatment algorithm is not described in the veterinary literature, the institution of cardiopulmonary cerebral resuscitation (CPCR) with associated drug interventions is assumed in the face of sudden cardiac arrest.

Urinary Retention

The ability to void urine involves the complex interaction between afferent stretch receptor signaling and subsequent activation of sacral parasympathetic pathways that trigger detrusor muscle contraction and relaxation of the urethral sphincter (Choi et al. 2012). Urinary retention, defined as the inability to initiate urination or completely empty the bladder during urination, is reported to occur following the administration of either neuraxial local anesthetics or opioids. Blockade of sensory input to the spinal cord and micturition centers in the brain (from the use of local anesthetics) or impaired parasympathetic signaling caused by opioid receptor agonism (from the use of opioids) at the level of S2–S4 results in ***m. detrusor vesicae*** (detrusor muscle) relaxation and a decreased ability to detect bladder filling. Studies in dogs, humans, and rats demonstrate that the incidence and duration of impaired signaling are dependent on the physiochemical properties and dosing of the individual drugs, with the use of long-acting opioids (e.g. morphine) and/or local anesthetics (e.g. bupivacaine) resulting in longer times to return of normal bladder function when compared to shorter-acting drugs (Drenger et al. 1989; Choi et al. 2012).

In the case of opioids, effects on the bladder and urethra are inconsistent. Experiments in dogs examining pressure and compliance of the bladder following intrathecal opioids have shown that buprenorphine and methadone differ from fentanyl and morphine by causing no change or an increase in ***m. detrusor vesicae*** tone, respectively (Drenger et al. 1986; Drenger et al. 1989). Those authors hypothesized that buprenorphine and methadone may, therefore, be less likely to cause urinary retention than fentanyl or morphine.

The clinical significance of this potential complication is unknown. A systematic review in people determined that the incidence of urinary retention varies between 0% and 79.5%, depending on route (i.e. intrathecal versus epidural) and the drug(s) administered (Choi et al. 2012). However, there is a failed consensus regarding what constitutes urinary retention and the methods by which it is determined. Various studies have documented urinary retention using self-description by the patient, failure to urinate at designated timepoints (e.g. at 8, 12, or >24 hours) post-block, the presence of large bladder volume with inability to void, or an inability to completely void with larger than expected residual volumes (Choi et al. 2012).

Reports of urinary retention following neuraxial anesthesia in veterinary medicine are few, with reported incidences varying between 0% and 44% (Troncy et al. 2002; Campoy et al. 2012; Peterson et al. 2014; Sarotti et al. 2022). In two large retrospective studies that examined urinary retention following epidural opioids in small animals, the incidence was determined to be 2.8% and 3.3% in dogs, and 8.7% in cats (Troncy et al. 2002; Peterson et al. 2014). Interestingly, Peterson et al. (2014) found that the incidence of urinary retention (no spontaneous urination within 24 hours) in anesthetized dogs that received an epidural did not differ significantly from that in dogs that did not receive an epidural.

This emphasizes the importance of recognizing that micturition can be impaired following other routes of opioid administration. Malinovsky et al. (1998) demonstrated increased bladder capacities and altered ability to sense bladder fullness after IV administration of fentanyl, morphine, buprenorphine, and nalbuphine in humans. While there are no specific prospective studies in veterinary species, a study using 3D US to evaluate residual bladder volumes following anesthesia and surgery in dogs suggests this may be similar as all dogs receiving opioids ($n = 23$), regardless of route, had residual bladder volumes > $0.4\,ml\,kg^{-1}$ (Vasquez et al. 2021). Finally, other factors that may affect micturition following anesthesia and surgery should not be ignored. The amount of fluids administered, the effects of inhalant anesthetics, and the type of surgery being performed have also been implicated in the development of urinary retention (Choi et al. 2012).

Pruritis

Pruritis following epidural or intrathecal administration of full μ opioid agonists has been reported in dogs, cats, horses, sheep, rodents, nonhuman primates, and humans (Wagner et al. 1996; Troncy et al. 2002; Lee et al. 2007; Bauquier 2012; Iff et al. 2012; Gent et al. 2013; Evangelista et al. 2016; Nyugen et al. 2021; Wang et al. 2021). While this is a common adverse effect in humans (e.g. 30–85%, depending on the μ agonist used and the patient population examined), its incidence in dogs is documented as 0.8%, and in other species is not fully elucidated as accounts are limited to a handful of case reports (Troncy et al. 2002; Bauquier 2012; Iff et al. 2012; Gent et al. 2013; Nyugen et al. 2021). Several proposed mechanisms for opioid-induced pruritis following neuraxial administration exist, however, a central mechanism seems most likely based on recent studies in rodents. Using μ opioid receptor (MOR) knock out mice, Wang et al. (2021) concluded that μ opioid agonists block GABAergic inhibitory interneurons within the dorsal horn of the spinal cord, leading to excitation of pruriceptive neurons and the development of itch.

Treatments for opioid-induced pruritis following neuraxial anesthesia are numerous, with no current consensus. In humans, the use of MOR antagonists, κ receptor agonists, 5HT receptor antagonists, gabapentin, propofol, and D2 receptor agonists have all been reported, with variable degrees of success (Nyugen et al. 2021). Case reports in cats have reported amelioration of pruritis using subanesthetic doses of propofol (Gent et al. 2013), ondansetron (Bauquier 2012), and naloxone (Evangelista et al. 2016). Iff et al. (2012) reported the use of both buprenorphine and butorphanol when treating a dog with pruritis and myoclonus following intrathecal morphine, bupivacaine, and lidocaine. Their use resulted in decreased signs of distress, however, did not completely eliminate the dog's clinical signs. With its limited incidence, the development of effective treatment options for opioid-induced pruritis following neuraxial administration in veterinary medicine is restricted at this time to findings in humans, laboratory studies, and anecdotal reports.

Delayed Hair Regrowth

Delayed hair regrowth over the lumbosacral junction is occasionally observed following neuraxial anesthesia. While often implicated, studies have determined that epidural drug administration is not a causative factor of this complication. Guerrero et al. (2014) examined the incidence of delayed hair regrowth in 80 dogs who were assigned to either receive an epidural injection of bupivacaine, preservative-free morphine and bupivacaine, or saline. An additional group of 10 dogs served as controls who had the hair over the lumbosacral junction clipped, with no epidural performed. Delayed hair regrowth was observed in 12.2% of dogs, with no significant differences between groups indicating the act of clipping itself, along with other individual factors are more likely explanations. Nevertheless, advising owners that hair regrowth may take up to 6 months following clipping has been recommended.

Infection

Introduction of pathogens when performing any type of injection is possible, therefore, appropriate measures to achieve asepsis during regional anesthesia is of paramount importance. Serious sequelae caused by infection have been associated with neuraxial techniques, including epidural abscess formation, discospondylitis, and/or meningitis (Remedios et al. 1996; MacFarlane and Iff 2011; Liu et al. 2019). Incidence of infection in veterinary patients is presumed to be rare, with only a single case report and correspondence documenting its occurrence. Described risk factors include the use of overly long spinal needles (3.5 in.) that could pierce abdominal viscera and introduce bacteria, failure to use proper asepsis, immunocompromised patient status, and infection elsewhere in the body that could lead to hematogenous spread (MacFarlane and Iff 2011; Remedios et al. 1996). Clinical signs following epidural abscess formation and discospondylitis in dogs are described as extreme pain localized to the site of injection, weakness, and disuse muscle atrophy with or without the presence of fever (Remedios et al. 1996; MacFarlane and Iff 2011). In humans, the mortality rate following epidural abscess formation is 5–16% (Liu et al. 2019).

Diagnosis with culture and institution of appropriate long-term antibiotic therapy has been associated with a positive outcome in a dog (Remedios et al. 1996).

DAMAGE TO OTHER STRUCTURES

Targeted nerves or fascial planes often lie in close association with delicate structures or body cavities, making them subject to unintentional or inadvertent needle puncture. Case reports have documented the accidental puncture of the peritoneal or pleural cavities, resulting in pneumothorax, arrhythmias, hemorrhage, and/or damage to underlying viscera (Adami and Studer 2014; Bhalla and Leece 2015). In the veterinary literature, these reports have occurred primarily when performing blind, anatomically based blocks, or with the use of nerve stimulation. The use of US guidance has not been shown to preclude this risk in humans however, which may be explained by the presence of artefacts, challenging anatomy, steep needle angles, and poor image quality that can impair the ability of the operator to visualize the needle tip at all times (Neal 2016).

Some blocks do not lend themselves to US guidance, such as those used for dental or ocular procedures, potentially increasing the risk of complications when performing these techniques. For example, retrobulbar hemorrhage, globe rupture, and temporary blindness have all been reported following blind **maxillary nerve** blocks in veterinary species (Alessio and Krieger 2015; Perry et al. 2015; Loughran et al. 2016).

TOXICITY OF LOCAL ANESTHETICS (LAST, LOCAL ANESTHETIC SYSTEMIC TOXICITY)

Local anesthetic agents exert their principal actions by interrupting the generation and propagation of action potentials through Na^+ channel blockade. Unfortunately, this effect is not limited to the target peripheral nerve tissues. Once a sufficient plasma concentration of the agent has been attained, this same mechanism of action is responsible for the systemic toxic effects of local anesthetics.

High plasma levels of local anesthetics can occur following administration of an overdose or by unintentional intravascular administration. In addition, unanticipated high plasma levels of local anesthetics can be attained if biotransformation and/or elimination of the drug are impaired or diminished, as may occur in individuals with hepatic or renal insufficiencies. For example, in people, the clearance of lidocaine decreased from 10 to $6\,ml\,kg^{-1}\,min^{-1}$ in the presence of hepatic disease (Thomson et al. 1973). When the pharmacokinetic (PK) variables of lidocaine were calculated in dogs after partial hepatectomy and transplantation, the maximal plasma concentration and area under the curve increased by almost 100% when compared with normal individuals (Perez-Guille et al. 2011). Decreased biotransformation of local anesthetics is potentially more problematic when amide local anesthetics

are used for nerve blockade as they have longer and more involved metabolic pathways than do aminoesters. In addition to severe liver and renal disease, heart failure can compromise metabolism and excretion of local anesthetics and result in elevated plasma concentrations (Thomson et al. 1971). When local anesthetic systemic toxicity manifests, central nervous system (CNS) and cardiovascular system (CVS) complications are the most relevant and commonly recognized.

Central Nervous System Toxicity

Toxic effects from local anesthetics can affect the CNS, the autonomic ganglia, and the neuromuscular junction. CNS toxicity occurs after these lipid-soluble agents cross the blood–brain barrier. With most local anesthetics, CNS signs generally manifest before CVS toxicity occurs, giving the anesthetist the opportunity to detect, and treat, the complications before they become potentially fatal. Local anesthetics can cause depression of cortical inhibitory pathways, thereby allowing unopposed activity of excitatory neuronal pathways. This transitional stage of unbalanced excitation (i.e. seizure activity) is typically followed by generalized CNS depression.

The reported clinical signs of local anesthetic CNS toxicity, in order of increasing plasma concentrations, are:

- Drowsiness, lethargy
- Light-headedness
- Visual and auditory disturbances
- Restlessness
- Nystagmus
- Muscular twitching
- Tonic–clonic seizures
  - Lactic acid formation
  - Hypoxia
- Generalized CNS depression
  - Unconsciousness
  - Coma
  - Hypoventilation progressing to respiratory arrest (Groban 2003)

There are exceptions to this order, especially when there is an overdose of bupivacaine. With bupivacaine, cardiac toxicity usually occurs concurrently with the "warning" signs that are typical of CNS intoxication, without the classic dose-dependent relationships that are seen with other drugs (Sage et al. 1985). Unlike lidocaine, bupivacaine can cause arrhythmias at the same doses that produce seizures, and even at subconvulsive doses (de Jong et al. 1982).

Several studies have investigated the relative toxicity of local anesthetics in small animals (Feldman et al. 1989, 1991, 1996). When administered intravenously, lidocaine, ropivacaine, and bupivacaine can produce convulsions in dogs at 20, 4.9, and 4.3 mg kg^{-1}, respectively. When two times those doses were used, mortality resulted in 33%, 17%, and 83% of the dogs, with corresponding plasma levels of 47, 11, and 18 μg ml^{-1} for lidocaine, ropivacaine, and bupivacaine, respectively.

These data indicate that bupivacaine is the most dangerous of the commonly used local anesthetics by demonstrating that the toxic dose of bupivacaine is lower than that of other drugs, the early warning signs of toxicity that are usually seen prior to cardiovascular collapse do not occur, mortality rates are higher when there is an overdose, and mortality occurs with lower plasma concentrations of the drug. When bupivacaine is used, correct dosing must be ensured, and it should never be used by an intravenous route (i.e. intravenous regional anesthesia, IVRA).

Cardiovascular System Toxicity

With most local anesthetics, excluding bupivacaine, larger doses are required to produce signs of CVS toxicity than to produce signs of CNS toxicity.

The reported clinical signs of local anesthetic CVS toxicity are:

- Hypotension
  - Depressed myocardial function
  - Peripheral vasodilation
  - Arrhythmias
- ECG changes (stemming from slowed conduction through Purkinje system)
  - Prolonged P–R interval
  - Widening of QRS complex
  - T-wave inversion
  - Atrioventricular block
- Arrhythmias
  - Bradycardia
  - Ventricular premature complexes (VPC)
  - Ventricular tachycardia
  - Ventricular fibrillation
  - Sinus arrest

Cardiovascular signs are characterized by depression of myocardial automaticity and a reduction in the duration of the refractory period. Therefore, both myocardial contractility and conduction velocity of impulses through the heart would be expected to be depressed. Coyle et al. (1994) reported the electrocardiographic (ECG) and echocardiographic effects of a bupivacaine overdose in dogs. They reported markedly impaired systolic function and severe right-sided dilation

following a mean total intravenous bupivacaine dose of 14.0 ± 3.3 mg kg^{-1}. ECG changes included widening of the QRS complex, inversion, bradycardia, VPCs, or a combination of these effects. As the toxicity progressed, Wenckebach phenomenon (i.e. Mobitz type 1 second-degree AV block), and ventricular tachycardia were also observed.

The cardiotoxic effects of local anesthetics differ from one agent to another. For example, an overdose of lidocaine will likely result in hypotension and bradycardia, whereas toxic doses of bupivacaine and ropivacaine produce sudden cardiovascular collapse or ventricular dysrhythmias that are resistant to treatment. In fact, approximately one-third of LAST cases reported in humans are reported to produce CNS and CVS signs concurrently (Neal et al. 2018). For this reason, recent research into the cardiotoxicity of the different local anesthetics has focused on the more potent, lipid-soluble, and toxic agents such as bupivacaine, levobupivacaine, and ropivacaine (Table 28.1).

Arrhythmogenicity Prolongation of cardiac conduction is seen in a dose-dependent fashion when local anesthetics are administered to animals. This is evidenced by increases in the P–R interval as well as the QRS duration. Bradycardia and AV blocks result from the depression of SA and AV nodal function. Increasing doses of bupivacaine result in re-entrant arrhythmias such as ventricular tachycardia and fibrillation. When potent aminoamides are compared, the potential for toxicity is highest with bupivacaine, lowest with ropivacaine, and intermediate with levobupivacaine (Groban 2003).

Mechanical Activity Decreases in blood pressure and increases in left ventricular end-diastolic pressure reflect the myocardial depressant effects of local anesthetics. Bupivacaine and levobupivacaine cause decreased myocardial contractility at

Table 28.1 Summary of the relative potencies for toxicity of local anesthetic agents.

	Relative potency for CNS toxicity	[a] CVS: CNS ratio for toxicity
Esters		
Procaine	0.3	3.7
Chloroprocaine	0.3	3.7
Tetracaine	2.0	–
Amides		
Lidocaine	1.0	7.1
Mepivacaine	1.4	7.1
Ropivacaine	2.9	2.0
Levobupivacaine	2.9	2.0
Bupivacaine	4.0	2.0

[a] CVS: CNS denotes the ratio of local anesthetic dose that causes CVS collapse relative to the local anesthetic dose that causes seizures. Lower values represent greater cardiotoxicity.

subconvulsive doses when they are administered to sheep (Huang et al. 1998). In that study, the frequency of arrhythmias was highest with bupivacaine. In a study with pentobarbital anesthetized dogs, both lidocaine $16\,mg\,kg^{-1}$ and bupivacaine $4\,mg\,kg^{-1}$ depressed hemodynamic function (Bruelle et al. 1996). The doses of lidocaine, bupivacaine, levobupivacaine, and ropivacaine that induced cardiovascular collapse in dogs were 127, 22, 27, and $42\,mg\,kg^{-1}$, respectively (Groban et al. 2001). The mortality rates at these doses were 0% for lidocaine, 10% for ropivacaine, 30% for levobupivacaine, and 50% for bupivacaine, despite cardiac massage and advanced life support (Groban et al. 2001).

Liposomal Bupivacaine and LAST

A formulation of bupivacaine liposome injectable suspension (BLIS) is licensed for local infiltration and peripheral nerve block use in dogs and cats, respectively (Nocita™ Elanco, United States). After being injected into a patient, liposome particles that contain bupivacaine slowly degrade over time, releasing free bupivacaine into the surrounding tissues, reportedly resulting in an analgesic effect that lasts up to 72 hours (Nocita™ package insert 2021).

Other than the safety studies that were performed in order to obtain regulatory approval, minimal literature regarding Nocita™ and LAST exist in animals. Using a similar formulation that is licensed for use in humans (Exparel® Pacira Pharmaceuticals, United States), Joshi et al. (2015) performed dose studies comparing the safety and PK profiles of BLIS to bupivacaine HCl following intravenous (IV) administration in dogs. Those investigators determined that the maximum doses of each drug that did not result in severe adverse effects (e.g. convulsions, hypotension) after IV administration were $4.5\,mg\,kg^{-1}$ of liposome bupivacaine and $0.75\,mg\,kg^{-1}$ bupivacaine HCl, indicating a more favorable safety profile for the BLIS formulation. This observation was supported by concurrent PK analysis that determined that the C_{max} of BLIS was at least two-times lower than that of bupivacaine HCl when both were administered at $1.5\,mg\,kg^{-1}$ IV (Joshi et al. 2015).

PK studies in humans following surgical site infiltration found that BLIS has a bimodal release profile that produces two separate concentration peaks; one peak occurs approximately 1 hour following administration, and a second, later peak occurs 10–36 hours later (Hu et al. 2013). Though not reported in animals, this suggests that the monitoring period for patients receiving liposome bupivacaine should be extended following administration.

Further studies regarding the safety of BLIS in veterinary species are still needed, especially with regards to its coadministration with other local anesthetics. One study evaluated the effect of subcutaneous administration of BLIS into the same tissues following lidocaine administration in pigs (Richard et al. 2011). Those investigators found that administration of BLIS five minutes after lidocaine administration increased each drug's maximum plasma concentrations (C_{max}) by 1000% and 1060%, respectively. Interestingly, if BLIS was administered more than 20 minutes after the administration of lidocaine, this increase was not observed. The specific mechanism behind these massive increases in drug levels is unknown but was speculated to be the result of breakdown of the liposomes, resulting in rapid release of free bupivacaine and additional interactions between lidocaine and the liposome particles leading to its own plasma concentration increase (Richard et al. 2011). At this time, package inserts for BLIS (Exparel® Pacira pharmaceuticals, United States; Nocita™ Elanco, United States) do not recommend coadministration with other amide-type local anesthetics until further studies have been performed.

Treatment of LAST

It is expected that when using local anesthetics for locoregional techniques, the anesthetist should always be prepared for intervention should signs of toxicity occur. These signs can occur quickly following intravascular injection, however, depending on the route of administration, block location, and the dose of local anesthetic administered, signs may take up to 60 minutes to develop, requiring the anesthetist to be continually diligent (Neal et al. 2018). Rapid recognition and instillation of treatment protocols significantly impact recovery from cardiovascular collapse following LAST, so it is essential that patients undergoing nerve blocks have appropriate monitoring in place (i.e. ECG, blood pressure, end-tidal CO_2) to prevent any delay in recognition of this complication and initiation of appropriate treatments. Over the past decade, algorithms for treatment of LAST have been developed in human medicine (Neal et al. 2018; Macfarlane et al. 2021). A current adaptation of these guidelines is not available for veterinary patients; however, many of these published algorithms have been based on animal models and a degree of overlap is likely.

Treatment of local anesthetic systemic toxicities has historically consisted of supportive therapy and pharmacologic treatment of the different clinical signs. Recently, specific agents (i.e. IV lipid emulsions) have been developed that have the ability to chelate local anesthetics in plasma, reducing their circulating concentrations and minimizing their toxic effects. As a result, these have been recommended as first-line therapy in patients with evidence of cardio- and even neurotoxicity and it is strongly advised that individuals who perform locoregional anesthesia have lipid emulsion therapy available for emergency use in the part of the hospital where nerve blocks are typically performed (Figure 28.7) (Neal et al. 2018; Macfarlane et al. 2021).

Lipid Rescue/Lipid Emulsion Therapy Since its initial description in the literature, intravenous lipid emulsion therapy has been the subject of multiple investigations both alone and in concert with vasopressors for their ability to resuscitate people and animals from local anesthetic-induced cardiovascular collapse (Hicks et al. 2009; de Queiroz Siqueira et al. 2013; Gitman and Barrington 2018). While it has been long believed

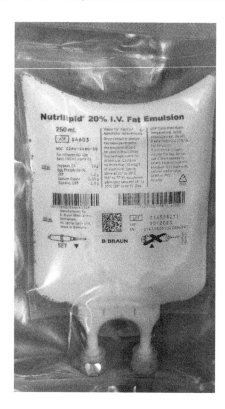

FIGURE 28.7 Ready-to-use lipid emulsion (lipid rescue) for treatment of local anesthetic systemic toxicity (LAST). In hospitals where locoregional blocks are being performed, lipid rescue should be kept in stock and in a location where it can be easily accessed, along with supplies to administer it and a written copy of a LAST treatment protocol. Source: Luis Campoy (Book Author).

that lipid emulsion therapy acts as a "lipid sink" that extracts highly lipid-soluble local anesthetics like bupivacaine from the plasma (i.e. making them unavailable to tissues), a recent study by Fettiplace et al. (2015) provided further insight to its mechanisms of action. Those investigators discovered that lipid emulsion therapy acts as transporter of lipid-soluble local anesthetics, quickly lowering tissue concentrations in the heart and brain and redistributing the drug(s) to the skeletal muscle and liver. In addition, lipid emulsion therapy has direct effects on the myocardium, producing inotropic effects that help to improve cardiac output and coronary blood flow which further increases delivery of the local anesthetic to the liver for detoxification (Fettiplace et al. 2015).

Lipid emulsion therapy has been used successfully to treat CNS and CVS toxicity following overdose of local anesthetics. In rats, administration of a 20% intravenous lipid emulsion (Intralipid®) has been shown to decrease mortality from 100% to 0% following bupivacaine toxicity (Weinberg et al. 1998). Similar findings were found after bupivacaine 10 mg kg^{-1} IV was used to induce cardiovascular collapse in dogs (Weinberg et al. 2003). Following 10 minutes of unsuccessful cardiac massage, a 20% lipid emulsion was administered as a bolus (4 ml kg^{-1}), followed by 0.5 ml kg^{-1} min for 10 minutes. This treatment resulted in 100% survival in treated

dogs, whereas administration of saline resulted in 100% mortality. A recent meta-analysis evaluated survival in animal models following LAST and treatment with lipid emulsion therapy (Fettiplace and McCabe 2017). Using data from 16 publications, the meta-analysis determined that administration of lipid emulsion therapy increases the odds-ratio of survival more than four-fold when compared to CPCR alone. They also reported that failure of lipid emulsion therapy to resuscitate patients occurred in studies where CPCR was not initiated or there was a delay in treatment (Fettiplace and McCabe 2017).

Propofol, the injectable anesthetic, is formulated in a 10% lipid solution and has been previously touted as a possible replacement for 20% lipid emulsion therapy. It should be noted that 2 mg kg^{-1} of propofol provides only 3% of the dose of lipid that would be administered based on the doses of Intralipid® that were administered in the aforementioned studies and only ~8% of the dose of lipid that would be found in the clinically recommended bolus dose of 1.5 mL kg^{-1} (Weinberg et al. 2003; Neal et al. 2018). Using propofol for this purpose, therefore, is unlikely to have the desired effect on LAST, in addition to the fact that as an injectable anesthetic, it will likely exacerbate the patient's preexisting hemodynamic instability. The use of propofol for treating LAST is, therefore, not recommended.

Vasopressor Use in Local Anesthetic Toxicity In the face of LAST, treatment of cardiovascular collapse with specific vasopressors, particularly epinephrine, has been controversial. Epinephrine, despite many of its positive effects on cardiac output and coronary circulation, has been shown to aggravate ventricular arrhythmias and increase lactic acid formation, exacerbating LAST and worsening patient outcomes (Weinberg et al. 2008; Hiller et al. 2009; Macfarlane et al. 2021). Not all studies show a negative effect of epinephrine, however, and its use is still recommended in people, albeit at low doses (e.g. 1 mcg kg^{-1}) to avoid its negative metabolic effects and significant increases in myocardial work (Neal et al. 2018). Vasopressin, on the other hand, while shown to have a positive effect in one study, is not advised due to its negative effects on cardiac output and tissue perfusion (Di Gregorio et al. 2009).

Current recommendations, adapted from those for humans, are listed in Table 28.2 (Neal et al. 2018; Macfarlane et al. 2021). Algorithms, such as this, can serve as an effective visual aid for anesthetists when facing a LAST crisis, and posting them in areas where locoregional blocks are performed is encouraged.

The current incidence of LAST is unknown in veterinary medicine, however, the popularity of locoregional techniques as well as the development of new blocks (e.g. fascial plane blocks) that require large doses and volumes of local anesthetics could result in an increase of reported cases. With this knowledge, what is just as important as knowing how to treat LAST is the initiation of practices that help to prevent it from occurring in the first place. In its most recent practice

Table 28.2 Treatment of local anesthetic systemic toxicity (LAST).

Management

Airway – Avoid hypoxemia, hypercapnia, and acidosis

- Intubate patient and secure airway
- Administer 100% oxygen
- Ventilate patient to maintain normocapnia (i.e. $ETCO_2$ 35–45 mmHg)

20% Lipid emulsion therapy – Start at onset of signs attributed to LAST

- **Bolus**: 1.5 ml kg^{-1} IV over one to two minutes; can be repeated every five minutes (three maximum)
- **Infusion**: After bolus, start constant rate infusion (CRI) at 0.25 ml kg^{-1} min^{-1}; increase to 0.5 ml kg^{-1} min^{-1} if no response
- Continue treatment for an additional 10–30 minutes following return of CNS and CVS stability
- Do not exceed 10–12 ml kg^{-1} in a 30-minute period

Seizure control

- Diazepam or Midazolam: 0.25–0.50 mg kg^{-1} IV
- Levetiracetam: 30–60 mg kg^{-1} IV
- Propofol: small incremental boluses IV; Not advised in patients with concurrent CVS depression

Cardiovascular collapse

Stop administration of any cardiodepressive drugs (i.e. inhalant anesthetic, opioids, etc.)

- Initiate cardiopulmonary cerebral resuscitation (CPCR) (e.g. chest compressions and ventilation in accordance with RECOVER guidelines (Fletcher et al. 2012))
- Epinephrine: 1 mcg kg^{-1} IV

  (Note: this dose is lower than recommended RECOVER guidelines of 10 mcg kg^{-1})
- Avoid use of vasopressin
- Administration of additional drugs to support blood pressure (e.g. inotropes) and heart rate (e.g. anticholinergics) may be indicated

Treatment of arrhythmias

- Arrhythmias **MAY** respond to administration of 20% lipid emulsion
- Do **NOT** administer local anesthetics (e.g. lidocaine, procainamide) for treatment of arrhythmias
- Avoid use of calcium channel blockers and beta blockers due to depressive effects on CVS
- Amiodarone (extra-label): 2 mg kg^{-1} IV over 10 minutes, followed by CRI of 0.8 mg kg^{-1} h^{-1} for 6 hours.

  (Note: use is recommended for treatment of arrhythmias that are not responsive to lipid emulsion in people)
- Defibrillation (0.5 J kg^{-1}) can be considered in patients with ventricular fibrillation

Once CNS and CVS stability is achieved

- Continue monitoring for a minimum of 6 hours and repeat treatments as indicated if signs of LAST return

advisory on LAST, The ASRA provided recommendations regarding prevention of LAST (Neal et al. 2018). US guidance for performing blocks is recommended whenever possible since direct visualization allows the anesthetist to see vasculature in the vicinity of the injection and more importantly, may allow early recognition of intravascular injection should local anesthetic not be observed exiting the needle tip. When injecting large volumes of local anesthetics, test doses (i.e. small aliquots) of local anesthetics are also recommended to help verify location and monitor for any adverse effects during injection. It is also always advised to ensure negative aspiration (i.e. absence of blood) prior to injection for any block and to use the lowest effective dose of local anesthetic whenever possible (Neal et al. 2018). Some publications also recommend preparation of a "LAST kit" containing necessary medications (i.e. IV lipid emulsion, epinephrine, etc.), syringes, needles, fluid lines, and a copy of the treatment protocol that can be easily accessed in case of emergency (Macfarlane et al. 2021). The use of these guidelines along with recognition and rapid instillation of treatment through diligence of monitoring and observation can be combined to hopefully minimize negative outcomes associated with LAST.

Neural Toxicity

Neurological deficits have been seen in humans following epidural and spinal anesthesia with chloroprocaine (Ravindran et al. 1980). It is not known whether those cases were the result of direct neural toxicity from the local anesthetic or from the preservatives that were present in the formulations used. Cauda equina syndrome has also been documented after repeated doses or infusions of epidurally administered 5% lidocaine (Schneider et al. 1993). It is speculated that this complication may have occurred due to pooling of the anesthetic around the cauda equina, with large concentrations causing direct neural damage.

Neurotoxicity in a rat spinal model has been shown for a variety of agents, including lidocaine, mepivacaine, and tetracaine (Takenami et al. 2000, 2005, 2009). In a recent investigation, ropivacaine proved to be less neurotoxic than levobupivacaine, procaine, and bupivacaine (Takenami et al. 2012). Although all of these agents showed varying degrees of histological changes (affecting mainly axons of the dorsal root entry zone), reports of neurological deficits following the use of modern local anesthetic agents in clinical veterinary practice are extremely rare.

Other Toxic Effects of Local Anesthetics

Local anesthetic agents can be used by several routes, and some toxic effects may be related, at least in part, to their route of administration and close proximity to certain tissues. Lidocaine and bupivacaine are frequently used in veterinary medicine to provide analgesia at the site of surgical incision, whether by local infiltration of the surgical site or by intraperitoneal administration for abdominal surgery. The efficacy of these techniques is questionable; some reports indicate an analgesic effect, whereas others have failed to detect such an advantage. Furthermore, improved postoperative pain relief in people has been demonstrated for some surgeries but not for others (Moiniche et al. 1998, 1999; Ng et al. 2002). However, an analgesic effect from a combination of intraperitoneal and incisional local anesthetics has been shown in dogs (Carpenter et al. 2004). Whether the presence of local anesthetics on the incision could impair wound healing has also been the focus of research for decades. *In vitro* evidence has been found against the use of local anesthetics for incisional analgesia: proliferation and differentiation of mesenchymal stem cells, which are implicated in wound healing, were impaired when exposed to increasing concentrations of lidocaine, bupivacaine, and ropivacaine (Lucchinetti et al. 2012). Early studies in rats demonstrated delayed healing five to seven days after lidocaine infiltration at the site of incision (Morris and Tracey 1977). Similar results were found when procaine was studied (Morris and Appleby 1980). Interestingly, infiltration with sterile water also caused delayed healing at five days when compared with rats who had not been infiltrated. When lidocaine and bupivacaine infiltration was evaluated in rabbits, no differences were found between treated animals and those that were infiltrated with saline (Vasseur et al. 1984). When studied in guinea pigs, infiltration with 1% lidocaine caused histopathological changes; however, no differences were seen when breaking strength was evaluated (Drucker et al. 1998). In a recent study, no differences in wound healing were found between lidocaine, bupivacaine, and saline when tested in rats (Waite et al. 2010).

There is some controversy regarding the use of intra-articular administration of local anesthetics in people. Although there are investigations that favor this route of administration because of improved analgesia following surgery, there is concern about potential toxic effects, especially in specific joints such as the shoulder. Intra-articular bupivacaine and ropivacaine have been shown to improve patient comfort and functionality after a variety of surgical procedures in both people and dogs (Sammarco et al. 1996; Hoelzler et al. 2005; Gomez-Cardero and Rodriguez-Merchan 2010; Dobrydnjov et al. 2011). Other investigators have found either weak evidence to support the use of intra-articular local anesthesia (Moiniche et al. 1999), or no advantages at all (Rosen et al. 2010). Several investigations have documented the potential for toxic effects of local anesthetics on chondrocytes and stem cells (Farkas et al. 2010; Haasters et al. 2011). A study in dog cadavers examined the exposure of cartilage explants to different concentrations of lidocaine (0.5%, 1%) and bupivacaine (0.25%, 0.125%, 0.0625%) (Sherman et al. 2015). Other than bupivacaine at 0.0625%, all other cartilage samples demonstrated complete chondrocyte death. These findings are consistent with those published in a recent systematic review which determined that toxic effects are agent, time, and concentration dependent (Kreuz et al. 2018). This review identified that bupivacaine and lidocaine are the most, mepivacaine intermediate, and ropivacaine, the least chondrotoxic. This could vary somewhat based on the concentration, however, with some studies demonstrating that bupivacaine at concentrations between 0.0625% and 0.125% and ropivacaine concentrations less than 0.5% may maintain cell viability.

HYPERSENSITIVITY REACTIONS

The incidence of serious anaphylactic and anaphylactoid reactions during anesthesia in people has been estimated to range between 1:3500, and 1:20000. The majority of these reactions are attributed to the use of muscle relaxants (69%), latex (12%), and antibiotics (8%) (Hepner and Castells 2003). Local anesthetic agents were implicated in less than 3% of these reactions. Most commonly, the toxic effects that result from high plasma levels of a local anesthetic are misdiagnosed as being a hypersensitivity reaction. When hypersensitivity reactions do occur, they are often limited to causing minor clinical signs such as skin redness, edema of the skin, or injection of mucous membranes. It has been estimated that from all of the adverse reactions associated with the use of local anesthetics, allergic reactions represent less than 1% (Brown et al. 1981).

Aminoester local anesthetics are derivatives of paraminobenzoic acid (PABA). During metabolism, these drugs undergo hydrolysis and the PABA molecule is produced. For this reason, aminoesters are more likely to cause severe hypersensitivity reactions (Type I; IgE-mediated) as a result of potential previous exposure of the patient to environmental products containing PABA, such as some foods, creams, sulfonamide agents, and methylparaben (a preservative) (Finucane 2003). Type I reactions involve the release of large amounts of histamine, serotonin, and leukotrienes from mast cells, resulting in profound bronchospasm and vasodilatation, constituting a medical emergency.

Allergic reactions to aminoamide local anesthetic agents occur much less frequently, although reports of these do exist (Brown et al. 1981). In people, the most common type of hypersensitivity to local anesthetics is a type IV reaction, which commonly has a slower onset and is associated with histamine release that is not mediated by immunoglobulin. The severity of these reactions can range from mild contact dermatitis to anaphylactoid shock.

The treatment of allergic reactions to local anesthetics is no different from that of any other type of allergic reaction and involves:

- oxygen administration;

- securing the airway;

- removal of the agent where possible;

- administration of epinephrine;

- administration of bronchodilators (i.e. albuterol);

- administration of H_1 (i.e. diphenhydramine) and H_2 (i.e. famotidine) blocking agents;

- administration of corticosteroids.

There is no known cross-sensitivity between amide and ester local anesthetics. A patient that is known to be hypersensitive to an aminoester can safely receive an aminoamide agent (and vice versa) as long as the alternative drug is preservative-free.

SUMMARY

When performing locoregional anesthetic techniques, a thorough understanding of the potential for complications is necessary. This allows for the rational instillation of precautions prior to performing blocks, as well as an informed basis by which to determine outcomes and treatment should they arise. The use of US guidance has decreased the incidence of vascular injections of local anesthetics during peripheral nerve blocks in humans, however, direct nerve trauma continues to occur at a similar rate, and its effect on the incidence of other complications has not been fully determined (Neal et al. 2015). Fortunately, reports of severe complications remain low in veterinary species at this time, however, as the use of locoregional anesthesia and the complexity of blocks continues to increase, the incidence of complications may follow suit.

REFERENCES

Adami C, Studer N (2014) A case of severe ventricular arrhythmias occurring as a complication of nerve-stimulator guided brachial plexus location [letter to the editor]. Vet Anaesth Analg 42, 230–231.

Alaman M, Bonastre C, de Blas I et al. (2022) Description of a novel ultrasound-guided approach for a dorsal quadratus lumborum block: a canine cadaver study. Vet Anaesth Analg 49, 118–125.

Alessio TL, Krieger EM (2015) Transient unilateral vision loss in a dog following inadvertent intravitreal injection of bupivacaine during a dental procedure. J Am Vet Med Assoc 246, 990–993.

Baeriswyl M, Taffe P, Kirkham KR et al. (2018) Comparison of peripheral nerve blockade characteristics between non-diabetic patients and patients suffering from diabetic neuropathy: a prospective cohort study. Anesth 73, 1110–1117.

Bauquier SH (2012) Hypotension and pruritus induced by neuraxial anaesthesia in a cat. Aust Vet J 90, 402–403.

Bhalla RJ, Leece EA (2015) Pneumothorax following nerve stimulator-guided axillary brachial plexus block in a dog [letter to the editor]. Vet Anaesth Analg 42, 658–659.

Bosmans T, Schauvliege S, Gasthuys F et al. (2009) Influence of a preload of hydroxyethylstarch 6% on the cardiovascular effects of epidural administration of ropivacaine 0.75% in anaesthetized dogs. Vet Anaesth Analg 38, 494–504.

Brown DT, Beamish D, Wildsmith JA (1981) Allergic reaction to an amide local anaesthetic. Br J Anaesth 53, 435–437.

Bruelle P, LeFrant JY, de La Coussaye JE et al. (1996) Comparative electrophysiologic and hemodynamic effects of several amide local anesthetic drugs in anesthetized dogs. Anesth Analg 82, 648–656.

Campoy L, Martin-Flores M, Ludders JW et al. (2012) Comparison of bupivacaine femoral and sciatic nerve block versus bupivacaine and morphine epidural for stifle surgery in dogs. Vet Anaesth Analg 39, 91–98.

Carpenter RE, Wilson DV, Evans AT (2004) Evaluation of intraperitoneal and incisional lidocaine or bupivacaine for analgesia following ovariohysterectomy in the dog. Vet Anaesth Analg 31, 46–52.

Chambers DJ, Bhatia K (2018) Horner's syndrome following obstetric neuraxial blockade – a systematic review of the literature. Int J Obstet Anesth 35, 75–87.

Choi S, Mahon P, Awad IT (2012) Neuraxial anesthesia and bladder dysfunction in the perioperative period: a systematic review. Can J Anesth 59, 681–703.

Choquet O, Morau D, Biboulet P et al. (2012) Where should the tip of the needle be located in ultrasound-guided peripheral nerve blocks? Curr Opin Anesthesiol 25, 596–602.

Choquette A, del Castillo JRE, Moreau M et al. (2017) Comparison of lidocaine and lidocaine-epinephrine for the paravertebral brachial plexus block in dogs. Vet Anaesth Analg 44, 317–328.

Claudio R, Hadzic A, Shih H et al. (2004) Injection pressures by anesthesiologists during simulated peripheral nerve block. Reg Anesth Pain Med 29, 201–205.

Coyle DE, Porembka DT, Sehlhorst CS et al. (1994) Echocardiographic evaluation of bupivacaine cardiotoxicity. Anesth Analg 79, 335–339.

De Jong RH, Ronfeld RA, DeRosa RA (1982) Cardiovascular effects of convulsant and supraconvulsant doses of amide local anesthetics. Anesth Analg 61, 3–9.

De Queiroz Siqueira M, Chassard D, Musard H et al. (2013) Resuscitation with lipid, epinephrine, or both in levobupivacaine-induced cardiac toxicity in newborn piglets. Brit J Anaesth 112, 729–734.

Di Gregorio G, Schwartz D, Ripper R et al. (2009) Lipid emulsion is superior to vasopressin in a rodent model of resuscitation from toxin-induced cardiac arrest. Crit Care Med 37, 993–999.

Dobrydnjov I, Anderberg C, Olsson C et al. (2011) Intraarticular vs. extraarticular ropivacaine infusion following high-dose local infiltration analgesia after total knee arthroplasty: a randomized double-blind study. Acta Orthop 82, 692–698.

Drenger B, Magora F, Evron S et al. (1986) The action of intrathecal morphine and methadone on the lower urinary tract in the dog. J Urol 135, 852–855.

Drenger B, Magora F (1989) Urodynamic studies after intrathecal fentanyl and buprenorphine in the dog. Anesth Analg 69, 348–353.

Drucker M, Cardenas E, Arizti P et al. (1998) Experimental studies on the effect of lidocaine on wound healing. World J Surg 22, 394–397.

Estrella JS, Nelson RN, Sturges BK et al. (2008) Endoneurial microvascular pathology in feline diabetic neuropathy. Microvasc Res 75, 403–410.

Evangelista MC, Steagall P, Garofalo NA et al. (2016) Morphine- induced pruritus after epidural administration followed by treatment with naloxone in a cat. J Feline Med Surg Open Rep 1–3.

Farkas B, Kvell K, Czompoly T et al. (2010) Increased chondrocyte death after steroid and local anesthetic combination. Clin Orthop Relat Res 468, 3112–3120.

Feldman HS, Arthur GR, Covino BG (1989) Comparative systemic toxicity of convulsant and supraconvulsant doses of intravenous ropivacaine, bupivacaine, and lidocaine in the conscious dog. Anesth Analg 69, 794–801.

Feldman HS, Arthur GR, Pitkanen M et al. (1991) Treatment of acute systemic toxicity after the rapid intravenous injection of ropivacaine and bupivacaine in the conscious dog. Anesth Analg 73, 373–384.

Feldman HS, Dvoskin S, Arthur GR et al. (1996) Antinociceptive and motor-blocking efficacy of ropivacaine and bupivacaine after epidural administration in the dog. Reg Anesth 21, 318–326.

Fettiplace MR, Lis K, Ripper R, et al. (2015) Multi-modal contributions to detoxification of acute pharmacotoxicity by a triglyceride micro-emulsion. J Control Release 198, 62–70.

Fettiplace MR, McCabe DJ (2017) Lipid emulsion improves survival in animal models of local anesthetic toxicity: a meta-analysis. Clin Toxicol 55, 617–623.

Finucane BT (2003) Allergies to local anesthetics – the real truth. Can J Anaesth 50, 869–874.

Fitzmaurice M (2020) The autonomic nervous system. In: Miller and Evans' Anatomy of the Dog, 5th edition. Hermanson JW, de Lahunta A, Evans HE (eds.) Elsevier, USA. pp. 663–678.

Fletcher DJ, Boller M, Brainard BM et al. (2012) RECOVER evidence and knowledge gap analysis on veterinary CPR. Part 7: clinical guidelines. J Vet Emerg Crit Care 22, S102-S131.

Franco CD, Sala-Blanch X (2019) Functional anatomy of the nerve and optimal placement of the needle for successful (and) safe nerve blocks. Curr Opin Anesthesiol 32, 638–642.

Gadsden JC (2021) The role of peripheral nerve stimulation in the era of ultrasound-guided regional anaesthesia. Anaesthesia 76, 65–73.

Gent T, Iff I, Bettschart-Wolfensberger R et al. (2013) Neuraxial morphine induced pruritus in two cats and treatment with sub anaesthetic doses of propofol. Vet Anaesth Analg 40, 517–520.

Gitman M, Barrington MJ (2018) Local anesthetic systemic toxicity: a review of recent case reports and registries. Reg Anesth Pain Med 43, 124–130.

Gomez-Cardero P, Rodriguez-Merchan EC (2010) Postoperative analgesia in TKA: ropivacaine continuous intraarticular infusion. Clin Orthop Relat Res 468, 1242–1247.

Gorgi AA, Hofmeister EH, Higginbotham MJ et al. (2006) Effect of body position on cranial migration of epidurally injected methylene blue in recumbent dogs. Am J Vet Res 67, 219–221.

Groban L, Deal DD, Vernon JC et al. (2001) Cardiac resuscitation after incremental overdosage with lidocaine, bupivacaine, levobupivacaine, and ropivacaine in anesthetized dogs. Anesth Analg 92, 37–43.

Groban L (2003) Central nervous system and cardiac effects from long-acting amide local anesthetic toxicity in the intact animal model. Reg Anesth Pain Med 28, 3–11.

Guerrero KSK, Guerrero TG, Schwizer-Kolliker M et al. (2014) Incidence of delayed hair re-growth, pruritis, and urinary retention after epidural anaesthesia in dogs. Tierarzt Prax Kleintiere 2, 94–100.

Haasters F, Polzer H, Prall WC et al. (2011) Bupivacaine, ropivacaine, and morphine: comparison of toxicity on human hamstring-derived stem/progenitor cells. Knee Surg Sports Traumatol Arthosc 19, 2138–2144.

Hadzic A, Dilberovic F, Shah S et al. (2004) Combination of intraneural injection and high injection pressure leads to fascicular injury and neurologic deficits in dogs. Reg Anesth Pain Med 29, 417–423.

Hepner DL, Castells MC (2003) Anaphylaxis during the perioperative period. Anesth Analg 97, 1381–1395.

Hicks SD, Salcido DD, Logue ES et al. (2009) Lipid emulsion combined with epinephrine and vasopressin does not improve survival in a swine model of bupivacaine-induced cardiac arrest. Anesthesiology 111, 138–146.

Hiller DM, Di Gregorio G, Ripper R et al. (2009) Epinephrine impairs lipid resuscitation from bupivacaine overdose: a threshold effect. Anesthesiology 111, 498–505.

Hoelzler MG, Harvey RC, Lidbetter DA et al. (2005) Comparison of perioperative analgesic protocols for dogs undergoing tibial plateau leveling osteotomy. Vet Surg 34, 337–344.

Holte K, Foss NB, Svensen C et al. (2004) Epidural anesthesia, hypotension, and changes in intravascular volume. Anesthesiology 100, 281–286.

Hu D, Onel E, Singla N et al. (2013) Pharmacokinetic profile of liposome bupivacaine following a single administration at the surgical site. Clin Drug Inves 33, 109–115.

Huang YF, Pryor ME, Mather LE et al. (1998) Cardiovascular and central nervous system effects of intravenous levobupivacaine and bupivacaine in sheep. Anesth Analg 86, 797–804

Iff I, Moens Y (2008) Two cases of bradyarrhythmia and hypotension after extradural injections in dogs. Vet Anaesth Analg 35, 265–269

Iff I, Valeskini K, Mosing M (2012) Severe pruritis and myoclonus following intrathecal morphine administration in a dog. Can Vet J 53, 983–986.

Joshi GP, Patou G, Kharitonov V (2015) The safety of liposome bupivacaine following various routes of administration in animals. J Pain Res 8, 781–789.

Kapur E, Vuckovic I, Dilberovic F et al. (2007) Neurologic and histologic outcome after intraneural injections of lidocaine in canine sciatic nerves. Acta Anaesthesiol Scand 51, 101–107.

Kinsella SM and Tuckey JP (2001) Perioperative bradycardia and asystole: relationship to vasovagal syncope and the Bezold-Jarisch reflex. Brit J Anaesth 86, 859–868.

Kreuz PC, Steinwachs M, Angele (2018) Single-dose local anesthetics exhibit a type-, dose-, and time-dependent chondrotoxic effect on chondrocytes and cartilage: a systematic review of the current literature. Knee Surg Sports Traumatol Arthrosc 26, 819–830.

Lacey JR, Dubowitz JA, Riedel B (2022) Asystole following spinal anaesthesia: the hazards of intrinsic cardiac reflexes. Anaesth Rep 10, e12198.

Laredo FG, Belda E, Soler M et al. (2020) Short-term effects of deliberate subparaneural or subepineural injections with saline solution or bupivacaine 0.75% in the sciatic nerve of rabbits. Front Vet Sci 7: 217.

Lee H, Naughton NN, Woods JH et al. (2007) Effects of butorphanol on morphine-induced itch and analgesia in primates. Anesthesiology 107, 478–485.

Lee I, Yamagishi N, Oboshi K et al. (2004) Distribution of new methylene blue injected into the lumbosacral epidural space in cats. Vet Anaesth Analg 31, 190–194.

Limongi JAG and Lins RSAM (2011) Cardiopulmonary arrest in spinal anesthesia. Rev Bras Anestesiol 61, 110–120.

Lirk P, Verhamme C, Boeckh R et al. (2015) Effects of early and late diabetic neuropathy on sciatic nerve block duration and neurotoxicity in Zucker diabetic fatty rats. Brit J Anaesth 114, 319–326.

Liu H, Brown M, Sun L et al. (2019) Complications and liability related to regional and neuraxial anesthesia. Best Pract Res Clin Anaesthesiol 33, 487–497.

Loughran CM, Raisis AL, Haitjema G et al. (2016) Unilateral retrobulbar hematoma following maxillary nerve block in a dog. J Vet Emerg Crit Care 26, 815–818.

Lucchinetti E, Awad AE, Rahman M et al. (2012) Antiproliferative effects of local anesthetics on mesenchymal stem cells: potential implications for tumor spreading and wound healing. Anesthesiology 116, 841–856.

Macfarlane AJR, Gitman M, Bornstein KJ et al. (2021) Updates in our understanding of local anaesthetic systemic toxicity: a narrative review. Anaesthesia 76, 27–39.

MacFarlane P, Iff I (2011) Discospondylitis in a dog after attempted extradural injection. Vet Anaesth Analg 38, 272–273.

Malinovsky JM, Le Normand L, Lepage JY et al. (1998) The urodynamic effects of intravenous opioids and ketoprofen in humans. Anesth Analg 87, 456–461.

Mizisin AP, Weerasuriya A (2011) Homeostatic regulation of the endoneurial microenvironment during development, aging and in response to trauma, disease, and toxic insult. Acta Neuropathol 121, 291–312.

Moiniche S, Mikkelsen S, Wetterslev J et al. (1998) A qualitative systematic review of incisional local anaesthesia for postoperative pain relief after abdominal operations. Br J Anaesth 81, 377–383.

Moiniche S, Mikkelsen S, Wetterslev J et al. (1999) A systematic review of intra-articular local anesthesia for postoperative pain relief after arthroscopic knee surgery. Reg Anesth Pain Med 24, 430–437.

Moll X, Garcia F, Ferrer I et al. (2014) Distribution of methylene blue after injection into the epidural space of anaesthetized pregnant and non-pregnant sheep. PLoS One 9, e92860.

Monticelli P, Fitzgerald E, Viscasillas J (2018) A sonographic investigation for the development of ultrasound-guided paravertebral brachial plexus block in dogs: cadaveric study. Vet Anaesth Analg 45, 195–202.

Morgan MJ, Vite CH, Radhakrishnan A et al. (2008) Clinical peripheral neuropathy associated with diabetes mellitus in 3 dogs. Can Vet J 49, 583–586.

Mornjaković Z, Dilberović F, Cosović E et al. (2005) Histological changes of the sciatic nerve in dogs after intraneural application of lidocaine-relation to the established application pressure. Bosn J Basic Med Sci 5, 8–13.

Morris T, Tracey J (1977) Lignocaine: its effects on wound healing. Br J Surg 64, 902–903.

Morris T, Appleby R (1980) Retardation of wound healing by procaine. Br J Surg 67, 391–392.

Mosing M, Iff IK, Nemetz W (2008) Cardiopulmonary arrest and resuscitation following an extradural injection in a normovolemic dog. J Vet Emerg Crit Care 18, 532–536.

Myers RR, Heckman HM (1989) Effects of local anesthesia on nerve blood flow: studies using lidocaine with and without epinephrine. Anesthesiology 71, 757–762.

Neal JM, Barrington MJ, Brull R et al. (2015) The second ASRA practice advisory on neurologic complications associated with regional anesthesia and pain medicine. Reg Anesth Pain Med 40, 401–430.

Neal JM (2016) Ultrasound-guided regional anesthesia and patient safety: update of an evidence-based analysis. Reg Anesth Pain Med 41, 195–204.

Neal JM, Barrington MJ, Fettiplace MR, et al. (2018) The third American society of regional anesthesia and pain medicine practice advisory on local anesthetic systemic toxicity: executive summary 2017. Reg Anesth Pain Med 43, 113–123.

Ng A, Swami A, Smith G et al. (2002) The analgesic effects of intraperitoneal and incisional bupivacaine with epinephrine after total abdominal hysterectomy. Anesth Analg 95, 158–162, table of contents.

Nocita™ (2021) Package Insert. Greenfield, IN: Elanco US, Inc.

Nyugen E, Lim G, Ross SE (2021) Evaluation of therapies for peripheral and neuraxial opioid-induced pruritus based on molecular and cellular discoveries. Anesthesiology 135, 350–365.

Pascarella G, Stumia A, Costa F (2021) Triple monitoring may avoid intraneural injection during interscalene brachial plexus block for arthroscopic shoulder surgery: A prospective preliminary study. J Clin Med 10, 781.

Perez-Guille BE, Villegas-Alvarez F, Toledo-Lopez A et al. (2011) Pharmacokinetics of lidocaine and its metabolite as a hepatic function marker in dogs. Proc West Pharmacol Soc 54, 62–65.

Perlas A, Niazi A, McCarney C et al. (2006) The sensitivity of motor response to nerve stimulation and paresthesia for nerve localization as evaluated by ultrasound. Reg Anesth Pain Med 31, 445–450.

Perry R, Moore D, Scurrell E (2015) Globe penetration in a cat following maxillary nerve block for dental surgery. J Fel Med Surg 17, 66–72.

Peterson NW, Buote NJ, Bergman P (2014) Effect of epidural analgesia with opioids on the prevalence of urinary retention in dogs undergoing surgery for cranial cruciate ligament rupture. J Am Vet Med Assoc 244, 940–943.

Portela DA, Otero PE, Biondi M et al. (2013) Peripheral nerve stimulation under ultrasonographic control to determine the needle-to-nerve relationship. Vet Anaesth Analg 40, E91–99.

Pratheep KG, Sonawane K, Rajasekaran S et al. (2022) Transient paraplegia in lumbar spine surgery – a potential complication following erector spinae plane block. Eur Spine J 31, 3719–3723.

Prats-Galino A, Capek M, Reina MA et al. (2018) 3D reconstruction of peripheral nerves from optical projection tomography images: a method for studying fascicular interconnections and intraneural plexuses. Clin Anat 31, 424–431.

Rambhia M, Gadsden J (2019) Pressure monitoring: the evidence so far. Best Pract Res Clin Anaesthesiol 33, 47–56.

Ravindran RR, Bond VK, Tasch MD et al. (1980). Prolonged neural blockade following regional analgesia with 2-chloroprocaine. Anesth Analg 95, 447–451.

Raw RM, Read MR, Campoy L (2013) Peripheral nerve stimulators. In: Small Animal Regional Anesthesia and Analgesia. Campoy L, Read MR (eds.) Wiley, USA. pp. 65–76.

Remedios A, Wagner R, Caulkett NA et al. (1996) Epidural abscess and discospondylitis in a dog after administration of a lumbosacral epidural analgesic. Can Vet J 37, 106–107.

Rice ASC, McMahon SB (1992) Peripheral nerve injury caused by injection needles used in regional anaesthesia: influence of bevel configuration, studied in a rat model. Brit J Anaesth 69, 433–438.

Richard BM, Rickert DE, Doolittle D, et al. (2011) Pharmacokinetic compatibility study of lidocaine with EXPAREL in Yucatan miniature pigs. Int Scholar Res Net 2011, 582351, 1–6.

Rosen AS, Colwell CW, Jr., Pulido PA et al. (2010) A randomized controlled trial of intraarticular ropivacaine for pain management immediately following total knee arthroplasty. HSS J 6, 155–159.

Sage DJ, Feldman HS, Arthur RG et al. (1985) The cardiovascular effects of convulsant doses of lidocaine and bupivacaine in the conscious dog. Reg Anesth Pain Med 10, 175–183.

Sammarco JL, Conzemius MG, Perkowski SZ et al. (1996) Postoperative analgesia for stifle surgery: a comparison of intra-articular bupivacaine, morphine, or saline. Vet Surg 25, 59–69.

Sarotti D, Ala U, Franci P (2022) Epidural anesthesia in dogs undergoing hindlimb orthopedic surgery: effects of two injection sites. J Vet Med Sci 84, 457–464.

Savvas I, Anagnoustou T, Papazoglou G et al. (2006) Successful resuscitation from cardiac arrest associated with extradural lidocaine in a dog. Vet Anaesth Analg 33, 175–178.

Schneider M, Ettlin T, Kaufmann M et al. (1993) Transient neurologic toxicity after hyperbaric subarachnoid anesthesia with 5% lidocaine. Anesth Analg 76, 1154–1157.

Selander D, Dhuner KG, Lundborg G (1977) Peripheral nerve injury due to injection needles used for regional anesthesia. Acta Anaesthesiol Scand 21, 182–188.

Sherman SL, James C, Stoker AM et al. (2015) In vivo toxicity of local anesthetics and corticosteroids on chondrocyte and synoviocyte viability and metabolism. Cartilage 6, 106–112.

Smith RL, West SJ, Wilson J (2021) Using the BBraun BSmart™ pressure manometer to prevent unsafe injection pressures during simulated peripheral nerve blockade: a pilot study. Open Anesth J 15, 49–59.

Son W, Jang M, Yoon J et al. (2014) The effect of epidural injection speed on epidural pressure and distribution of solution in anesthetized dogs. Vet Anaesth Analg 41, 526–533.

Son W, Jang M, Jo S et al. (2015) The volume effect of lidocaine on thoracic epidural anesthesia in conscious Beagle dogs. Vet Anaesth Analg 42, 414–424.

Steinfeldt T, Nimphius W, Werner T et al. (2010a) Nerve injury by needle nerve perforation in regional anaesthesia: does size matter? Brit J Anaesth 104, 245–253.

Steinfeldt T, Nimphius W, Wurps M et al. (2010b) Nerve perforation with pencil point or short bevelled needles: histological outcome. Acta Anaesthesiol Scand 54, 993–999.

Stundner O, Meissnitzer M, Brummett CM et al. (2016) Comparison of tissue distribution, phrenic nerve involvement, and epidural spread in standard- vs low-volume ultrasound-guided interscalene plexus block using contrast magnetic resonance imaging: a randomized controlled trial. Brit J Anaesth 116, 405–412.

Takenami T, Yagishita S, Asato F et al. (2000) Neurotoxicity of intrathecally administered tetracaine commences at the posterior roots near entry into the spinal cord. Reg Anesth Pain Med 25, 372–379.

Takenami T, Yagishita S, Murase S et al. (2005) Neurotoxicity of intrathecally administered bupivacaine involves the posterior roots/posterior white matter and is milder than lidocaine in rats. Reg Anesth Pain Med 30, 464–472.

Takenami T, Yagishita S, Nara Y et al. (2009) Spinal procaine is less neurotoxic than mepivacaine, prilocaine and bupivacaine in rats. Reg Anesth Pain Med 34, 189–195.

Takenami T, Wang G, Nara Y et al. (2012) Intrathecally administered ropivacaine is less neurotoxic than procaine, bupivacaine, and levobupivacaine in a rat spinal model. Can J Anaesth 59, 456–465.

Thomson PD, Rowland M, Melmon KL (1971) The influence of heart failure, liver disease, and renal failure on the disposition of lidocaine in man. Am Heart J 82, 417–421.

Thomson PD, Melmon KL, Richardson JA et al. (1973) Lidocaine pharmacokinetics in advanced heart failure, liver disease, and renal failure in humans. Ann Intern Med 78, 499–508.

Troncy E, Junot S, Keroack S, et al. (2002) Results of preemptive epidural administration of morphine with

or without bupivacaine in dogs and cats undergoing surgery: 265 cases (1997-1999). J Am Vet Med Assoc 221, 666–672.

Tsui BCH, Li LXY, Pillay JJ (2006) Compressed air injection technique to standardize block injection pressures. Can J Anesth 53, 1098–1102.

Vasquez EJ, Kendall A, Muslulin S et al. (2021) Three-dimensional bladder ultrasound to measure daily urinary bladder volume in hospitalized dogs. J Vet Intern Med 35, 2256–2262.

Vasseur PB, Paul HA, Dybdal N et al. (1984) Effects of local anesthetics on healing of abdominal wounds in rabbits. Am J Vet Res 45, 2385–2388.

Veering B (2006) Hemodynamic effects of central neural blockade in elderly patients. Can J Anesth 53, 117–121.

Vettorato E, Bradbrook C, Gurney M, et al. (2012) Peripheral nerve blocks of the pelvic limb in dogs: a retrospective clinical study. Vet Comp Orthop Traumatol 25, 314–320.

Vettorato E and Corletto F (2016) Retrospective assessment of peripheral nerve block techniques used in cats undergoing hindlimb orthopaedic surgery. J Feline Med Surg 18, 826–833.

Wagner AE, Dunlop CI, Turner AS (1996) Experiences with morphine injected into the subarachnoid space in sheep. Vet Surg 25, 256–260.

Wang Z, Jiang C, Yao H et al. (2021) Central opioid receptors mediate morphine-induced itch and chronic itch via disinhibition. Brain 144, 665–681.

Waite A, Gilliver SC, Masterson GR et al. (2010) Clinically relevant doses of lidocaine and bupivacaine do not impair cutaneous wound healing in mice. Br J Anaesth 104, 768–773.

Weinberg GL, VadeBoncouer T, Ramaraju GA et al. (1998) Pretreatment or resuscitation with a lipid infusion shifts the dose-response to bupivacaine-induced asystole in rats. Anesthesiology 88, 1071–1075.

Weinberg G, Ripper R, Feinstein DL et al. (2003) Lipid emulsion infusion rescues dogs from bupivacaine-induced cardiac toxicity. Reg Anesth Pain Med 28, 198–202.

Weinberg GL, Di Gregorio G, Ripper R et al. (2008) Resuscitation with lipid versus epinephrine in a rat model of bupivacaine overdose. Anesthesiology 108, 907–913.

Zwueste DM, Grahn BH (2019) A review of Horner's syndrome in small animals. Can Vet J 60, 81–88.

Index

Small Animal Regional Anesthesia and Analgesia, Second Edition. Edited by Matt Read, Luis Campoy, and Berit Fischer.
© 2024 John Wiley & Sons, Inc. Published 2024 by John Wiley & Sons, Inc.